EM Fundamentals

The Essential Handbook for Emergency Medicine Residents

Laura Welsh, MD
Editor-in-Chief

Associate Editors
Emily Aaronson, MD
John Eicken, MD
Brian Geyer, MD, PhD

Disclaimer

This handbook is intended only as a general guide to patient care. It does not replace formal training. It should not be interpreted as clinical direction. The publisher, authors, editors, reviewers, and sponsoring organizations specifically disclaim any liability for any omissions or errors found in this handbook or for treatment errors.

Additional copies of this publication are available from:
Emergency Medicine Residents' Association
1125 Executive Circle
Irving, TX 75038-2522
972.550.0920
emra.org

Reviewers

Preface

We are excited to present *EMRA'S EM Fundamentals: The Essential Handbook for Emergency Medicine Residents*, a reference guide from the residents of the Harvard Affiliated Emergency Medicine Residency at Massachusetts General Hospital and Brigham and Women's Hospital in Boston, Massachusetts. The purpose of this handbook is to serve as a compact resource that is easily accessible during a busy shift. Emergency medicine is a unique specialty where a resident can find him or herself managing multiple sick patients simultaneously with additional patients awaiting care. As emergency physicians we pride ourselves on providing consistent, high-quality care no matter what the clinical situation or how busy the ED may be. It is our hope that this handbook will improve your ability to provide outstanding care whether it saves you time through easy access to reference material or it prompts you to consider a potentially life-threatening diagnosis, which you may not have otherwise considered. It is by no means comprehensive and should rather be used as a guide to construct a foundation on how to approach and manage the emergencies encountered in the ED.

The organization of the book is chief complaint based, as that is often all an emergency physician is given prior to evaluating a patient. The design was created with a busy junior resident in mind. Each chapter begins with a one-page "Quick Guide," which is a focused summary on the initial approach to the chief complaint and the "can't miss" emergency diagnoses. Consult the Quick Guides just prior to entering a patient's room or when leaving a patient's room after you find yourself asking "What could I be missing or forgetting?" Within each chief complaint chapter are disease-specific sections intended to serve as a practical guide to utilize during a shift.

Acknowledgments

The creation of this book would not have been possible without the contributions and expertise of numerous Massachusetts General Hospital and Brigham and Women's Hospital faculty members who teach us and guide us every day in the emergency department. We would like to thank **Dr. Eric Nadel**, **Dr. Kriti Bhatia**, and **Dr. Christian Arbelaez** for all of their mentorship. We cannot thank our faculty mentors enough, **Dr. David Peak** and **Dr. Kimo Takayesu**, who offered steadfast support and continual guidance throughout the creation of this book. Their extraordinary dedication to resident education has made this and many other projects possible.

FACULTY EDITORS

We would also like to thank our faculty editors:

Christopher Kabrhel, MD, MPH	David F.M. Brown, MD, FACEP
Michael Cole, MD	Thomas F. Burke, MD, FACEP
Michael Filbin, MD, FACEP	William Binder, MD
John T. Nagurney, MD, FACEP	Thomas O. Stair, MD
Daniel Lindberg, MD	Michael B. Stone, MD, RDMS, FACEP
Susan Elizabeth Farrell, MD	Kelli N. O'Laughlin, MD
Benjamin A. White, MD	Peter C. Hou, MD

We would like to recognize and thank the Massachusetts General Hospital Medicine residents for their advice and guidance as well as their selfless contribution to medical learning. Their own Housestaff Manual served as an inspiration for this book, and they continue to set the benchmark for resident-directed reference books.

Finally, we would like to thank our co-residents as well as the nurses and physician assistants with whom we work every day. What you have, and continue to teach us while on shift, is immeasurable and could never be captured in a book.

Abbreviations Used in this Book

AAA	Abdominal aortic aneurysm	ED	Emergency department
ABC	Airway, Breathing, Circulation	EDH	Epidural hematoma
ABG	Arterial blood gas	EEG	Electroencephalography
Abx	Antibiotics	EF	Ejection fraction
ACE	Angiotensin converting enzyme	EKG	Electrocardiogram
ACLS	Advanced cardiac life support	Epi	Epinephrine
AED	Antiepileptic drugs	ESR	Erythrocyte sedimentation rate
AKI	Acute kidney injury	EtOH	Ethanol
AMS	Altered mental status	ETT	Endotracheal tube
ARDS	Acute respiratory distress syndrome	FFP	Fresh frozen plasma
		FSBS	Fingerstick blood sugar
AV	Atrioventricular	GCC	Gonorrhea and chlamydia
BCx	Blood cultures	GCS	Glasgow coma scale
BID	Twice a day	GERD	Gastroesophageal reflux disease
BiPAP	Bilevel positive airway pressure	GI	Gastrointestinal/Gastroenterology
BMP	Basic metabolic panel	GIB	Gastrointestinal bleed
BNP	Brain natriuretic peptide	HCT	Hematocrit
BP	Blood pressure	HD	Hemodynamically
BPPV	Benign positional paroxysmal vertigo	HCG	Human chorionic gonadotropin
		HHS	Hyperosmolar hyperglycemia syndrome
BUN.	Blood urea nitrogen		
BVM	Bag valve mask	HLD	Hyperlipidemia
CAD	Coronary artery disease	HOB	Head of bed
CBC	Complete blood count	HTN	Hypertension
CHF	Congestive heart failure	IBD	Irritable bowel disease
CKD	Chronic kidney disease	ICP	Intracranial pressure
CMT	Cervical motion tenderness	ICU	Intensive care unit
CNS	Central nervous system	IM	Intramuscular
CO	Carbon monoxide	IO	Intraosseous access
CPK	Creatinine phosphokinase	IOP	Intraocular pressure
CRP	C-reactive protein	IR	Interventional radiology
CT	Computed tomography	IUP	Intrauterine pregnancy
CTA	Computed tomography angiography	IV	Intravenously
CVA	Cerebrovascular accident	IVC	Inferior vena cava
Cx	Culture	IVDU	Intravenous drug use
CXR	Chest X-ray	IVF	Intravenous fluids
Ddx	Differential diagnosis	JVP	Jugular venous pressure
DIC	Disseminated intravascular coagulation	LAD	Left anterior descending artery
		LBBB	Left bundle branch block
DKA	Diabetic ketoacidosis	LBO	Large bowel obstruction
DM	Diabetes mellitus	LE	Lower extremity
DTR	Deep tendon reflex	LFTs	Liver function tests
DVT	Deep venous thrombosis	LLE	Left lower extremity
Echo	Echocardiogram	LLQ	Left lower quadrant

LMA	Laryngeal mask airway	RBBB	Right bundle branch block
LMN	Lower motor neuron	RCA	Right coronary artery
LMP	Last menstrual period	RLE	Right lower extremity
LMWH	Low molecular weight heparin	RLQ	Right lower quadrant
LOC	Level (or loss) of consciousness	ROM	Range of motion
LP	Lumbar puncture	RSI	Rapid sequence intubation
LUE	Left upper extremity	RUE	Right upper extremity
LUQ	Left upper quadrant	RUQ	Right upper quadrant
LV	Left ventricle	RV	Right ventricle
MDI	Metered dose inhaler	RVR	Rapid ventricular response
MRI	Magnetic resonance imaging	SAH	Subarachnoid hemorrhage
MRA	Magnetic resonance angiography	SBO	Small bowel obstruction
MSK	Musculoskeletal	SBP	Systolic blood pressure
MVC	Motor vehicle collision	SCD	Sickle cell disease
NC	Nasal cannula	SDH	Subdural hemorrhage
NGT	Nasogastric tube	SIADH	Syndrome of inappropriate
NIPPV	Non-invasive positive pressure		antidiuretic hormone
	ventilation	SIRS	Systemic inflammatory response
NRB	Non-rebreather mask		syndrome
NS	Normal saline	SQ	Subcutaneous
NSAID	Non-steroidal anti-inflammatory	SSRI	Selective serotonin reuptake
	drug		inhibitors
NSTI	Necrotizing soft tissue infections	STD	ST segment depression
OCP	Oral contraceptive pill	STE	ST elevations
OD	Overdose	STI	Sexually transmitted infection
PCN	Penicillin	TCA	Tricyclic antidepressants
PCI	Percutaneous intervention	TB	Tuberculosis
PCP	Primary care doctor	TBI	Traumatic brain injury
PCR	Polymerase chain reaction	TBSA	Total body surface area
PE	Pulmonary embolism	TID	Three times a day
PEEP	Positive end expiratory pressure	TPA	Tissue plasminogen activator
PFO	Patent foramen ovale	TOA	Tuboovarian abscess
PID	Pelvic inflammatory disease	TPN	Total parenteral nutrition
PNA	Pneumonia	Trop	Troponin
PO	By mouth	TTP	Thrombotic thrombocytopenia
POC	Products of conception	TVUS	Transvaginal US
PPI	Proton pump inhibitor	UA	Urinalysis
PPx	Prophylaxis	UMN	Upper motor neurons
PRN	As needed	US	Ultrasound
PTA	Peritonsillar abscess	UTI	Urinary tract infection
PTH	Parathyroid hormone	VBG	Venous blood gas
PUD	Peptic ulcer disease	VF	Ventricular fibrillation
PR	Per rectum	VS	Vital signs
Pt(s)	Patient(s)	VT	Ventricular tachycardia
PTX	Pneumothorax	WCT	Wide complex tachycardia
PVI	Pulmonary vein isolation	WPW	Wolff-Parkinson-White syndrome

Contents

Section XVII. Weak and Dizzy

Section XVIII. Procedure Guide

Section 1
Abdominal Pain

1 ▶ Abdominal Pain Quick Guide

- ALWAYS: IV, O2, COMPLETE VS (including temperature and pulse oximetry), consider EKG (ACS can present as epigastric pain), abdominal exam (if obtain STAT portable upright CXR to assess for free air and obtain surgery consult).
- Can't-miss diagnoses in first 2 minutes: Ruptured AAA (hypotension, abdominal, or back pain), aortic dissection (tearing back pain, unequal pulses), mesenteric ischemia (pain out of proportion to exam), perforated hollow viscous (peritonitis), or acute myocardial infarction.

EVALUATION

- **High Yield History**: Previous surgeries (SBO), EtOH (hepatitis, pancreatitis, cirrhosis), pregnancy status (OB/GYN pathology), recent Abx use (C. diff), relation to food (gallbladder disease, ischemic colitis, ulcer), GI bleed (upper/lower), trauma, last bowel movement (obstruction, constipation).

Associated Symptoms	Quality of the Pain
Absence of flatus/bowel movements: SBO	Worse with meals: Biliary colic
Anorexia: Pancreatitis, appendicitis	Radiation to back: Pancreatitis, AAA
Diarrhea: C.Diff	Diffuse, severe, colicky: SBO
Bloody diarrhea: Infection or mesenteric ischemia	Pain out of proportion: Mesenteric ischemia
Nausea/vomiting: Important to ask about, can support certain diagnoses (gastroenteritis if with diarrhea, SBO if alone)	Radiation to groin: Renal colic
Shortness of breath: PNA/PE (lower lobes)	
Vaginal bleeding: Ectopic, abortion	

- **Exam**: Assess location of tenderness, rebound/guarding (surgical abdomen/perforation), distention (SBO), fluid wave (ascites), bowel sounds (high pitched/absent for SBO), pelvic exam for females with pelvic pain: adnexal tenderness (ovarian cyst, torsion, ectopic, TOA, appendicitis), rectal exam + guaiac (GI bleed, diverticulitis, colitis), subcutaneous/mediastinal air (esophageal rupture)
- **Special Signs** (all low sensitivity/specificity, but useful in larger context):
  — Murphy's: Patient ceases inspiration while you palpate the RUQ at mid-clavicular costal margin → associated with cholecystitis

- — McBurney's point: Tenderness to palpation 2/3 between umbilicus and ant. superior iliac spine → associated with appendicitis
- — Obturator: Pain with flexion and internal rotation of right leg → associated with appendicitis
- — Psoas: Patient on left side, pain with hyperextension of right hip→ associated with appendicitis
- — Rovsing: Pain in RLQ with palpation of LLQ → associated with appendicitis
- **Initial Workup**
  - — Labs: UA (infection, blood), HCG, CBC, BMP, LFTs, Lipase (if concern for pancreatitis), lactate (if sick)
  - — EKG: Always think about cardiac cause in elderly, women, and diabetics, also to assess arrhythmias in mesenteric ischemia
  - — Imaging
    - ▪ X-ray: Upright CXR to assess for free air in perforate viscus or KUB to evaluate for dilated loops of bowel for bowel obstruction.
    - ▪ CT: IV contrast to help visualize vasculature, abscesses, masses, and oral contrast to visualize hollow viscous structures
    - ▪ RUQ US: Imagining modality of choice for the biliary system
    - ▪ Pelvic US: If concern for GYN pathology such as ovarian cysts, torsion, or TOA.

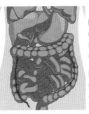

Epigastric: Gastritis, pancreatitis, ACS, PUD, biliary colic

RUQ: Biliary colic, cholecystitis, GERD, hepatitis, ulcer, cholangitis, RLL pneumonia, PE

LUQ: Gastritis, splenic pathology (infarction/rupture), pericarditis, myocarditis, LLL PNA, pleural effusion, PE

RLQ: Appendicitis, Meckel's, diverticulitis, ectopic, ovarian torsion/cyst, PID, endometriosis, psoas abscess, UTI, TOA, kidney stone

LLQ: Sigmoid diverticulitis, hernia, ectopic, ovarian torsion/cyst, PID, endometriosis, psoas abscess, UTI, TOA, kidney stone

Diffuse: Early appendicitis, gastroenteritis, SBO, LBO, SBP, IBD, DKA, mesenteric ischemia, AAA

MANAGEMENT

- Pain control: Consider morphine or hydromorphone IV for pain if not tolerating PO. Famotidine or viscous lidocaine for GERD or gastritis.
- Treat nausea and vomiting
  - — 1st line agent for nausea and vomiting: Ondansetron: 4mg IV q8h
  - — 2nd line agents for nausea and vomiting:
    - ▪ Metoclopramide: 10mg PO/IV q6h
    - ▪ Prochlorperazine: 10mg PO/IVq6h/25mg PR x1
    - ▪ Diphenhydramine: 25-50mg PO/IVq6h

- Haloperidol: 0.5-4mg PO/IVq6h
- Lorazepam: 1-2mg IV q6h
- Dexamethasone: 4-10mg PO q6h

BEWARE...

(!) Consider an EKG, especially in elderly patients as abdominal pain can be an angina equivalent

(!) Have lower threshold to obtain imaging in the elderly, immunosuppressed patients, and patients who had previous surgery, especially gastric bypass, which puts patients at risk of internal hernia.

Sources

Zane RD, Kosowsky JM, et al. Pocket Emergency Medicine. 2nd ed. Philadelphia, PA: Lippincott Williams & Wilkins; 2011.

Ma OJ, Cline D, Tintinalli J, et al. Emergency Medicine Manual. 6th ed. New York, NY: McGraw-Hill Professional; 2003.

Marx J, Hockberger R, Walls R. Rosen's Emergency Medicine: Concepts & Clinical Practice. 5th ed. Maryland Heights, MO: Mosby; 2002.

Hans L, Mawji Y. The ABCs of Emergency Medicine. 12th edition. Toronto, Canada: University of Toronto; 2012.

Medscape News & Perspective. New York, NY: http://emedicine.medscape.com.

Notes

2 ▶ Abdominal Aortic Aneurysm

- Dilation of abdominal aorta (all 3 layers) > 3cm
- Non-ruptured (often incidental and non-emergent), ruptured (lethal emergent condition)
- The diagnosis of AAA requires a high degree of suspicion in any patient with abdomen or back pain.
- Because some tears can be temporarily contained in the retroperitoneum, the patient may initially look clinically well.

Ddx
Renal colic
Back strain
Cholecystitis
Pancreatitis
Gastritis
Gastroenteritis
GI bleed (if aortoenteric fistula)
Diverticulitis

RUPTURED

- Lethal, with mortality of 65-90%. Survival requires prompt diagnosis and vascular surgery consultation for operative repair.
- Intraperitoneal ruptures are almost universally fatal.
- Retroperitoneal ruptures can be temporarily contained, allowing a window of time for repair.

EVALUATION

- **High Yield History**: Stereotypical patient is older male with history of HTN and smoking.
  - The triad of abdominal pain, pulsatile mass, and hypotension/syncope occurs in approximately 50% of ruptured AAA.
  - Abdominal pain (initially dull; however, once ruptured can be acute and increasing)
  - Can also have back, flank, or groin pain.
- **Exam**
  - Assess for pulsatile mass, flank ecchymosis and hypotension.
  - Perform full pulse exam though decreased femoral pulses has low sensitivity/specificity.
  - Extremity ischemia (from emboli of thrombus in aneurysm).
  - GI bleed (aortoenteric fistula is rare but devestating).
  - Neuro deficits (occlusion of the artery of Adamkiewicz also rare).
- **Once you suspect a ruptured AAA**
  - Confirm the diagnosis usually via imaging. Choice of imaging depends on the stability of your patient and whether the AAA is known. However, bedside US for aortic visualization and performance of a FAST can expedite management.
  - Concurrently resuscitate the patient
- **Diagnostics**
  - Labs: Consider CBC, BMP, LFTs, lipase, UA, trop, coags, and type and screen.
  - If unstable, then obtain type and cross match for blood.
  - Overview of imaging:
    - Abdominal US: Very sensitive (100% with skilled technician) and specific for UNRUPTURED infrarenal AAA. Limited ability to detect rupture and decreased yield with obesity and bowel gas. However, cannot exclude ruptured AAA.

- Abdominal CTA: Able to visualize rupture and guide surgical managment. Does not neccesarily require IV contrast (difficult in pts with renal failure, contrast allergy) and requires pt to be stable enough to go to CT scanner.

General Approach	
Patient stable, AAA known (followed as outpatient)—DO NOT waste your time with a formal ultrasound here. The ultrasound will show a AAA, but unless you have an intraperitoneal rupture with a positive FAST (rare to see in the ED, as most of these people die before they can get to you), *the US will give you no new information because it cannot detect retroperitoneal hematomas.* You need a CT with IV contrast to demonstrate the retroperitoneal hematoma.	**Patient unstable, AAA known**—Emergent surgical consultation. If stable for CT, go to the scanner. If too unstable, do a bedside US to evaluate size of aneurysm, look for intramural hematoma (specific but not sensitive), and to detect intraperitoneal rupture (again, specific but not sensitive). If + AAA and hypotension, surgeons may take the patient emergently to the OR.
Patient stable, AAA unknown—Bedside or radiology-performed US to detect presence of AAA then CT to assess for possible rupture.	**Patient unstable with abd/back pain, AAA unknown** – Bedside US to detect presence of AAA +/- free fluid in abdomen. If +, emergent surgical consultation. Be sure to consider other causes of abdominal pain and hypotension (sepsis, bowel perforation, GI bleed, aortoenteric fistula, etc.)

MANAGEMENT

- Resuscitate and mobilize your surgical team ASAP! This is a true emergency.
- Order 4-6 units of emergency release blood (O+ or O-), platelets, and FFP, as you will likely be doing massive transfusion.
- Two large bore IVs (18 gauge or larger). In line with the principle of "permissive hypotension" that we use in trauma, shoot for a goal SBP of approx 90mmHg and titrate to mental status.
- Consider placement of arterial catheter for continuous BP monitoring.
- Get your surgeons to the bedside and your patient to the OR STAT.
  *One of the few instances where A does not come before C. If patient loses the airway, it is because s/he is bleeding to death. Therefore, resuscitate first and only intubate if trouble oxygenating or your patient is frankly obtunded. Induction will cause further hypotension, the ventilator will decrease preload, and the loss of sympathetic tone may just be the straw that breaks the camel's back and causes the patient to go into a PEA arrest. Of course, have all intubation supplies ready at the bedside and intubate if you need to for transport, but if possible, avoid this until the patient is prepped and draped in the OR.

DISPOSITION

- OR, then the SICU

BEWARE...

(!) Aortic disease in elderly patients can present with vague complaints; maintain a high level of suspicion.

(!) Ensure that your ultrasound visualizes the entire aorta. Do not confuse an indeterminate ultrasound with a "rule out."

(!) The aorta is a retroperitoneal structure; the patients who live long enough to reach the ED likely have a contained retroperitoneal hematoma and will likely not have free fluid on their FAST exam.

Sources

Reed KC, Curtis LA. Aortic Emergencies – Part II: Abdominal Aneurysms and Aortic Trauma. *Emergency Medicine Practice.* March 2006:3.

Jim J, Thompson RW. Management of Symptomatic (Non-Ruptured) and Ruptured Abdominal Aortic Aneurysm. In: Mills JL, Eidt JF, Mohler ER. *UpToDate.* Waltham, MA: 2014;2-14.

Notes

3 ▶ Acute Appendicitis

- Inflammation of appendix secondary to obstruction by fecalith (adults), lymphoid hyperplasia (children), or neoplasm (elderly).
- Lifetime risk of experiencing appendicitis is 8.6% for men and 6.7% for women.
- Most common between 10–30 years, but no age is exempt.
- Patients at extremes of age have increased atypical presentations, complications, and mortality.
- Complications include perforation, periappendiceal abscess, suppurative peritonitis, and septic thrombophlebitis.
- Mortality for non-perforated appendicitis is <1%, perforated appendicitis 3%.

Ddx
Gastroenteritis
Crohn's disease (IBD)
Diverticulitis
AAA
Ovarian cyst
Ovarian torsion
PID/TOA
Pyelonephritis
Nephrolithiasis
Ectopic pregnancy
SBO

EVALUATION

- **High Yield History**: Classic symptoms are periumbilical colicky pain that intensifies in the first 24 hrs, becoming constant and sharp, migrating to the RLQ. Typical presentation occurs in only 50% of patients.
  — Patient may also report nausea and vomiting AFTER the onset of pain.
  — There is no single sign, symptom, or laboratory test to reliably identify or exclude acute appendicitis.
- **Exam**: Look for peritoneal signs (rebound, guarding, percussion tenderness). A GU/pelvic exam should also be performed to evaluate for alternative diagnoses (CMT does NOT exclude appendicitis).
  — McBurney's point: Point of maximal tenderness lying two-thirds of the way along a line drawn from the umbilicus to the anterior superior iliac spine.
  — Psoas sign: Pain with hyperextension of right leg.
  — Obturator sign: Pain with internal rotation of flexed right hip.
  — Rovsing's sign: RLQ pain with palpation of LLQ.
  — Hop test (in children): Patient asked to hop but refuses due to pain.
- **Diagnostics**
  — Labs: CBC (leukocytosis), CRP (CRP >8 *and* WBC ≥10 is HIGHLY suggestive of appendicitis while CRP <8 *and* WBC <10 virtually excludes appendicitis only in LOW pretest probability patients), BMP, LFTs HCG (rule out ectopic), UA (stone, infection), guaiac (invasive colitis)
    ▪ Repeat WBC is not beneficial.
    ▪ A significantly elevated WBC does not exclude the diagnosis of acute appendicitis.
  — Overview of imaging:
    ▪ US is the initial imaging modality of choice in children and pregnant patients and patient's non-obese patients.

- US is helpful if positive; however, it is not as reliable at excluding acute appendicitis or identifying rupture.
- In patients deemed to have a high probability of acute appendicitis based on assessment, appendectomy without imaging is appropriate.

Imaging Modality	Diagnostic Criteria	Evidence	Notes
Ultra-sonography	Aperistaltic, blind-ending tubular, and non-compressible structure with diameter >6mm. In transverse view may have "target-like" appearance.	Sensitivity 66% to 100%; (increased with duration of pain but decreased with pregnancy); specificity 83% to 96%	• Use in young, non-obese patients or in pregnancy • Highly operator dependent • REMEMBER: If appendix not visualized the study is INCONCLUSIVE
CT	Abnormal appendix identified or calcified appendicolith seen in association with periappendiceal inflammation or diameter >6mm	Sensitivity of 90% to 100%; specificity 91% to 99%	• If broad Ddx consider adding oral contrast • If patient is thin consider adding IV contrast • REMEMBER: If appendix not visualized acute appendicitis can be EXCLUDED
MRI	Enlarged appendix >7mm, appendiceal wall >2mm, periappendiceal inflammation	Sensitivity of 97% to 100%; specificity of 92% to 98%	• Consider in pregnancy if diagnostic uncertainty persists despite ultrasonography

MANAGEMENT

- Keep the patient NPO and start IVF.
- Treat pain: Consider morphine: 0.05-0.1mg/kg.
- Treat nausea: Consider ondansetron 4mg IV.
- Surgical consultation (for appendectomy vs. antibiotics in acute UNCOMPLICATED appendicitis; percutaneous drainage of abscess with antibiotics and delayed appendectomy in acute PERFORATED appendicitis).
- Antibiotics without surgery can be used safely as primary treatment in patients presenting with acute UNCOMPLICATED appendicitis
- PERFORATED appendicitis merits initiating antibiotics once recognized. Abx choice depends on the patient's comorbidities.
- In UNCOMPLICATED appendicitis use of perioperative antibiotics has shown to decrease the rates of post-operative wound infections and abscess.

Appendix	Timing	Antibiotics
Non-perforated	Start within 1hr of surgery	Cefoxitin 2g IV QID **OR** ciprofloxacin 400mg IV Q12H + metronidazole 500mg IV Q6H
Perforated	Start as soon as recognized	*Mild-Mod Risk Patients:* Cefoxitin 2g IV QID **OR** ciprofloxacin 400mg IV Q12H **OR** + metronidazole 500mg IV Q8H *High Risk Patients:* Cefepime 2g IV Q12H + metronidazole 500mg IV Q8H **OR** Piperacillin-tazobactam 4.5g IV QID **OR** Imipenem 500mg Q6H

DISPOSITION

- Per discussion with your surgical team, most often to the OR.
- Rarely, a select group of very low-risk patients can be discharged home.
- RETURN IF: Pain persists or gets worse, you have high fevers, persistent nausea, vomiting, or any new or concerning symptoms.

BEWARE...

(!) Do not be falsely reassured by the absence of leukocytosis.

(!) The presence of CMT does not exclude the possibility of appendicitis.

(!) Post-appendectomy patients can still get "stump appendicitis," which is inflammation of the residual appendiceal stump. Rare.

Sources

Andersson RE. Meta-analysis of the clinical and laboratory diagnosis of appendicitis. *Br J Surg.* 2004;91(1):28-37.

Daskalakis K, Juhlin C, Pahlman L. The use of pre- or postoperative antibiotics in surgery for appendicitis: a systematic review. *Scand J Surg.* 2014;103:14-20.

Humes DJ, Simpson J. Acute appendicitis. *BMJ.* 2006;333(7567):530-4.

Varadhan KK, Neal KR, Lobo DN. Safety and efficacy of antibiotics compared with appendectomy for treatment of uncomplicated acute appendicitis: meta-analysis of randomised controlled trials. *BMJ.* 2012;344:e2156.

Vissers RJ, Lennarz WB. Pitfalls in appendicitis. *Emerg Med Clin North Am.* 2010;28(1):103-18, viii.

Notes

4 ▶ Bowel Obstruction

- Two types: SBO and LBO. Occurs due to blockage of forward flow of intestinal contents. Mortality rate as high as 30% when strangulation occurs.

EVALUATION

- **High Yield History**: Characterized by crampy, intermittent abdominal pain (often poorly localized), distention, nausea, and vomiting with the absence of flatus and bowel movements.
  - Past medical history for prior abdominal surgeries, hernia repair, malignancy, inflammatory bowel disease, immunocompromised state
- **Exam**
  - Abdominal distension, tympany, hyperactive/hypoactive or absent bowel sounds
  - Check for hernias. *IF* present: Tender to palpation? Able to be reduced? Appearance of overlying skin?
  - Peritoneal signs are concerning for strangulation or perforation.
  - Fever, tachycardia, tachypnea, hypotension are concerning for possible sepsis.
- **Diagnostics**
  - Labs: CBC (leukocytosis may indicate translocation of intestinal bacteria), BMP, lipase (pancreatitis), LFTs, lactate (ischemia)
  - EKG in patients to evaluate for MI presenting as abdominal pain and nausea
  - Imaging:
    - Upright and supine abdominal x-ray (diagnostic in 60% of cases, but only order if pt. is high pretest probability or you suspect perforation): Assess for free air under the diaphragm in the upright (indicates perforation), air-fluid levels (obstruction), or in the supine for dilated loops of bowel proximal to the site of obstruction with a lack of air distal to the obstruction. If negative and high degree of suspicion, obtain CT.
    - CT (PO/IV contrast): 90% sensitive and can identify the location of the obstruction by the presence of a transition point. Absence of contrast in the rectum is a sign of complete obstruction.
    - Abdominal US (88% sensitive, 96% specific): Assess for dilated loops of fluid filled bowel with back-and-forth peristalsis.

Ddx
Ascites
Mesenteric ischemia
Perforated viscous
Intra-abdominal sepsis
Post-operative ileus
Appendicitis
Cholecystitis
Gastroenteritis
Diverticulitis

Etiologies	
SBO	**LBO (less common)**
Adhesions from prior surgery (50%)	Volvulus
Malignancy	Malignancy
Crohn's disease	Diverticular abscess
Intestinal herniation	Pseudo-obstruction (autonomic dysfunction causing decreased bowel motility)

MANAGEMENT

- ABCs. Make patient NPO for bowel rest.
- Pain and nausea control.
- Consider placement of NGT to decompress bowel and provide relief of nausea and vomiting.
- IVF: These patients are generally hypovolemic from vomiting and third spacing into their bowel. Consider Foley catheter to monitor urine output in response to resuscitation.
- Correct metabolic derangement. Patients may be hypokalemic from vomiting.
- Antibiotics only indicated if concern for bowel strangulation or perforation. Consider ciprofloxacin (400mg IV BID) and metronidazole (500mg IV TID).
- Surgical consultation for conservative vs. operative management.

DISPOSITION

- Admit for trial of bowel decompression with NGT followed by surgical intervention if resolution of symptoms does not occur.
- Some patients with history of recurrent SBO may present with a partial obstruction that resolves while they are in the ED. Strict return precautions should be discussed with and given to the patient.
- RETURN IF: Your symptoms return, you have persistent vomiting, severe pain, fever, or any other new or concerning symptoms.

BEWARE...

- ⓘ A small bowel obstruction in a patient without history of abdominal surgeries is concerning for a malignancy.
- ⓘ Always have a high degree of suspicion for cardiac process in elderly patients who present with abdominal pain.
- ⓘ The absence of flatus or bowel movement is not always present in partial/early obstruction.
- ⓘ Note that hypertonic CT contrast agents (gastrograffin) may be somewhat therapeutic by reducing bowel edema and promoting peristalsis.

Source

American College of Radiology Appropriateness Criteria: Suspected Small-Bowel Obstruction. http://www.acr.org/~/media/832F100277004BC69A8C818C7C9BFF33.pdf. Published 2013.

5 ▶ Clostridium difficile Colitis (C.diff)

- The presence of symptoms (usually diarrhea) AND stool test positive for *C. diff* or its toxins
- Patients are either colonized or newly exposed with the bacteria. *C.diff* is normally metabolically inactive in healthy hosts, but antibiotics kill gut flora, leading to an overgrowth of *C.diff* and enterotoxin release.
- Most commonly associated with recent fluoroquinolone, cephalosporin, carbepenem, or clindamycin use.
- Majority of patients will have had antibiotics in past 14 days, almost all within past 3 months.

Ddx
Abx or chemo induced diarrhea
Viral/protozoan/bacterial diarrhea
Traveler's diarrhea
Food poisoning
IBD
Ischemic colitis
Malabsorption
Hepatitis

EVALUATION

- **High Yield History:** Foul-smelling pseudomembranous diarrhea associated with fever, cramping, abdominal discomfort, and recent antibiotic use. Diarrhea may have mucus or trace blood, but reports of melena are rare.
  - Patients with severe disease may have colonic ileus or toxic dilatation → presents as abdominal pain and distension but minimal diarrhea, this is a surgical emergency.
  - Assess for risk factors: elderly, inhibition of gastric acid secretion by PPI, recent antibiotic use and which ones, last hospitalization/ICU/nursing home, chemotherapy, IBD, immunosuppression, previous C. diff (25% recurrence)
- **Exam**: Fever, tachycardia, lower abdominal tenderness, large-volume watery stools
- **Diagnostics**
  - Labs: CBC, BMP, LFTs, lactate, *C. difficile* toxin assay (confirm with antigen assay vs. PCR), fecal leukocytes. Stool being sent for testing should conform to shape of container; if it is solid it is highly unlikely to be *C. difficile*.
  - EKG: Especially in elderly patients with abdominal pain
  - Imaging: Consider CT to evaluate for complications. Radiographic findings: Colonic wall thickening, colonic dilation, free fluid, or free air

Category	Criteria	Treatment
Mild-Moderate	Low grade temp, WBC <15, Cr <1.5x patient's baseline, no sepsis, no peritoneal signs, and age <65	Metronidazole 500mg PO Q8hr x10 days
Severe	High fever, WBC >15, Cr >1.5x baseline or age >65	Vancomycin 125-500mg PO Q6hr x10days; Consider surgical consult
Severe with complications	At least one: >12 BM/day, T >103, WBC >25, sepsis, intense and constant abdominal pain, ileus, or ICU care for C.diff	Vancomycin125-500mg PO Q6hr AND metronidazole 500mg IV Q8hr Surgical consultation

MANAGEMENT

- Medications
  - Antibiotics: Treatment depends on severity of presentation. PO/IV metronidazole, PO Vancomycin (see above)
  - Stop offending antibiotics as well as all other nonessential antibiotics if possible.
  - Avoid anti-motility agents such as loperamide and if possible stop medications such as PPI (can alter intestina; pH) or opiates (constipating).
- Surgical consultation for severe cases and especially in the presence of ileus, peritonitis, or concern for toxic megacolon
- Colectomy indicated for cases of toxic megacolon, colonic perforation, acute abdomen, or in some cases of septic shock
- Provide IVF and supportive treatment. Consider probiotics, but their utility is unclear.

DISPOSITION

- Admission indicated for most patients. Consider ICU admission for patients with severe disease, age greater than 70, WBC >35 or <4, bands > 10%, or complications due to the high mortality associated with these conditions.
- Consider discharge in otherwise young, healthy patients without severe disease and who are able to obtain close follow up.
- RETURN IF: You have high fevers, severe pain, symptoms are not improving, you stop passing stool, or any other concerning symptoms.

BEWARE...

(!) Many patients will have antibiotic-associated diarrhea that is not *C.diff.*

(!) Always thoroughly wash hands after treating patients with suspected or confirmed *C.diff*, as the spores are not killed with hand sanitizer.

Sources

Cohen SH, Gerding DN Johnson S, et al. Clinical practice guidelines for Clostridium difficile infection in adults: 2010 update by the Society for Healthcare Epidemiology of America (SHEA) and the Infectious Disease Society of America (IDSA). *Infect Control Hosp Epidemiol.* 2010;31(5):431-455

Debast SB, Bauer MP, Kuijper EJ, Committee. European Society of Clinical Microbiology and Infectious Diseases: update of the treatment guidance document for Clostridium difficile infection. *Clin Microbiol Infect.* 2014; 20 Suppl 2:1.

Linsky A, Gupta K, Lawler EV, Fonda JR, Hermos JA. Proton pump inhibitors and risk for recurrent Clostridium difficile infection. *Arch Intern Med.* 2010 Jul 12;170(13):1100.

6 ▶ Diverticulitis

- Colonic diverticula generally occur in the descending and sigmoid colon. When fecal material hardens within a diverticulum, the diverticulum becomes inflamed, resulting in focal necrosis with a microperforation.

- Classification: Uncomplicated (microperforation) vs. complicated (macroperforation). Complicated implies the regional spread of inflammatory process. Complications include abscess formation, peritonitis, obstruction (from inflammation or strictures), and fistula formation.

Ddx
SBO
Hernia
Ischemic colitis
Colorectal CA
IBD
Appendicitis
Infectious colitis
TOA
Nephrolithiasis
Cystitis
Ectopic

EVALUATION

- **High Yield History:** Typical symptoms include LLQ pain, fever, and change in bowel function (diarrhea or constipation). Nausea and vomiting do occur but are less common symptoms.

  — Patients may report dysuria or urgency from irritation to bladder from the inflamed diverticula.

  — Many patients will have recurrent episodes of diverticulitis. Ask about prior episodes and any complications.

- **Exam:** The most common signs are fever and LLQ tenderness to palpation.

  — Tachycardia and hypotension are uncommon and suggest a complicated case.

  — Peritoneal signs are also concerning for complicated diverticulitis.

- **Diagnostics**

  — Labs: CBC, BMP, LFTs, UA. If concerned for complicated case, consider lactate and pre-op labs including type and screen

  — Imaging: CT abdomen and pelvis with IV/PO contrast for all new cases and if concerned for complicated diverticulitis

    ▪ Goal to determine the extent of disease, if an abscess is present, to aid in possible surgical planning, and to exclude other etiologies

    ▪ Most common findings are pericolic fat standing, colonic diverticuli, and bowel wall thickening.

MANAGEMENT

- NPO/bowel rest, IVF, and pain control.
- Antibiotics: Based on hospital practice and resistance patterns. Examples: combination fluoroquinolone and metronidazole, Ampicillin/sulbactam, ticarcillin/clavulanate, or ertapenem.
- Surgical consult: Indicated for unstable patients, peritonitis, and special populations such as the elderly or immunocompromised. Also for patients with concern for complicated case based on exam, labs, or imaging.

DISPOSITION

- Admit patients who are older, immunosuppressed, have significant comorbidities, have high fever (>102.5°F/39°C), or significant leukocytosis.
- To the OR: If unstable, peritonitis, obstruction, clinically significant fistula, or abscess. Many abscesses are amenable to IR guided drainage.
- If uncomplicated case and otherwise healthy patient, consider discharge home.
- Criteria for outpatient treatment
    — Ability to return for medical reevaluation if condition worsens.
    — Ability to comply with outpatient treatment plan (ability to pick up prescriptions, is a reliable patient, etc.).
    — Pain is controlled and able to tolerate PO intake without nausea or pain and advance diet based on symptoms.
    — Afebrile or low-grade temps only.
    — No significant comorbidities.
- Discharge instructions
    — 10-14 day course of PO antibiotics. Example course: ciprofloxacin 500mg BID and metronidazole 500mg TID x14days.
    — Clear diet for 2-3 days (or symptomatic improvement) and slowly advance diet at home. A high fiber and low residue diet is without much evidence but still recommended.
    — Follow up with PCP for possible colonoscopy after symptoms are resolved to exclude malignancy and evaluate extent of diverticular disease.
    — Patients with recurrent episodes should be referred to a surgeon to discuss possible elective surgical interventions.
- RETURN IF: You develop high fevers, severe pain, constipation, are unable to take your antibiotics, or develop any other concerning symptoms.

BEWARE...

(!) Patient can have RLQ pain if they have a redundant sigmoid or right-sided diverticulitis (less common, higher prevalence in Asian populations).

(!) Diverticulitis can occur in the small bowel, but it is rare.

(!) Young patients (<40 years old) are more likely to have recurrent episodes.

Sources

Byrnes MC, Mazuski JE. Antimicrobial therapy for acute colonic diverticulitis. *Surg Infect (Larchmt)*. 2009;10(2):143-54.

Touzios JG, Dozois EJ. Diverticulosis and acute diverticulitis. *Gastroenterol Clin North Am*. 2009;38(3):513-25.

Biondo S, Golda T, Kreisler E, et al. Outpatient versus hospitalization management for uncomplicated diverticulitis: a prospective, multicenter randomized clinical trial (DIVER Trial). *Ann Surg*. 2014;259(1):38-44.

7 ▶ Biliary Disease

Several disease processes can affect the biliary tract (gallbladder and bile ducts), and they can have similar presentations.

Evaluation

Ddx
Hepatitis
Pancreatitis
Peptic ulcer
Esophagitis
Renal colic
Pneumonia
Pulmonary embolism
ACS
Aortic dissection

- **High Yield History**: Dull, achy epigastric or RUQ pain that may radiate to right shoulder and is associated with eating large meal of fatty foods. Patient may also have nausea, vomiting.
    - Risk factors for gallstones include female gender, older age, obesity, rapid weight loss, parity, family history, TPN, diabetes. Small ratio of stones are composed of calcium bilirubinate and are typically due to intravascular hemolysis (ie, sickle cell disease).
- **Exam**: Fever occurs in cholecystitis or cholangitis. Assess for RUQ tenderness, Murphy's sign (inspiratory arrest on deep palpation of RUQ), and any signs of jaundice.
    - Charcot's triad: Fever, RUQ pain, and jaundice→ cholangitis
    - Reynold's Pentad: Fever, RUQ pain, jaundice, shock, and altered mental status → severe cholangitis

- ## Diagnostics
    - Labs: CBC, BMP, LFTs, lipase, UA, and HCG
    - EKG: Cardiac illness and biliary pathology have a large overlap in symptoms.
    - Ultrasound is the imaging modality of choice for RUQ symptoms. Assess for gallstones, biliary sludge.
        - Signs of cholecystitis: Pericolic fluid, gallbladder wall thickness >3mm and sonographic Murphy's sign
        - Signs of obstruction: common bile duct (CBD) >6mm
    - HIDA scan: If high suspicion for cholecystitis but indeterminate US
    - MRCP: To further characterize biliary duct obstructions
    - ERCP: Diagnostic means to characterize a biliary duct obstruction such as choledocholithiasis and to also intervene with a sphincterotomy

Other Etiologies

- Acalculous cholecystitis: More common in elderly and critically ill patients (particularly those on TPN); common complication of AIDS as a result of CMV or cryptosporidium. Associated with long-term TPN. Fever may be only symptom. Higher acuity and greater mortality than calculous cholecystitis.
- Emphysematous cholecystitis: Characterized by gas in gallbladder wall, thought to be due to invasion of mucosa by gas producing organisms (eg, *E. coli, Klebsiella, Clostridium*). Common in diabetic patients, males, and up to 50% acalculous cholecystitis cases.

	Presentation	Work-Up	Treatment/Disposition
Biliary Colic	— Transient gallstone impaction at cystic duct or ampulla of Vater — Epigastric or RUQ pain that can be intermittent or constant. Pain can radiate to left shoulder — Exam generally benign — Associated with eating (fatty foods), nausea, and vomiting	**Labs:** Generally normal **US:** Gallstones	• Pain and nausea control • Majority discharged home on low-fat diet • If impacted stone, symptoms are less likely to resolve → surgery consult • Consider outpatient cholecystectomy
Acute Cholecystits	— Sudden inflammation of the gallbladder, likely due to obstruction of cystic duct (any cause) — May occur with or without bacterial infection — RUQ pain, fever, nausea and vomiting — + Murphy's sign - inspiratory arrest on deep palpation of RUQ	**Labs:** WBC (normal/↑); AST/ALT, Tbili and Alk phos (normal/↑) **US:** Gallstones, thick-ened GB wall (>3mm) pericholecystic fluid (PPV >90%) **HIDA scan:** Gallbladder fails to fill (most sensitive, specific)	• NPO, start IVF as indicated • Pain and nausea control • **Abx:** Piperacillin/Tazobactam, 3rd gen cephalosporin, or ampicillin + gentamicin • Surgical consult – for cholecystectomy • If significant inflammation may admit for delayed cholecystectomy
Choledocholithiasis	— Obstruction of CBD by gallstone — If uncomplicated has similar presentation and exam to cholelithiasis — Complications include gallstone pancreatitis and cholangitis	**Labs:** ↑Alk Phos, ↑Bili, ↑AST/ALT — If complicated ↑lipase or ↑WBC **US:** CBD >6mm	• Symptom control • ERCP for high risk patients • MRCP and endoscopic US for low or intermediate risk patients
Cholangitis	— Obstruction, elevated intraluminal pressure, and bacterial infection — **Charcot's triad:** Fever, jaundice, RUQ pain (all not consistently present) — +/- Fever, nausea, vomiting, signs of sepsis, jaundice	**Labs:** ↑WBC, ↑Bili, ↑Alk Phos,↑AST/ALT **US:** Ductal dilation, stones **ERCP:** For pt with high suspicion	• IVF +/- pressors • **Abx:** Piperacillin/Tazobactam, imipenem, or ampicillin/sulbactam + flagyl • Biliary tract decompression (ERCP, surgery)

MANAGEMENT

- IVF, NPO, pain control, and antiemetics.
- If concerned for cholecystitis or cholangitis give antibiotics.
  - Piperacillin/Tazobactam, 3rd gen cephalosporin, or ampicillin + gentamycin
- Surgery consultation for all cases of cholecystitis and choledocholithiasis.
- GI consult for choledocholithiasis and cholangitis for ERCP.
- Patients with cholangitis need urgent biliary tract decompression with ERCP or percutaneous interventional radiology drainage.

DISPOSITION

- Admit cases of cholecystitis, cholangitis, and choledocholithiasis for antibiotics and definite treatment.
- Discharge home patients with uncomplicated cholelithiasis with pain control and antiemetics. Patients should be advised to eat a low-fat diet and to follow up with a general surgeon for an outpatient cholecystectomy.
- RETURN IF: You have high fevers, persistent severe pain, your skin or eyes turn yellow, or any other new or concerning symptoms.

BEWARE...

- ⚠ Patients who have had a cholecystectomy can still develop choledocholithiasis.
- ⚠ CBD 6mm and can increase 1mm every decade after 60yo. Also, CBD usually dilated after cholecystectomy.
- ⚠ Consider gallstone pancreatitis in patients who presents with pancreatitis (lipase > 3 times the normal level).
- ⚠ Must keep biliary disease on differential in patients with atypical presentation (eg, elderly, septic).
- ⚠ Always ensure adequate work-up to exclude other pathologies; namely, get an EKG!
- ⚠ In patients who present with post-op pain after laproscopic surgery, always consider retained stone or bile leak.

Source

Privette TW, Carlisle MC, Palma JK. Emergencies of the liver, gallbladder, and pancreas. *Emerg Med Clin North Am.* 2011;29(2):293-317.

Notes

8 ▶ Pancreatitis

- Diagnosis established by the presence of 2 out of 3 criteria: 1) Abdominal pain consistent with the disease, 2) Lipase or amylase > 3x the upper limit of normal, 3) Characteristic findings from abdominal imaging
- Classified as: *mild* (absence of organ failure and/or necrosis), *moderately severe* (≤48h organ failure and/or local complication), and *severe disease* (>48hrs organ failure).
- Local complications include: peripancreatic fluid collections, pancreatic and peripancreatic necrosis, pseudocysts, and walled-off necrosis.
- Overall mortality 5%; in severe disease increases to 25-35%.
- No scoring system accurately predicts severity of disease.

Etiologies of Pancreatitis				
Toxic	**Metabolic**	**Obstructive**	**Infectious**	**Other**
EtOH*, methanol **Drugs:** ACEi, azathioprine, calcium, cisplatin, corticosteroids, estrogen, erythromycin, furosemide, mercaptopurine, metronidazole, macrobid, pentamide, propofol, octreotide, ranididine, salicylates, sulfa, tamoxifen, tetracycline, thiazide, valproate	Hypercalcemia Hyperlipidemia Hypertriglyceridemia DKA	Gallstones* Ampullary tumors Pancreas Divisum ERCP Postpacreatography Neuroendocrine tumors Pancreatic carcinoma Sphincter of Oddi fibrosis, stricture, tumor	**Viral:** Adenovirus, coxsackievirus, CMV, EBC, HIV, HepABC, echovirus, varicella, rubella **Other:** Aspergillus, campylobacter, cryptococcus, mumps, TB, mycoplasma, Salmonella, Streptococcus, Legionella	DKA, Crohn's, cystic fibrosis, emboli, hemochromatosis, hypothermia, vasculitis, lupus, ischemia (hypoperfusion), pregnancy, Reye's, trauma, uremia, scorpion bites, idiopathic*, trauma

*Most common causes

EVALUATION

- **High Yield History**: Rapid onset of epigastric or LUQ abdominal pain; often radiates to back and can be persistent and severe in nature. Associated with nausea and vomiting.
  - Assess for possible precipitants; most common are gallstones and EtOH.
- **Exam:** May present with SIRs criteria (fevers, tachycardia, and hypoxia).
  - Epigastric tenderness, jaundice
  - Hemorrhagic pancreatitis: Cullen sign (periumbilical ecchymosis) or Grey Turner sign (flank ecchymosis)

Lab Pattern
↑WBC
↑Lipase (>2-3x nl)
↑ALT/AST/AlkPhos
↑Lactate
↓Albumin
↓PaO2

- **Diagnostics**
  - Labs: CBC, BMP, LFTs lipase (more sensitive than amylase), lactate (if sick). ALT >150IU/L suggests biliary pancreatitis. Draw blood/urine cultures prior to antibiotics for suspected extrapancreatic infection (ie, PNA, UTI, cholangitis, bacteremia)
  - EKG: For patients with upper abdominal pain
  - Imaging
    - US: Identify gallstones, dilated CBD (3mm at 30 years old; then add 1mm for each 10 years after; BUT varied size post-cholecystectomy); first line if pancreatitis is suspected.

ED independent variables that correlate with severity
Persistent SIRS
Age> 55
Obesity, BMI>30
HCT>44%
Pulmonary insufficiency/hypoxemia, PaO2 < 60
Rising BUN, Cr >2 (after rehydration)
Pleural effusions/infiltrates
Multiple or extensive extrapancreatic collections

    - CT w/contrast: Not normally needed—can help if diagnosis is uncertain or if local complications suspected. Current recommendation: Obtain a CT scan for evaluation of necrosis in a patient with evidence of ongoing pain, fever, persistent SIRS, or organ dysfunction *after 48-72hrs of admission.*
    - CXR: Concern for pleural effusion/infiltrates

MANAGEMENT

- NPO, IVF
  - Aggressive IV hydration (250-500mL/hr or 5-10mL/kg/hr) over the first 12-24 hrs (LR preferred over NS). Note: Fluid choice is often controversial and very region-dependent.
  - Reassess resuscitation (aim for a decrease in BUN, normal Cr) within 6 hrs and for the next 24-48 hrs.
  - Complications of aggressive hydration: volume overload, pulmonary edema, abdominal compartment syndrome.
- Replete electrolytes, especially Ca^{2+} (drops due to saponification).
- Control pain and nausea/vomiting
- Start appropriate antibiotics for suspected extrapancreatic infections (ie, cholangitis, PNA, UTI, bacteremia). Discontinue if cultures are negative.
- If suspected or confirmed pancreatic necrosis, give abx (eg, imipenem 500mg IVQ6H; known to penetrate pancreatic necrosis).
- Biliary pancreatitis: If acute cholangitis-early ERCP. Consider MRCP or endoscopic US instead of ERCP if no signs of obstruction in order to screen for choledocholithiasis.

DISPOSITION

- ICU: Presence of severity factors (see table), sepsis, multiple co-morbidities, oliguria.
- Uncomplicated patients can be admitted to the floor.
- These patients rarely are discharged from the ED.
- RETURN IF: You have high fevers, persistent severe pain, or any other new or concerning symptoms.

BEWARE...

(!) Patients with recurrent pancreatitis may have normal or minimally elevated lipase.

(!) Always search for an etiology

Sources

Wu BU, Conwell DL. Acute pancreatitis part I: approach to early management. *Clin Gastroenterol Hepatol.* 2010;8(5):410-6

Schepers NJ, Besselink MG, Van santvoort HC, et al. Early management of acute pancreatitis. *Best Pract Res Clin Gastroenterol.* 2013;27(5):727-43.

Tenner S, Baillie J, Dewitt J, Vege SS. American College of Gastroenterology guideline: management of acute pancreatitis. *Am J Gastroenterol.* 2013;108(9):1400-15.

Notes

9 ▶ Mesenteric Ischemia

- Occluded blood flow in mesenteric vessels, resulting in bowel ischemia and infarction.
- Arterial: Low flow states (sepsis, hypovolemia-CHF); thrombotic (HTN, DM, CAD, PVD); embolic (a-fib); iatrogenic (medication adverse effect-epinephrine; procedural complication); trauma.

Evaluation

- **High Yield History**: Acute onset abdominal pain that is persistent, poorly localized, colicky, and severe. "Pain out of proportion to exam." Associated with nausea, vomiting, and diarrhea. "Intestinal angina" (pain with eating).

  — Assess for risk factors: Atrial fibrillation, PVD, valvular heart disease, or aortic aneurysm.

- **Exam**: May have low-grade temp, tachycardia. Patients often are described as "writhing in pain."

  — Abdominal exam is generally benign unless significant ischemia has occurred → peritoneal signs

  — Guaiac positive stool may be present (sloughing of dead bowel).

  — Assess for risk factors including irregular heart rate, murmurs, signs of peripheral vascular disease, or hypotension

- **Diagnostics**

  — Labs: CBC (leukocytosis), BMP (metabolic acidosis), LFTs (increased AST, Alk phos), lipase, lactate (highly sensitive, not specific), LDH, phosphate, CPK, and amylase maybe elevated. Obtain coags. Troponin (r/o ACS).

  — Imaging

    - Upright and supine KUB may have signs of bowel obstruction, free air, or pneumatosis intestinalis.
    - CT (PO/IV contrast of abdomen): Edema of bowel wall, intramural gas, ascites. Note: Can have mesenteric ischemia with a negative CT. If suspicion is high, obtain angiography (catheter directed or CTA).
    - EKG

Ddx
Infectious colitis
IBD
Diverticulitis
Radiation Enteritis
C. diff
Cholecystitis
Perforated Bowel
Nephrolithiasis
Bowel Obstruction

Celiac artery	Superior mesenteric artery	Inferior mesenteric artery
Esophagus, stomach, proximal duodenum, liver, gallbladder, pancreas, spleen	Distal duodenum, jejunum, ileum, colon up to splenic flexure	Descending colon, sigmoid colon, rectum

MANAGEMENT

- **Emergent surgical consultation**: Patients with peritoneal signs require exploratory laparotomy.
- Correct underlying causes
  — Hypovolemia or hypotension: fluid resuscitation +/- pressors (avoid alpha agonists such as phenylephrine)

- — Control arrhythmias (avoid digoxin, beta blockers).
  - — Stop all vasoconstrictive medications.
- NGT for enteral decompression.
- Broad spectrum antibiotics to cover gut flora.
  - — Piperacillin/tazobactam or third-generation cephalosporin plus metronidazole
- For embolic or thrombotic ischemia, consider systemic anticoagulation with heparin.
- Consider IR for angiography and catheter directed antithrombotic therapy.

Causes of Mesenteric Ischemia		
Etiology	**Pathogenesis**	**Risk Factors**
Arterial embolus (40-50%)	Emboli from the heart	CAD (post PCI), valvular disease, Afib
Arterial thrombus (25%)	Chronic visceral atherosclerosis → plaque rupture	Atherosclerosis, "abdominal angina'
Non-occlusive (20%)	Mesenteric vasoconstriction or low flow states leading to decreased perfusion to watershed areas	Hypotension, splanchnic vasoconstriction from (pressors or cocaine)
Venous thrombosis (5-10%)	Relative venous stasis	Hypercoaguable states, trauma, polycythemia Vera, inflammatory states

DISPOSITION

- All these patients are admitted or go directly to the OR.

Sources

Sise MJ. Acute mesenteric ischemia. *Surg Clin North Am*. 2014;94(1):165-81.

Acosta S, Björck M. Modern treatment of acute mesenteric ischaemia. *Br J Surg*. 2014;101(1):e100-8.

Bobadilla JL. Mesenteric ischemia. *Surg Clin North Am*. 2013;93(4):925-40, ix.

Notes

10 ▶ Ovarian Torsion

- Can occur at any age, but most commonly occurs in women of reproductive age.
- Generally associated with benign tumors or large cysts that are >5cm.
- Torsion of a normal ovary is rare but does occur (more common in premenarchal girls).
- Progression is venous/lymphatic obstruction → edema → ischemia and necrosis of the ovary → peritoneal irritation.
- Ovarian ischemia can lead to necrosis and peritoneal irritation.
- No pathognomonic sign or symptom and is therefore frequently confused with other conditions.

Ddx
Appendicitis
Ruptured ovarian cyst
UTI/renal colic
PID/TOA
Diverticulitis
Ectopic
Pregnancy
Endometriosis

EVALUATION

- **High Yield History**: Acute onset low abdominal/pelvic pain, often associated with nausea +/- vomiting. (Nausea and onset of pain usually occur simultaneously.) May have history of recent exertion.
  — Tends to occur on R>L but can occur on either side. Pain can be sharp/stabbing and can radiate to flank, back, or groin. Pain is generally constant from time of onset but intermittent symptoms may represent intermittent torsion.
  — Risk factors: Known ovarian mass, cysts, fertility treatment, and early pregnancy (due to enlarging corpus luteum).
- **Exam**: May be hypertensive and tachycardic due to pain. Fever can indicate alternative diagnosis but fever can occur in the setting of tissue necrosis. Abdominal exam ranges from benign to peritoneal (with ovarian necrosis).
- **Diagnostics**
  — Labs: No specific lab will diagnose torsion, but lab data can be useful to exclude alternative diagnosis. Always get HCG and UA, CBC. Consider STI testing.
  — Imaging: Bedside US can be used to assess for free fluid or IUP.
    ▪ TVUS: will typically show enlarged ovary (due to edema and vascular congestion) with associated mass
      ◆ Ovary may have altered position (normally lateral to uters).
      ◆ Classically heterogeneous stroma and small peripherally displaced follicles are seen.
      ◆ Decreased or absent venous flow. May see "whirlpool" sign indicating twisted vessels.

MANAGEMENT

- NPO, IV fluids
- Emergent gynecology consult for diagnostic laparoscopy and surgical de-torsion.
- Rapid diagnosis is key to preserving ovarian tissue.
- Provide adequate pain control and supportive care.

DISPOSITION

- Patients with diagnosis should be admitted to the gynecology service or go directly to the OR.
- If pain resolved but large cyst is visible on US, consider admission for observation for intermittent torsion.
- If alternate diagnosis made but patient had large cyst noted on US, she needs close GYN follow-up.
- RETURN IF: You have severe pelvic pain, especially on the side of the cyst, persistent vomiting, or any other new or concerning symptoms.

BEWARE...

(!) Failure to consider the diagnosis.

(!) Torsion can occur with anatomically normal ovaries, particularly in pediatric patients.

(!) Ultrasound demonstrating arterial flow does not rule out torsion (especially intermittent torsion). If you have high clinical suspicion, request emergent gynecology consult.

Sources

Houry D, Abbott JT. Ovarian torsion: a fifteen-year review. *Ann Emerg Med*. 2001;38(2):156-9.

Cass DL. Ovarian torsion. *Semin Pediatr Surg*. 2005;14(2):86-92.

Notes

Section II.
Altered Mental Status

1 ▶ Altered Mental Status Quick Guide

- ALWAYS: IV, O2, Monitor, COMPLETE VS (including temperature and pulse oximetry), EKG (arrhythmias or specific patterns consistent with toxic ingestion), fingerstick glucose, airway equipment close nearby if needed
- Can't-miss diagnoses in first 2 minutes:
  - Hypoglycemia → D50 IV or oral glucose if able to take PO.
  - Hypoxemia → Manage airway and ventilation (pulse ox and EtCO2). O2 (BVM, NIV, or intubate prn); naloxone 0.4-2mg IV/IM/IN.
  - Bacterial Meningitis → Antibiotics +/- antivirals +/- steroids.
  - Shock → Identify etiology and resuscitate
  - Ischemic or Hemorrhagic CVA → Identify; interventions as indicated by local protocols.

Assess need for immediate intervention by overall appearance		
Confused	**Agitated**	**Unresponsive**
Maintain airway, oxygenation, ventilation. If GCS<8 or rapidly declining, consider RSI.	Keep yourself and staff safe: security standby, remove items that could be used as weapons prior to approaching pt (ie, stethoscope from around neck). Manage environment: minimize stimuli, keep voice volume low and tone calm, avoid sudden movements, keep an exit between pt and yourself.	**Status epilepticus or post-ictal**: Supine, airway maintenance, O2, IV/IM benzos (midazolam, lorazepam, diazepam) fo sz. If ineffective, consider fosphenytoin IV.
Reassure patient and use family members to provide comfort to the patient	Consider antipsychotic 5-10mg if willing to take sublingual and history suggests primary psych etiology	**Apneic / hypoxic/GCS <8**: Naloxone 0.4-2mg, IV/IM/IN; intubate prn
Consider sitter as well as physical and chemical restraints	**Tremulous**: Consider repeat dosing of benzos if history of EtOH and no concern for hepatic encephalopathy **Violent**: Antipsychotics (ziprasidone, haloperidol) +/- benzos)	**Head trauma**: Hypotensive, bradycardic, irregular respirations, anisocoria: — Intubate (RSI) — Call nerosurgery — Consider hypertonic saline and mannitol — Hyperventilation to EtCO2 ~30 (as last resort only)

EVALUATION

- **High Yield History**: Acute vs. chronic, PMH, meds (esp. opiate, anticholinergic, but many others can cause this), time "last seen at baseline mental status"
- **Exam**: VS! Focused neurologic exam (key: level of consciousness, pupils, reflexes, localizing signs):
  — Response to pain (pen in nail bed, sternal rub)
  — Hypoventilation or inability to protect airway
  — Pupils, posturing
  — Reflexes: Corneal, dolls' eyes, gag
  — Look for asymmetric responses.
- Other evidence of toxicological syndromes, "wet or dry," meningeal signs, rash, bitten tongue, incontinence, evidence of trauma (esp. to head)
- **Initial Workup (based on Hx/Exam)**: UA, urine/serum tox, ABG or VBG, CBC, BMP, LFTs, NH3, TSH, RPR, B12, serum osmolarity, drug levels if applicable, CSF studies (LP).
  — Imaging: CXR, head CT, MRI, EEG (in consultation with neurology)
  — EKG: Assess for QTc, ischemia, hypo/hyperkalemia and calcemia, arrhythmia, or evidence of toxic ingestions.

Differential (Extensive!)			
Primary Intracranial	**Systemic Disease**	**Drugs/Toxins**	**Withdrawal**
Trauma (contusion/bleed/ herniation)	Electrolyte/acid-base abnormalities (DKA)	EtOH	EtOH
Tumor	Arrhythmia/HTN	Opioids	Opiates
ICH	Hyper/Hypoglycemia	Toxic alcohols	BZDs
Seizure/non-convulsive status	Hepatic encephalopathy	Prescribed meds	
Psych	Uremia	Street drugs	
Stroke	Thyrotoxicosis/Myxedema coma	CO	
Infectious	Infection: UTI/PNA/Sepsis/ SBP/etc.	Heavy metals	
	Hyper/Hypocortisol	Toxidromes	
	Hypercapnea		

MANAGEMENT OF ACUTE EtOH INTOXICATION

- May be able to observe until pt is clinically sober and is able to ambulate independently without extensive testing.
  - Smells like alcohol or admits to EtOH
  - Denies other ingestions or suicidal ideation
  - Normal vital signs, normal glucose
  - Reassuring exam: No signs of trauma and moving all extremities
- Otherwise consider labs +/- head CT, +/- cervical spine protection, and evaluation

BEWARE...

(!) Get collateral information and complete medication list from family and EMS.

(!) Send the urine early!

(!) Don't accept incomplete sets of vital signs.

(!) Get an EKG after the first 10mg of Haldol to evaluate for prolonged QTc.

GCS		
Eye Opening	Spontaneous	4
	To voice	3
	To pain	2
	None	1
Verbal	Oriented	5
	Confused	4
	Inappropriate words	3
	Incomprehensible	2
	None	1
Motor	Obeys commands	6
	Localizes Pain	5
	Withdraws to pain	4
	Decorticate	3
	Decerebrate	2
	None	1

Notes

2 ▶ Agitated Patient

- The first priority is the safety of you and your staff.
- Patients may present with agitation or may develop during an ED stay.
- Identify escalating behaviors and utilize de-escalation techniques.

EVALUATION

- **High Yield History**: Assess for organic causes of agitation: drugs, alcohol, delirium (esp. in elderly).
  - History from EMTs, family, friends, neighbors, PCP.
  - Any drug use, psychiatric illness or trauma?
  - Any medical illness or complaints prior to onset of symptoms?
- **Exam**: VS, FS blood glucose
  - Any toxidromes or evidence of drug use?
  - Complete neurologic exam and trauma survey.
- **Diagnostics**
  - EKG on all patients.
  - Labs and imaging → driven by history, exam and collateral information:
    - CBC, chem 7, LFTs, NH3, VBG, lactate, UA, troponin, UDS, EtOH, LP, TSH, ASA/acetaminophen/other drug levels, HCG
    - CXR, CT brain

Ddx
Hypoxia
Hypoglycemia
Hyperthermia
Psychiatric disorders
HTN emergency
EtOH withdrawal
Anticholinergic
Brain-injury
Stimulant overdose
Seizure
ICH
Brain tumor
Delirium/sepsis
Meningitis/encephalitis
Hypercarbia
Thyrotoxicosis

MANAGEMENT

- ENSURE PERSONAL AND STAFF SAFETY.
- Place patient in a private but not isolated room. Notify security, remove patient's possessions (including medications and weapons). Anything that can be used as a weapon should be removed from the room and your person, including your stethoscope (do not wear around your neck) and large earrings. Should secure long hair.
- **Verbal de-escalation:** For patients who are agitated but cooperative. Not for patients who are violent, uncooperative, or delirious. A calm, non-confrontational but firm demeanor should be adopted. Provide comfort with warm blankets, food, or drink (no hot water or anything that could be used as a weapon, such as soda cans, forks, etc.).
- **Physical restraints:** Document necessity/what else was tried/end-point. ALL PATIENTS WHO ARE PHYSICALLY RESTRAINED MUST ALSO BE CHEMICALLY RESTRAINED. Should repeatedly reassess need for restraints and de-escalate as soon as able.

- **Chemical restraints/sedation (as per facility policy):**
  - Oral: Haloperidol (5mg po, 0.5-1mg po if elderly) or olanzapine (5-10mg po; comes as oral dissolving tab), or lorazepam 1-2mg po.
  - Injectable: Benzos (lorazepam 1-2mg IV/IM; haloperidol 0.5-10mg IV/IM; ziprasidone 10-20mg IM).
  - For extrapyramidal sx: Diphenhydramine (25-50mg PO/IV/IM) or benztropine (1mg PO/IV/IM).
  - Check EKG for prolonged QT if any antipsychotics

DISPOSITION

- Disposition depends on the underlying etiology as agitation is generally a symptom of another process. Many of these patients will be admitted for the underlying disease process.
- Consider discharge if a clear etiology is discovered and treated (ie, EtOH intoxication). Pt must be safe for discharge and unlikely to have imminent recurrence of sx.
- RETURN IF: You have any severe headaches, seizure activity, develop high fevers, have chest pain or shortness of breath, feel unsafe, have thoughts of hurting yourself, or have any other new or concerning symptoms.

BEWARE...

! Learn to identify escalating behaviors early.

! Always consider a medical explanation for agitation.

! Fully search patient and remove meds/weapons.

! Physical restraints without adequate chemical sedation → musculoskeletal/nerve injury or aspiration.

Notes

3 ▶ Alcohol Withdrawal

- A potentially life-threatening syndrome that occurs in the setting of abrupt decrease or discontinuation of alcohol use in habitual drinkers. EtOH acts as a GABA agonist. In the setting of abrupt cessation of chronic EtOH there is decreased GABA signaling and unopposed NMDA (excitatory) simulation.

- **Kindling:** The phenomena that occurs when repeat events of alcohol withdrawal lead to an increased severity of subsequent withdrawal episodes.

- All patients in the ED are at risk for withdrawal. Be especially cautious with patients being monitored until clinically sober, those with prolonged ED stays (including transfer patients), and all trauma patients.

Ddx
Head trauma
CNS infection
Hypoglycemia
Epilepsy
Psychiatric disease
Toxic alcohols
Stimulants
Anticholinergic intoxication
Sepsis
Hepatic encephalopathy
Thyrotoxicosis

EVALUATION

- **High Yield History**
  - EtOH use: Type of alcohol, amount per day, last drink, how long the patient has been drinking, and any recent attempts to cut back.
  - Any history of withdrawal symptoms or history of withdrawal seizures.
  - Why has the patient stopped drinking (is there underlying infection or other medical symptoms)?
  - Other ingestions?
  - Any history of trauma?

- **Tremulousness**: Occurs early (12-18 hrs) and is associated with hypertension, tachycardia, nausea, vomiting, diaphoresis, anxiety, tremors.

- **Withdrawal seizures**: Can be the presenting symptom of alcohol withdrawal or anytime in the first 24-48 hrs. Can be a single seizure or a brief flurry with short post-ictal states; usually are generalized tonic-clonic.

- **Hallucinosis**: Occurs early (<48 hrs) and is associated with tremulousness, hallucinations (usually visual/tactile but can be auditory).

- **Delirium tremens**: Occurs late (2-10 days) and is associated with hallucinosis (agitation, confusion, visual hallucinations) and autonomic instability (↑ temp, ↑ resp, ↑ pulse, HTN). High mortality, up to 20-40%.

- **Exam**: Vital Signs, mental status, and neurologic abnormalities.
  - Any diaphoresis, tremors, asterixis?
  - Assess for underlying infections or any signs of trauma.

- **Diagnostics**
  - Labs: Serum EtOH level is not indicative of risk for withdrawal.
    - Consider EtOH level, urine/serum tox, BMP, CBC, lipase, CPK, LP, Mag level, LFTs. If concern for toxic alcohol obtain serum osmolarity.
  - Imaging: Consider CXR, head CT, and EKG for all patients.

MANAGEMENT

- ABCs: Start with IV access, IVF, and telemetry to assess for arrhythmias as indicated. Intubate for airway protection as indicated.
- Benzodiazepines are the standard treatment for treating both withdrawal symptoms and seizures. May require large doses; monitor the airway. Use institutional withdrawal protocol (ie, "CIWA," etc.).
  - Lorazepam: Start with 2mg IV/PO Q2 hrs for mild cases, up to 6-8mg IV every 15-60min in severe cases.
  - Diazepam: 20mg PO or IV Q2hrs up to 15-20mg Q30-60min in severe cases.
  - Consider chlordiazepoxide 50mg PO in mild cases.
- If refractory to benzodiazepines→ can consider barbiturates such as phenobarbital for status epilepticus, severe symptoms or in special populations where another agent is required.
- If refractory to benzodiazepines and phenobarbitol→ intubate and start propofol infusion.
- For hallucinations consider haloperidol or ziprasidone or dexmedetomidine (Load: 1 mcg/kg IV over 10min; then start infusion of 0.2-0.7 mcg/kg/hr).
- For all patient replete fluids and electrolytes as well as thiamine and folate (may need large doses of thiamine: 300-500mg/day). Consider initiating a "Banana Bag" (multivitamins 1-2 amps; thiamine 100-500mg, folate 1mg, Magnesium 2gms in 1 liter IV fluids x1).

DISPOSITION

- Patients who have had a seizure or DTs should be admitted to the ICU.
- Uncomplicated withdrawal or hallucinosis can be admitted to the medical floor vs. ICU.
- Mild cases (mild tremulousness that can be controlled in the ED) can be discharged with a detox referral. Consider prescribing short course of oral benzos for symptom management UNLESS pt is going to continue drinking.
- RETURN IF: You have a seizure or develop tremors or hallucinations and do not have access to alcohol, vomiting, chest pain, shortness of breath, abdominal pain, thoughts of self-harm, or any other new or concerning symptoms..

BEWARE...

- (!) Identify and treat early, but be sure not to miss sepsis, trauma, or any co-ingestion.
- (!) Alcohol withdrawal affects all socioeconomic groups; consider in **everyone** who presents with first-time seizure.
- (!) Give sufficient quantities of benzodiazepines in ED to control symptoms. These patients will have a high tolerance.

Sources

Mayo-Smith MF, et al. Management of alcohol withdrawal delirium: an evidence-based practice guideline. *Arch Intern Med.* 2004;164(13):1405-1412.

Amato L, Minozzi S, Vecchi S, Davoli M. Benzodiazepines for alcohol withdrawal. *Cochrane Database Syst Rev.* 2010;(3):CD005063.

Pitzele HZ, Tolia VM. Twenty per hour: altered mental state due to ethanol abuse and withdrawal. *Emerg Med Clin North Am.* 2010;28(3):683-705.

Marx J, Hockberger R, Walls R. Rosen's Emergency Medicine: Concepts & Clinical Practice. 5th ed. Maryland Heights, MO: Mosby; 2002.

Notes

4 ▶ Toxic Alcohol Ingestion

- Toxic alcohols: Ethylene glycol, methanol, and isopropyl alcohol
- Sometimes patients will present with the report of ingestion, but most don't. Maintain high suspicion.
- The combination of an osmolar gap of >10-25 mosm AND a high anion gap metabolic acidosis (anion gap >12) suggests toxic alcohol ingestion. The osmolar gap and anion gap change over time. Initially there is a high osmolar gap due the toxic alcohol itself. As it is metabolized the osmolar gap decreases and the anion gap increases because of the presence of metabolites.

Ddx
EtOH intoxication
Uremia
DKA
Alcoholic ketoacidosis
Hepatic Encephalopathy
Lactic acidosis
Salicylate or acetaminophen OD

EVALUATION

- **High Yield History**: Type, amount, co-ingestion, last ingestion, container, accidental vs. recreation vs. self-harm
  — Review the bottle if it is brought in by family or EMS.
  — If found down, determine time frame and assess for evidence of trauma.
  — Clues to ingestion include the smell of acetone (isopropanol), the presence of hematuria or flank pain (ethylene glycol), and visual symptoms (methanol).
  — Consider the diagnosis in patients who present with EtOH ingestion but do not improve with observation.
- **Exam**: Secure airway, look for evidence of trauma
- **Labs**: FSBS, BMP, anion gap, serum osmolarity, osmolar gap (calculated), toxic alcohol levels, EtOH level, serum/urine tox, calcium, VBG, UA, serum ketons (if hyperglycemic), lactate, ASA/acetaminophen levels, LFTs.

	Osmolar gap	Anion gap
EtOH	+	If ketoacidosis
Ethylene glycol	+	+
Methanol	+	+
Isopropyl alcohol	+	-

  — Anion Gap: $Na^+ - [Cl^- + HCO_3^-]$
  — Serum osmolarity: $2 [Na+] + [BUN]/2.8 + [glucose]/18 + [EtOH]/4.6$
  — Osmolar gap = Measured – Calculated
    ▪ <10 usually normal
    ▪ Can be >25 with large methanol or ethylene glycol ingestions
- Osmolar gap is from parent alcohols and may be absent with late presentation after metabolism of the parent alcohol to toxic metabolites.
- Note that EtOH ingestion can have an anion gap acidosis in the case of alcoholic ketoacidosis and can also have an elevated lactate.

ETHYLENE GLYCOL

- Metabolized by alcohol dehydrogenase (ADH) to glycolate, glyoxylate, and then oxalic acid.
- Parent alcohol is relatively nontoxic, causing CNS sedation similar to EtOH.
- Toxicity from the metabolites → renal failure (from oxalic crystal precipitation), hypocalcemia, and pulmonary edema.
- Found in antifreeze, de-icing solutions and industrial solvents.
- Clinical syndrome: 4 stages, characterized by myocardial, cerebral, and renal damage.
  — Stage I: Acute neurologic (30 minutes-12 hrs post-ingestion): Parent alcohol causes intoxication.
  — Stage II: Cardiopulmonary (12-24 hrs): Tachycardia, hypertension, tachypnea, ARDS.
  — Stage III: Renal (24-72 hrs): Flank pain, hematuria, proteinuria, oliguria, and anuria.
  — Stage IV: Delayed neurologic (6-12 days): Cranial neuropathy most common finding.
- Rapid absorption with peak levels in 1-4 hrs, half-life 3-9 hrs. Toxic dose 0.2 mL/kg and lethal dose 1.4 mL/kg.
- Diagnosis: "Double gap" (anion + osmolar gaps), renal failure, calcium oxalate crystalluria, hypocalcemia all suggestive of diagnosis.
- Anion gap acidosis present only when acid metabolites have accumulated, usually within 4-8 hrs but may be delayed for more than 12 hrs if EtOH co-ingestion. Often profound acidosis with HCO_3^- <8.
- Lactate may be artificially elevated due to lab interference.
- Obtain a level to confirm ingestion but if concern is high enough to test, start treatment.

Seizure Ddx
Syncope
Hypoglycemia
Hyponatremia
Myoclonus
Atypical migraine
Movement disorder
TIA
Conversion Disorder

METHANOL

- Metabolized by ADH to formic acid and formaldehyde.
- Parent alcohol is similar to EtOH but with less CNS depression.
- Found in moonshine, windshield washer fluid, toner, canned heat, paint solvents, gasoline additives, home heating fuels. Also occupational exposure (painting, glazing, varnishing, printing; inhalational exposure often leads to toxic serum levels).
- Peak levels in 30-60 minutes. Half life of 24-30 hrs. Doses as small as 4ml can cause blindness and death.
- ADH has low affinity for methanol → latency period of 12-24 hrs between ingestion and presentation of symptoms or metabolic abnormalities.
- Will get delayed symptoms with EtOH co-ingestion.
- Toxicity from formic acid results in GI, CNS, and ophthalmologic symptoms.
  — Necrosis of the putamen → parkinsonism: rigidity, tremor, and monotonous speech; confusion, headache, and seizures.
  — Retinal damage→ blurring, blindness, central scotoma described as a "snowstorm."
  — Also causes nausea, vomiting, anorexia, and abdominal pain.

- **Diagnosis**: Made based on the history, presence of visual symptoms as well as the "double gap" (anion and osmolar).
  — Note, the anion gap may be delayed 12-24hrs.

ISOPROPYL ALCOHOL

- Metabolized by ADH to acetone, which is a ketone.
- Parent alcohol has twice the CNS depression effect of EtOH.
- Acetone is less toxic than isopropanol with mild CNS sedation.
- Found in rubbing alcohol (70-90% isopropanol), paint thinner, solvents, skin products.
- Peak levels in 30min-3 hrs. $T^{1/2}$ 3-7h. Potential lethal dose is 2-4mL/kg, but ingestions of 1L are survivable.
- Toxicity is possible following dermal exposure (infants).
- Presents with intoxication, abdominal pain, nausea/vomiting, fruity odor (significant ketosis). With massive ingestion can develop hypotension, tachycardia, peripheral and myocardial depression as well as hematemesis and pulmonary edema.
- **Diagnosis**: Osmolar gap without anion gap (metabolite is a ketone not an acid), and presence of urine ketones.
  — Pseudo renal failure: serum creatinine increases 1mg/dL for every 100mg/dL acetone.
  — Pursue alternative diagnoses if clinical symptoms fail to improve steadily over a few hours.

MANAGEMENT

- Airway evaluation→intubate if indicated, resuscitate with IVF.
- No role for gastric decontamination as these are all rapidly absorbed.
- **For methanol and ethylene glycol**:
  — Inhibit alcohol dehydrogenase from creating further toxic metabolites (if low osmolar gap, generally too late in course for this to be effective):
    ▪ Fomepizole 15mg/kg IV load then 10mg/kg Q12hrs.
    ▪ Alternative is EtOH but is difficult to dose, sedating, and irritating to veins.
  — Hemodialysis for severe acidosis, renal failure, or other evidence or end-organ damage.
  — Administer cofactors: Thiamine 100mg IV Q6H and pyridoxine 50mg IV Q6H x 2 days. This promotes metabolism of folic acid in methanol poisoning, unclear effects in ethylene glycol poisoning.
  — Consider sodium bicarbonate in patients with pH< 7.3 to promote urinary excretion.
- Monitor and replete calcium in ethylene glycol poisoning.
- Isopropyl alcohol treatment is generally supportive as acetone is less toxic than the parent alcohol.
  — No role for fomepizole as you want to encourage metabolism.
  — If hypotension, use IVF and pressors as needed. Consider dialysis in the rare cause of refractory hypotension.

DISPOSITION

- EtOH: Can discharge home when able to ambulate unassisted. If withdrawing, must admit.
- Isopropyl alcohol: If small ingestion and no symptoms after 2-3 hrs of observation and no co-ingestion, can discharge home as long as there is no concern for safety such as a suicide attempt or pediatric exposure.
- Admit all patients with methanol or ethylene glycol ingestion.

BEWARE...

ⓘ A lower osmolar gap does not exclude toxic alcohol ingestion. Pt may be presenting later into the ingestion, and the parent alcohol may already be metabolized.

ⓘ Test for toxic alcohols, but if suspicious enough to be testing, start treatment.

ⓘ Always suspect toxic alcohol exposure in patients who do not fit the typical EtOH ingestion profile or are not improving as expected.

Notes

5 ▶ Hepatic Encephalopathy

Normally ammonia (NH3) is processed to urea in the liver but in hepatic disease there is increased NH3 because of portosystemic shunting of NH3, with endogenous GABAergic BZD-like neurotransmitters accounting for encephalopathy.

EVALUATION

Ddx
Infection (SBP)
Meningitis
Encephalitis
Head trauma
Hypoglycemia
Electrolyte abnormalities
Uremia
Ingestions
EtOH withdrawal

- **High Yield History**: Consider in any patient with liver disease who presents with changes in mental status, behavior, or personality
  - Assess for precipitants: Infection such as spontaneous bacterial peritonitis (SBP), GIB, new hepatocellular carcinoma, electrolyte abnormalities, diuretics, sedatives, benzos, opioids or portosystemic shunts (TIPS), constipation/dehydration/high protein diet
- **Exam**: Altered mental status, asterixis, jaundice, hepatic fetor
  - Stage 1: Disordered sleep, irritable, depressed, mild cognitive dysfunction
  - Stage 2: Lethargy, confusion, disorientation, asterixis, personality changes
  - Stage 3: Stupor, somnolent, confused speech, unable to follow commands
  - Stage 4: Coma
- **Diagnostics**: Serum ammonia levels do not correlate with the severity of encephalopathy; primarily a clinical diagnosis
  - Labs: CBC, BMP, LFTs, coags, tox screen, NH3, blood cultures if febrile, peritoneal fluid analysis troponin PRN.
  - Ammonia: >200µg/dL associated with cerebral edema/herniation.
  - Diagnostic paracentesis if patient febrile, has abdominal tenderness, or is significantly altered.
    - 30-60cc of fluid is usually sufficient.
    - Send for cell count, culture, and differential.
    - Fluid PMN count >250cells/mm^2 is diagnostic of SBP.
    - Consider patient's level of coagulopathy before any invasive procedure.
    - Do not perform tap if no pockets of fluid >4cm deep on ED Ultrasound.
  - Obtain RUQ US with Doppler if patient is post TIPS procedure to evaluate patency.
  - Consider head CT.

MANAGEMENT

- Airway protection, consider OGT/NGT for lactulose administration if patient unable to take PO (versus PR).
- Correct electrolyte abnormalities.
- Completely avoid sedatives if possible.

- Rule out other causes of AMS → see AMS Quick Guide.
- Medications:
  - Lactulose poorly absorbed in GI tract and converts to lactic acid by GI bacteria → fecal stream acidotic → traps NH_3 as NH_4^+ in stool
    - 30-60gm PO, NGT or 300gm PR, titrate to 2–4 loose stools/day.
    - Improves mental status but does not improve survival.
  - Rifaximin 400mg TID to decrease colonic bacteria that produce NH_3
  - Alternative to rifaximin is neomycin 500-1000mg Q6hrs
  - SBP: Antibiotics should cover bowel bacteria that have translocated across bowel wall: *E. coli, Klebsiella*, and rarely *Strep* and *Staph*
    - Third generation cephalosporin: Cefotaxime 2gm IV q8h or Ceftriaxone 2gm IV q24h
    - If PCN allergic: Levofloxacin (750mg IV Q24h) or ciprofloxacin (400mg IV BID) or Pip/Tazo (4.5gm IV TID).

DISPOSITION

- Admit stage 2 or above, or stage 1 with poor compliance/no home support.
- Low protein diet on discharge (30-40g/day).
- Home lactulose.
- RETURN IF: You experience declining mental status, confusion, high fevers, black tarry stool, inability to take fluids, or any other concerning symptoms.

BEWARE...

ⓘ Don't give hepatic metabolized meds or meds that can worsen encephalopathy (ie, lorazepam).

ⓘ Don't miss GI bleed, electrolyte disturbances, infection (watch for spontaneous bacterial peritonitis).

Sources

Albrecht J, Norenberg MD. Glutamine: a Trojan horse in ammonia neurotoxicity. *Hepatology*. 2006;44(4): 788-94.

O'beirne JP, Chouhan M, Hughes RD. The role of infection and inflammation in the pathogenesis of hepatic encephalopathy and cerebral edema in acute liver failure. N*at Clin Pract Gastroenterol Hepatol*. 2006;3(3):118-9.

Khungar V, Poordad F. Hepatic encephalopathy. *Clin Liver Dis*. 2012;16(2):301-20.

Ong JP, Aggarwal A, Krieger D, et al. Correlation between ammonia levels and the severity of hepatic encephalopathy. *Am J Med*. 2003;114(3):188-93.

6 ▶ DKA/HHS

- **Diabetic Ketoacidosis (DKA)**: Acute onset (24 hrs). Absolute or severe relative insulin deficiency resulting in decreased utilization of glucose and increase gluconeogenesis (excess counter regulatory hormones). This results in hyperglycemia and ketosis. DKA predominantly seen in type I diabetics but is possible in type II DM.

  — Characterized by severe relative or absolute insulin deficiency leading to hyperglycemia (>250mg/dL), ketonemia, and metabolic acidosis (pH<7.3, bicarbonate <15mEq/L).

Ddx
Alcoholic Ketoacidosis
Infection/ Sepsis
Ingestions
Toxic alcohol ingestion
Uremia
Gastroenteritis
Appendicitis
Pancreatitis

- **Hyperosmolar Hyperglycemic State (HHS):** Insidious onset (days). Relative insulin deficiency → increased osmolarity and osmotic diuresis → urine output → PO intake → dehydration and hyper viscosity → insulin inhibits lipolysis → mild ketonemia (predominantly occurs in type II DM).

  — Characterized by hyperglycemia (>600mg/dL), hyperosmolarity (serum osm>300) and significant hypovolemia. Less acidosis and ketosis than in DKA (pH >7.3, bicarbonate >15mEq and minimal ketonuria/ketonemia).

EVALUATION

- **High Yield History**: Both can present with polydipsia and polyuria.

  — DKA patients will often present with nausea, vomiting, abdominal pain, weight loss, weakness, visual changes, and AMS.

  — Patients with HHS are more likely to have AMS (mild to comatose) and/or neurological sx or deficits.

  — Assess for precipitants including infection,* first presentation of new onset type I DM* (*account for two-thirds of cases), MI, CVA, non-adherence/change in insulin dose, EtOH, trauma, GI bleed, pancreatitis, pregnancy, Cushing syndrome, hyperthyroidism, and medications (steroids, HCTZ, atypical anti-psychotics, cocaine).

- **Exam**

  — DKA: AMS, tachypnea with Kussmaul respirations, tachycardia, orthostatic/frank hypotension, fruity (acetone) breath, and signs of dehydration.

  — HHS: CNS findings (ie, focal deficits, seizure), extreme dehydration, orthostatic/frank hypotension, tachycardia.

- **Diagnostics**: Both processes are nursing intensive because of the frequent medication titration and lab draws.

  — Labs: FSBS, CBC, BMP, (remember: correct Na ↑ 1.6 mEq/L for every 100 mg/dL that the glucose is >100 mg/dL), UA, urine and serum ketones, ABG/VBG, serum β-hydroxybutyrate, LFTs, lipase, TSH, Mg, and Phos. Consider troponin, HCG. Calculate anion gap.

  — EKG and imagining if indicated by precipitating event.

MANAGEMENT

- VS, EKG, IVFs. Monitor UOP, and treat precipitant (ie, infection).
- Check FSBS Q1 hour and check BMP and VBG Q1-2 hrs.
- Goal is to treat precipitant, replete fluids and electrolytes, and lower the blood sugar. Do not start insulin until potassium level is known.
- **Electrolytes**: Total body K⁺ deplete. Must check K⁺ prior to insulin (causes large cellular shifts and rapid hypokalemia → life-threatening arrhythmias).
  - K⁺ < 3.3: No insulin. Give 20-30mEq/hr IV until K+ >/= 3.3 mEq/L (will need central IV line for >10mEq/hr).
  - 3.3< K⁺< 5.0: Give 20mEq K⁺ in 1L IVF, start insulin drip.
  - K⁺>5.0: Start insulin drip. Do not supplement K⁺.
  - *Only replete phos if ≤ 1.0.
  - Maintain K+ = 4-5mEq/L. Check Q2hrs.
- **Dehydration**: Fluid deficit in HHS (average >8L) vs. DKA (3-6L)
  - **Step 1:** Bolus IVF
    - Replete 1-2L NS over first 1-2hrs
    - Pediatrics: 20mL/kg NS over first hour; *don't exceed 45mL/kg in first 4 hrs* to avoid cerebral edema
  - **Step 2**: Maintenance IVF. After initial bolus, change to ½ NS (250-500 mL/hr) IF corrected serum Na⁺ (add *1.6mEq Na⁺ for every 100mEq/dl glucose above normal levels*) is high or normal. If corrected serum Na+ is:
    - Hi or nl → 1/2NS (250-500 ml/hr) until volume is restored.
    - Low → NS (250-500 ml/hr) until volume is restored.
  - **Step 3**: After glucose <250, change to D5 ½ NS (150-250 mL/hr) until anion gap resolves. Titrate rate of fluids based on age, cardiac status, and degree dehydration. UOP goal 1-2ml/kg/hr. In HHS more IVF is required. The goal is to replace ½ fluid deficit in first 8 hrs, the rest over next 24 hrs.
- **Hyperglycemia**: Fluid alone will start to decrease glucose in patients with HHS. Do not start insulin if K+ <3.3 mEq/L. Peds: NEVER BOLUS; use IV drip only.
  - Regular insulin: Start drip at 0.14U/kg/hr (no need for bolus); peds: Start drip @ 0.1U/kg/hr. Goal to decrease glucose by 50-70mg/dL/hr. If not meeting goal, double insulin drip. Optional bolus method for adults only. Regular insulin 0.1 u/kg IV bolus (or ½ dose IV and ½ SQ) then begin insulin drip @ 0.1 u/kg/hr.
  - Continue insulin drip until glucose <250. Then decrease insulin drip to 0.05U/kg/hr to maintain glucose 150-200.
  - If glucose<150, give D50, but do not stop insulin drip. Continue insulin drip until ANION GAP closed, glucose < 200 mg/dL (or osm<315, glucose <300, and pt alert in HHS) and converted to SQ dosing.
  - To convert to SQ: Change insulin drip to 1-4 U/h and start intermediate/long-acting insulin (0.2-0.4 U/kg/d). Overlap IV/SQ insulin by 2-4 hrs. To convert to SQ pt must be taking PO; if NPO cont. IV insulin and D5 IVF.

- **Acidosis**: Bicarbonate only indicated in severe acidemia (pH <6.9) and is controversial. NaHCO3 100 mEq in sterile H2O 400 ml +/- KCl 20 mEq: infuse over 2 hrs.

DISPOSITION

- Many of these patients will be admitted to the ICU due to nursing needs. Also consider level of acuity based on the underlying precipitant.
- If the anion gap is closed or mild case of DKA, can consider admission to the floor.

BEWARE...

⚠ Treatment complications: hypoglycemia, hypokalemia, hypophosphatemia, and cerebral edema (more common in children, monitor IVF).

⚠ Slight acidosis present in HHS due to lactate, starvation ketosis, or renal hypoperfusion but still less acidotic than DKA.

⚠ Do not forget to treat underlying issue/precipitant.

⚠ UA "ketones" tests for acetoacetate. Beta-hydroxybutyrate → acetoacetate with treatment so ketonuria may *seem* to worsen. Therefore you can't "trend" UA ketones but could follow serum beta-hydroxybutyrate (not typically done).

Sources

Kitabchi AE, Umpierrez GE, Miles JM, Fisher JN. Hyperglycemic crises in adult patients with diabetes. *Diabetes Care*. 2009;32(7):1335-43.

Goyal N, Miller JB, Sankey SS, Mossallam U. Utility of initial bolus insulin in the treatment of diabetic ketoacidosis. *J Emerg Med*. 2010;38(4):422-7.

Notes

7 ▶ Seizure

- Generalized seizures (abnormal neuronal activity throughout both hemispheres — always causes an alteration in mental status).
- Convulsive (tonic-clonic/"grand mal") and nonconvulsive (absence).
- Partial seizure (a limited or confined area of neuronal involvement).
- Partial seizure subtypes: Simple (no impairment of consciousness) vs. Complex (involves some degree of impaired consciousness).
- Status epilepticus: seizure activity lasting >10 minutes or recurrent seizures without regaining full consciousness.

Etiology Ddx
CVA
Head bleed
Trauma
Tumor
Infection
Hyponatremia
Eclampsia
Toxin ingestion
Febrile
EtOH withdrawal
Hypoglycemia
Hypocalcemia
Hypomagneseemia
Subtherapeutic or supratherapeutic AED levels

EVALUATION

- **High Yield History**: Important to obtain details from patient and witnesses to distinguish between alternative diagnoses.
  - Timeline leading up to event, description of motor activity, duration, loss of urine or tongue biting, any fall with head strike?
  - Any history of prior strokes or head trauma, infectious symptoms, seizure disorder, cardiac illness, diabetes, HIV, or cancer?
  - Medications: Anticoagulation? Antiepileptics? Any changed or missed doses? New meds that lower seizure threshold?
  - EtOH or other substance abuse. Any preceding trauma?
- **Exam**: VS, signs of head trauma or meningitis, and any toxidromes. Look for gravid uterus — if pregnant, this is eclampsia (see OB section).
  - Full neuro and mental status exam; look for automatisms that could be sign of partial seizures and status.
  - Persistent AMS or neuro deficit can be difficult to distinguish from post-ictal state or Todd's paralysis.
- **Diagnostics**
  - EKG (syncope from an arrhythmia).
  - Minimum: Glucose, Na+ and HCG. Consider antiepileptics levels, full toxic-metabolic workup, and additional labs based on comorbidities (sepsis labs, troponin, etc.). CK if prolonged or repeated sz.
  - Consider lactate and prolactin, which may help distinguish seizure from volitional etiology.
  - Head CT for 1st time seizure, pts with history of trauma/cancer/anticoagulation, or focal abnormality.
  - If febrile or immunocompromised, consider LP.
- Consult neurology if persistent symptoms, concern for status epilepticus, or need for EEG.

MANAGEMENT

- Evaluate ABCs and place pt in position to reduce self-harm (on side, bedrails up, padded if possible), supplemental O_2.

- May need cooling if hyperthermic.
- Hypoglycemia → (1amp D50 IV or glucagon 1mg IM), Pregnancy → (2-4gm $MgSO_4$ IV).
- Initial: Lorazepam 2-4mg IV/IM, repeat prn (max – 0.1mg/kg).
- Refractory (>5min): fosphenytoin (20-30 PE/kg @ 150 PE/min IV) or levetiracetam (20mg/kg IV to max 60mg/kg) or valproic acid (20-40mg/kg @ 7.5mg/min IV) or phenobarbital (20mg/kg IV @ 50-100mg/min).
- Persistent/Status (>30min): Propofol (induction dose 1-2mg/kg; maintenance infusion: 30-200mcg/kg/min), intubation, STAT EEG. CAUTION: If intubation is required, may be hyperkalemic, so consider alternative to succinylcholine. Do not use long-acting paralytics (ie, vecuronium) in sz pts (masks ongoing sz activity).
- Immediate resuscitation of status epilepticus requires simultaneous efforts to terminate seizure activity and support ABCs while also identifying the etiology.

DISPOSITION

- Patients with persistent symptoms, not returning to baseline, or positive workup will need admission.
- Head injury, SAH: seizure prophylaxis x 1week – (ie, levetiracetam 1g IV then 500mg BID)
- ICH (SDH/parenchymal blood) = controversial: Neurosurgery consult STAT.
- First-time seizures: If clinically at baseline, workup negative, no comorbidities, and can arrange rapid neuro follow up — ok for discharge to safe home situation and accompanied by a responsible person who will drive.
  - Patients with a normal neuro exam and a structurally normal brain do not need antiepileptics initiated in the ED, patients with structural lesion may benefit from initiation of antiepileptics in ED after discussion with physician who will follow outpatient.
  - Counsel to refrain from driving until outpatient evaluation.
- Patients with known seizure disorder: Load if subtherapeutic antiepileptics levels, discuss med changes with their neurologist, most likely discharge.
- RETURN IF: You have severe headache, high fever, persistent vomiting, changes in vision, severe muscle pain, dark (tea-colored) urine, recurrent seizures, or any other new or concerning symptoms.

BEWARE...

- ⚠ Account for duration of sedating effect of lorazepam and monitor closely.
- ⚠ Immunocompromised patients who seize need an LP.
- ⚠ Alcohol withdrawal can present with seizure (without usual withdrawal prodrome).
- ⚠ If intubated and paralyzed or receiving aggressive therapy will need STAT EEG to rule out nonconvulsive status.

Source

Shearer P, Park D. Seizures and Status Epilepticus: Diagnosis and Management in the Emergency Department. *Emergency Medicine Practice*. August 2006;8(3).

8 ▶ Psychiatric Complaints

Psychiatric disease makes up a large portion of chief complaints and comorbidities of ED pts. While it is important to acknowledge the patient's psychiatric concern, our role is to ensure the patient is medically cleared for treatment (no active medical issues requiring further emergent workup or treatment or organic causes of psychiatric symptoms requiring medical interventions acutely).

Evaluation: ALWAYS MAKE SAFETY OF SELF AND STAFF THE TOP PRIORITY. IF THERE IS ANY CONCERN FOR UNPREDICTABLE, ERRATIC, OR VIOLENT BEHAVIOR ON THE PART OF THE PATIENT, ADDRESS IT FIRST.

Ddx
— Broad differential based on the history, ROS and examination.
— Do not forget medication side effects and ingestions.

EVALUATION

- **High Yield History**: History of psych hospitalizations or suicide attempts, presence of suicidal/homicidal thoughts or plans, presence of auditory/visual hallucinations, safety support at home
    - Medication compliance, drug/alcohol intake, substances ingested.
    - Collateral information from family, friends, outpatient physician/therapist and the patient's pharmacy.
- **Exam**
    - Full physical exam; additional focused areas based on ROS.
    - Orientation questions are essential because most psychiatric patients remain oriented; if not, suspect other causes (trauma, meningitis, encephalitis, sepsis, delirium, metabolic disarray, etc.).
- **Diagnostics**
    - Based on your history and physical examination. Some hospitals have a policy to help reduce over testing that can be used to guide your evaluation, but it is always important to include the psych consultants, especially if inpatient admission is sought.
    - For patients who will not be held for safety, seen by psychiatry consultation, or admitted, this workup is based on the history and physical.
    - Urine: Drugs of abuse tests for suspected use, ingestions, or planned admission; HCG for all females of reproductive age.
    - Blood: For all adult patients getting admitted or held for safety BMP, CBC (diff not required), LFTs (coags not required), basic tox panel (full panel not required), any medication levels (lithium, phenytoin, valproic acid, etc.).
    - EKG: For all patients on medications that cause conduction abnormalities (TCAs, SSRIs, antipsychotics etc.) or those who took stimulants. Consider troponin, total CK.
    - Consider toxic/metabolic derangements, infectious workups, and TSH if patient has no prior history of anxiety/agitation or psychosis.

MANAGEMENT

- Many states have laws that permit you to detain individuals against their will for a specific amount of time if they meet certain criteria. Some of these may include: 1) The patient is at risk for self-harm (suicidal); 2) The patient is a risk for harm to others (homicidal); 3) The patient is unable to protect himself or herself; (eg, an acutely disorganized schizophrenic patient not safe if discharged).
- KNOW YOUR STATE'S LAWS. If able do not wait for the psychiatry consult to assess the patient; when a patient meets one of the safety criteria determined by your individual state, detain him/her until their evaluation is complete.
- If holding a pt against their will due to concern for psychiatric well-being, remove their belongings and arrange a 1:1 sitter at bedside.
- Assess pt's capacity to make medical decisions. If deemed not to have **capacity**, pt can be detained against their will and medicated and/or physically restrained for safety, if indicated.
- **Capacity** requires (all four): Ability to understand relevant information, communicate a stable choice, appreciate the situation and its consequences, and manipulate information provided in a rational manner. (Note: Only courts determine "competence"; physicians can determine "capacity.")

DISPOSITION

- If deemed unsafe for discharge, admit to appropriate psychiatric unit/facility after being medically cleared.
- Consider obtaining psychiatric consult, if available, when boarding psychiatric pt in ED waiting for placement (make sure to order ongoing medications for sx management) and when uncertain if safe for discharge.
- If acute or new medical issue are diagnosed while in the ED, make a clear treatment plan and communicate it to accepting facility.
- If minor depression, anxiety, or other psych complaint without SI or psychosis, can discharge to home with psych follow-up and clear safety plan.
- RETURN IF: You have thoughts of self-harm or harm to others, feel unsafe, or you have any new or concerning symptoms.

BEWARE...

- (!) Always order safety precautions and a sitter on patients who are held for safety, and reassess the need for same periodically, as per hospital policy..
- (!) Always perform a thorough history and physical exam. Acutely psychotic or severely depressed pts sometimes don't display typical symptoms or responses to pain/discomfort.
- (!) Remember that psychiatric patients get medical illnesses, and many medical illness can present with AMS → don't anchor!
- (!) For patients being boarded while bed placement is found, write for home medications.

Sources

Santillanes G, Donofrio JJ, Lam CN, Claudius I. Is medical clearance necessary for pediatric psychiatric patients? *J Emerg Med.* 2014;46(6):800-7.

Zun LS. Pitfalls in the care of the psychiatric patient in the emergency department. *J Emerg Med.* 2012;43(5):829-35.

Notes

Section III
Back Pain

1 ▶ Back Pain Quick Guide

- ALWAYS: IV, O2, complete VS, full neurologic exam, assessment for midline tenderness, and full history assessing for presence of red flag symptoms.
- Can't-miss diagnoses in first 2 minutes: Aortic dissection, ruptured aortic aneurysm, unstable vertebral fracture, cord compression (including epidural abscess, hematoma).
- Most back pain is mechanical low back pain, but differential diagnosis is broad, including aortic / vascular (AAA, dissection, retroperitoneal bleed), renal (pyelonephritis, stone, infarct), pancreatic, GYN (HCG), PNA, infection/inflammation of the spine/cord.

EVALUATION

- **High Yield History**: Chronicity, associated symptoms, previous similar episodes, "red flags," past medical history of DM, malignancy, anti-coagulation, autoimmune disorder, hyper-PTH, osteoporosis, sickle cell disease. IVDU, immunosuppression (abscess), or steroids (vertebral fracture).
- **Red flag signs/symptoms:** Document absence or presence in all back pain patients:

CAN'T-MISS DIAGNOSES			
Diagnosis	**Risk Factors/ Symptoms**	**Physical Exam**	**Next Step**
Aortic Dissection	Male, >40, HTN, DM, smoker (typical). Also: pg, trauma, Marfan's, aortic coarctation. C/O: Sudden onset, "tearing pain," syncope	Hypotension, unequal pulses, murmur, neuro deficits, diaphoresis	W/U:CTA TX: Beta-blockers +/- nitroprusside and surgical consult if Type A
Expanding/Ruptured AAA	Advanced age, male, cardiac risk factors. C/O: Pain in thoracic and lumbar spine, abdominal pain, syncope	Pulsatile mass (<50%), abdominal bruits, decreased LE pulses, dusky lower extremity, +FAST or AAA on US	W/U: FAST/US vs. CTA (most ruptures are retroperitoneal- FAST/ US will miss it unless free fluid also in abdomen), TX: Surgical consult and BP control

Spinal Infections — Epidural Abscess — Vertebral osteomyelitis — Discitis	DM, renal failure, IVDU, endocarditis, bacteremia, recent spinal surgery, skin/ soft tissue infection, immunocompromised. C/o: Spine pain, f/c/ weakness (focal, bilateral, generalized)	Fever (~50%), localized spinal tenderness (usually at least 3-4 vertebral levels), focal neuro symptoms (~50%)	W/U: CBC (2/3 have leukocytosis), blood cultures, ESR / CRP (almost universally positive), and STAT MRI with contrast. TX: IV abx (usually after neurosurgery consult)
Epidural Compression Syndromes — Cauda Equina — Conus Medularis (L2) — Cord Compression	Back pain with rapid progression to neuro symptoms (urinary retention with overflow incontinence, fecal incontinence, uni or bilateral leg pain)	Saddle anesthesia, LE weakness, UMN signs (compression above L1),): Clonus, hyperreflexia, spasticity, Babinski's sign, nl muscle mass. LMN signs (compression below L1): Atrophy, fasciculations, weakness, decreased muscle mass.	W/U: MRI of the entire spine as it is difficult to tell cord level based on initial exam and may be more than one area. TX: Neurosurgical consult
Malignancy	Known malignancy, age >50, symptoms > 1 month, unexplained weight loss	Usually nonspecific but may include pain on palpation	W/U: X-ray and consider MRI if negative and clinical suspicion is high. Detailed exam of for likely primary tumor. TX: Heme-onc and/or neurosurg consult

- **Exam**: VS! (Any abnormality is a red flag), full MSK exam for spine and extremities: (strength, sensation, tenderness, ROM, pulses, DTRs, gait-walk every patient), cardiac exam, neuro exam.
- **Initial workup**: Usually minimal for MSK pain unless abnormal finding, high risk, or "red flag" encountered. Focus on treatment and expectation setting.

BEWARE...

🅘 Be suspicious of NEW low back pain in elderly; have a low threshold to image.

🅘 Epidural abscess at any location can cause symptoms consistent with cauda equina. Get entire spine MRI, not just lumbar spine.

Notes

2 ▶ Mechanical Back Pain

- Incidence by location→ lumbosacral > cervical >> thoracic
- Of lumbosacral injuries, L4-5 and L5-S1 are by far most common.
- Musculoskeletal low back pain (most common cause of back pain) is a diagnosis of exclusion that is usually self-limited in 4-6 weeks and only requires conservative management. Patient education is crucial. Referral to PCP is useful for ongoing management and consideration of advanced imaging.

EVALUATION

- **High Yield History**: Assess pain as you would normally (cardinal features, etc.), then add a directed review of symptoms to make more or less likely the "can't-miss" diagnoses.
  - Recent trauma, malignancy, fever, weight loss, parasthesias or other focal neuro symptoms, bowel and/or bladder incontinence or retention, IVDU, steroid use, past back surgeries, spinal hardware, or pain that is constant, worse when supine, severe (malignancy, infection).
- **Exam**: Detailed musculoskeletal exam and neurologic exam evaluating strength, sensation, DTRs, range of motion, gait.
  - Check for spinal or paraspinal localization and reproducibility.
  - DRE for tone/sensation.
- **Imaging**: Consider lumbar and sacral radiographs for: Age <18 or >50, any history malignancy or unexplained weight loss, fever, history or evidence of trauma, bony tenderness, focal neuro deficits, duration of pain >4-6wks. Not indicated for suspected disc herniation or if emergent CT/MRI is planned.

Special Techniques	
Specific sensory deficit	L5 (first web space), S1 (lateral small toe)
Specific motor deficit	L5 (weakness with great toe extension), S1 (weakened plantar flexion)
Deep tendon reflexes	L5 (normal), S1 (weak ankle jerk)
Upper motor neuron lesion	Clonus, hyperreflexia, up-going toes (pathological Babinski sign)
Poor rectal tone, perianal sensory deficit	Highly specific for cord injury, but does not give level
Straight leg raise — dermatomal pain or shooting pain in lower leg (not back or thigh) with hip flexion < 90 degrees	Specific but not sensitive for nerve root irritation; pain with contralateral SLR is specific for sciatica.

MANAGEMENT

- In patients age 18-50 with acute low back pain and absence of history of trauma, fever, weight loss, malignancy, immunocompromised, bladder/bowel dysfunction, or radiculopathy, consider empiric treatment for musculoskeletal back pain. Regimen includes: acetominophen/NSAIDS (if no renal or GI issues), opiates only for initial/breakthrough pain control, referral to PCP for evaluation for physical therapy and detailed patient education, avoidance of strict bed rest. Consider benzodiazepines (but never with opiates) or cyclobenzaprine.

- Patients with isolated c-spine pain of musculoskeletal origin also require conservative management, as outlined above.

DISPOSITION

- Simple musculoskeletal low back pain or disc herniation may be discharged home with appropriate pain control and PCP follow-up. Patients should be active but avoid pain-causing activities and heavy lifting.

- Do not hesitate to give a cane or walker to a patient who appears to have an unsteady gait to prevent fall.

- Disposition of emergent conditions varies with etiology (see table in Quick Guide).

- RETURN IF: You develop worsening pain, fever, weakness, incontinence, you pass out, or have any other new or concerning symptoms.

BEWARE...

- ⓘ Ensure that you are not missing a potentially deadly emergent diagnosis; take a moment to mentally review the Can't-Miss Diagnoses (Quick Guide) and "red flags" when evaluating each pt.

- ⓘ Always refer to and involve the patient's PCP (useful to monitor and initiate team-based management. of refractory cases).

Notes

3 ▶ Nephrolithiasis

- Types: Calcium oxalate (most common), struvite (urea-splitters), uric acid, and cystine
- If unable to pass stone, there is risk of urosepsis, anuria, and renal failure.

EVALUATION

- **High Yield History**: Pain in flank radiating to groin; maximal at onset then becomes episodic and colicky
  - May also report gross hematuria, dysuria, urgency, frequency, nausea, and vomiting
  - History of prior stones, family hx of stones, any stones requiring urological intervention, renal transplant, UTIs (pyelonephritis).
  - Note: VERY rare for elderly pt without hx of stones to present with nephrolithiasis. Consider alternate dx.
- **Exam**: May be tachycardic, hypertensive, and tachypnic from pain. Fevers are concerning for infected stone.
  - Patient may be writhing in pain, diaphoretic, and unable to find comfortable position.
  - Exam should be non-focal; CVA or abdominal tenderness suggests alternative diagnosis.
  - Perform GU/gyn exam to exclude other potential diagnoses.
- **Diagnostics**
  - Labs: UA (for infection and hematuria), CBC, BMP (to assess renal function), HCG, UCx
  - Imaging:
    - US can be used for first presentation of nephrolithiasis. Consider its use especially in the case of subsequent presentations if concern for hydronephrosis or hydroureter.
    - Non-contrast abdominal CT to assess for complications or for other diagnosis such as AAA.
    - Consider KUB for ongoing outpatient monitoring if fail to pass stone (establish baseline location of stone)..

Prognosis		
Size	Mean days to pass stone	Likelihood of needing intervention
< 2 mm	8	3%
3 mm	12	14%
4-6 mm	22	50%
> 6 mm	—	99%

Size and **location** predict likelihood of spontaneous stone passage. Regardless of size, the lower the stone in the urinary system, the greater chance of passing (American Urological Association, 2014).

MANAGEMENT

- Pain control: Morphine (0.1mg/kg—Can start most pts with 4mg IV) and ketorolac (30mg IV) if no CKD.
- Anti-emetic: Ondansetron 4mg IV (EKG to evaluate QT).
- IVF if dehydrated. No conclusive evidence that hydration helps pass stone.
- Consult Urology for: solitary/transplanted kidney, concurrent infection, stone unlikely to pass (>6mm or proximal), renal insufficiency.
- Patients with nephrolithiasis and urinary tract infection can decompensate quickly. Provide antibiotics (ciprofloxacin or 3rd generation cephalosporin) and consult urology for definitive care.

DISPOSITION

- Admit: Intractable pain or vomiting, infection, obstruction, renal insufficiency, solitary/transplanted kidney, stone unlikely to pass (>6mm or proximal)
- Most discharged home with:
  - — Strainer to catch stone for analysis and outpatient urologic follow-up
  - — Analgesia: NSAIDs, oxycodone, and phenazopyridine (200mg TID after meals).
  - — Tamsulosin (0.4mg daily) x 14 days to help pass stone.
  - — Ondansetron 4mg Q4hrs as needed for nausea/vomiting (if no prolonged QT).
- RETURN IF: You develop fever, increased pain, refractory vomiting (unable to keep down fluids/meds), or any other new or worsening symptom.

BEWARE...

(!) Always assess for a concurrent infection as these patients can develop sepsis rapidly!

(!) It is atypical for a patient to present for a first-time kidney stone after the age of 65. Consider AAA in an older patient with back pain (often left side) and hematuria.

(!) Patient with high-grade obstruction and infection or known renal pathology should NOT be sent home without urology consult first.

Source

Smith-Bindman R, Aubin C, Bailitz J, et al. Ultrasonography versus Computed Tomography for Suspected Nephrolithiasis. *N Engl J Med*. 2014;371(12):1100–1110.

Notes

4 ▶ Epidural Abscess

- Can occur from contiguous spread (1/3 of cases), hematogenous dissemination (1/2 of cases), or direct inoculation.
- Affects both the posterior (more common) and anterior epidural space.
- Damage to spinal cord occurs via direct compression, thrombosis, and interruption of blood supply.
- Can happen at any spinal level or more than one. Most commonly occurs in the lumbar and thoracic spine followed by the cervical spine and rarely in the sacral spine.
- Common pathogens are S. aureus (60% of cases, MRSA 15-40%), S. epidermidis (in spinal procedures), E.Coli (in UTI), Klebsiella, Pseudomonas (in IVDU), Strep.

Ddx
DJD/arthritis
Metastasis
Discitis
Osteomyelitis (coexists in 80% of cases)
Meningitis
Zoster
Epidural hematoma
Low back strain

EVALUATION

- **High Yield History**: Suspect in any patient with severe progressive back pain, fever, and neurologic deficits (rare to have all 3).
  — Back pain (45-75%), fever (30-50%), radicular pain.
  — Risk factors: IVDU, history of spinal surgery, spinal trauma, spinal abnormality, spinal intervention (glucocorticoid injection, epidural, nerve stimulator placement), osteomyelitis, HIV, indwelling IV access, alcoholism, malignancy, DM, CKD/dialysis, sepsis, or older age.
- **Exam**: Fever, may be tachycardic from infection or pain.
  — Bony tenderness along the spine.
  — Full neuro exam for any focal neurologic deficits.
  — Check rectal tone and check post-void bladder volume.
- **Diagnostics**
  — Labs: CBC (leukocytosis), BMP, Increased CRP (87%) and ESR (94%), blood cultures (bacteremia) BEFORE antibiotics (but do not delay abx once dx is suspected).
  — LP NOT recommended because of increased risk of spread.
  — Imaging: MRI (most sensitive and non invasive, cord compression protocol, image entire spine as it can be difficult to determine location of abscess based on exam.
  — CT myelogram (rarely used).

MANAGEMENT

- Antibiotics (Use of antibiotics prior to neurosurgery consult is controversial but generally should not be delayed.):
  — Vancomycin 15-30mg/kg IV if suspected MRSA or nafcillin 2grams IV or oxacillin 2grams IV.
  — AND metronidazole 500mg IV.
  — AND cefotaxime 2grams IV or ceftriaxone 2grams IV or ceftazidime 2grams IV if suspected pseudomonas.

- Spinal surgery consult for possible surgical decompressive laminectomy (contraindicated if pt not surgical candidate, paralysis for 24-36hrs, or paraspinal infection).
- Will eventually need abx therapy to cover organisms based on either blood cultures, abscess cultures from operation, or if not surgical candidate CT guided needle aspiration of abscess.
- Steroids can be considered in patients with progressive neurologic deficits awaiting surgery (however has been associated with sporadic adverse outcomes).

DISPOSITION

- Admit to the floor or to the ICU for decompressive laminectomy.
- Patients with concerning presentation for epidural abscess should not be discharged.

BEWARE...

(!) Image the entire spine if unable to precisely locate lesion on your exam. Presentations can be variable and more than one lesion can exist.

(!) Obtain emergent imaging. MRI with contrast; this is one of the true emergencies. Advocate for your patient.

(!) Have a high suspicion for this diagnosis in any patient with history of IVDU who presents with back pain.

Sources

Shah NH, Roos KL. Spinal epidural abscess and paralytic mechanisms. *Curr Opin Neurol.* 2013;26(3):314-7.

Shweikeh F, Saeed K, Bukavina L, Zyck S, Drazin D, Steinmetz MP. An institutional series and contemporary review of bacterial spinal epidural abscess: current status and future directions. *Neurosurg Focus.* 2014;37(2):E9.

Arko L, Quach E, Nguyen V, Chang D, Sukul V, Kim BS. Medical and surgical management of spinal epidural abscess: a systematic review. *Neurosurg Focus.* 2014;37(2):E4.

Notes

Section IV
Bleeding/Hematologic Complaints

1 ▶ Epistaxis

— **Anterior epistaxis** (90%)—Occurs anteriorly along the nasal septum at Kiesselbach's plexus located at Little's area (lower part of the anterior nasal septum)- an area of arterial anastomosis. Most cases of anterior epistaxis are unilateral, and self-limited with adequate tamponade.

— **Posterior epistaxis** (10%)—Occurs posteriorly along the nasal septum or lateral nasal wall. Supplied by branches of the sphenopalatine artery. Often presents in elderly, with brisk bilateral bleeding.

Etiologies	
LOCAL CAUSES	**SYSTEMIC CAUSES**
Idiopathic (80-90%): Spontaneous rupture during valsalva, noseblowing, weightlifting, etc.	**Heme:** Hemophilia, ITP, TTP, HIT, DIC, ALF, platelet dysfunction (i.e. Bernard-Soulier), coagulopathy (Von Willibrands) etc.
Traumatic: Epistaxis digitorum, facial injury, foreign body	**Environmental:** Humidity, cold, altitude
Inflammatory: Infection, allergic rhinitis, nasal polyps	**Meds:** Anticoag (heparin, LMWH, Coumadin, anti-Xa), antiplatelet (ASA, clopidogrel, ginkgo, ginseng), chemo, chronic 02 use, inhaled corticosteroids
Neoplastic: Juvenile Angiofibroma (benign), SCC	**Organ failure:** Uremia, hepatic
Vascular: Hereditary Hemorrhagic Telangiectasia	**Other:** HTN, alcohol abuse
Iatrogenic: ORL/OMFS surgery, NG tube placement	
Structural: Septal spurs, deviation, perf., hematoma	
Drugs: Topical decongestants, cocaine	

EVALUATION

- **High Yield History:** Circumstances (ie, spontaneous, nose blowing, trauma, etc.), methods attempted to stop bleeding, prior episodes/frequency/severity, estimated blood loss, recent heating in home, upper respiratory symptoms, recent trauma.
    - Past medical history for intranasal procedures, coagulopathy, cancer, renal failure, hepatic failure, allergic rhinitis, sinusitis, HTN.
    - Medications: Anticoagulants or antiplatelet agents; also supplements (ginkgo, garlic, ginseng).

- — Family history of bleeding diathesis orcancers (intranasal).
- — Any drug use (specifically cocaine or anything else that can be snorted) or EtOH use (altered platelet function).
- **Exam:** Focus on localizing the bleeding by using a nasal speculum oriented to open vertically and a good light source. Have the pt blow his/her nose to evacuate clots to improve visualization. If actively bleeding, can use intranasal oxymetazoline or phenylephrine to facilitate exam. Note: It can be difficult to distinguish anterior from posterior bleeding on exam, and this may only become clear by risk factors for posterior bleed (elderly, coagulopathy, bilateral bleed), or once anterior packing has failed. Exam should also focus on stigmata of anemia, renal failure, and hepatic failure.
- **Diagnostics:** Labs are generally not needed for resolved cases of anterior epistaxis. Can consider:
  - — CBC, Type and screen: If patient is continuously bleeding during evaluation or if posterior epistaxis.
  - — Coags: Should be ordered only if pt is anticoagulated, bleeding diathesis suspected, or surgery anticipated.
  - — Chem7: If suspecting acute renal failure as contributing factor.
  - — LFTs: If stigmata of hepatic failure or suspect hepatic failure as contributing factor.
  - — EKG, cardiac biomarkers: Only if patient having chest pain or equivalent, especially with history of ACS.

MANAGEMENT (Note: Wear gloves, gown, eye/face protection)

- **Step 1–Assess ABCs:** If patient profusely bleeding or unstable, establish 2 large-bore IVs, IVFs, and consider blood products. Consider airway protection and early ENT consultation if profound posterior bleeding source identified. Control HTN if present.
- **Step 2–Position:** Have patient lean forward to expel blood out of the nose. Note: Ingested blood is quite irritating to the GI system and may induce vomiting, posing risk of aspiration.
- **Step 3–Pressure:** Apply pressure directly to the anterior nasal septum, not the bridge of the nose. Place a cold compress over the nose or have pt suck on ice; maintain for 10-20min. This step is often all that is needed to stop anterior epistaxis.
- **Step 4–Anesthetics/Vasoconstrictors:** If pressure alone has not stopped the bleed, apply topical vasoconstrictor (oxymetazoline or phenylephrine), intranasal spray, or cotton pledgets soaked in the vasoconstrictor and anesthetic (ie, viscous lidocaine 2% or lidocaine 4% topical solution with 0.5% phenylephrine). Leave in place 5-10min with direct pressure applied.
- **Step 5–Cautery/Thrombogenic Foams**
  - — Chemical cautery: Apply a silver nitrate stick to the bleed with firm pressure for 5-10 seconds.
  - — Thrombogenic foams and gels: These can be considered in lieu of nasal packing (step 6). They are bioabsorbable so don't need to be removed. (ie, a hemostatic gelatin matrix mixed with thrombin and injected into nasal cavity).
  - — Tranexamic acid (TXA) 25mg (0.25ml of IV formulation) slurry with sterile sponge topically.

— Electrical cautery: Using disposable electrical cautery device; should consult ORL first.
  Note: If bilateral epistaxis, this step should only be applied to one side to decrease risk of perforation.

- **Step 6–Nasal Packing**

Anterior Nasal Packing	Posterior Nasal Packing
a) Nasal tampons: Involves packing with sterile sponge. Insert carefully along the floor of the nasal cavity to the posterior nasal cavity. Some products require application of a few drops of either NS or topical vasoconstrictor to allow for expansion within the nare. Others have an inflatable cuff that should be inflated using a 10cc syringe after insertiondinsertion. b) Formal packing: Involves posterior to anterior packing with ribbon gauze impregnated with petrolatum jelly or antibiotic cream, using bayonet forceps and nasal speculum. Ribbon gauze laid down in an accordion-like fashion, pressing each layer down until the nasal cavity is filled. Note: Recommended number of days for leaving packing in place varies in the literature from 1–5 days. There is also controversy as to whether prophylactic antibiotics should be given during this time to decrease the risk of toxic shock syndrome. In any case, packing should be removed by a physician, therefore follow-up must be arranged.	Usually performed by ORL, but may be done under emergent conditions with sedation a) Formal packing: Typically done under anesthesia or deep sedation b) Foley balloon tamponade: Pass a Foley balloon through the nasopharynx until visualized in the oropharynx. Inflate Foley with 3-4cc water or air. Pull forward until balloon engages the posterior choana. The nasal cavity is then packed anteriorly as above. c) Other: Brighton balloon, Epistat nasal catheter, Simpson plug Note: All patients with posterior packing will need admission with telemetry (reflex bradyarrythmias) and antibiotics (cephalexin, amoxicillin or ampicillin) to prevent toxic shock syndrome.

- **Step 7–Surgery**: Includes septal surgery, sphenopalatine artery ligation, anterior/posterior ethmoidal artery ligation, maxillary artery ligation, external carotid artery ligation, angiographic embolization of selected vessels.

DISPOSITION

- Anterior epistaxis; resolved prior to intervention: Discharge home.
- Anterior epistaxis that requires cautery or packing; observation for continued bleeding while awaiting labs, likely discharge home.
- Anterior epistaxis; unresolved despite above interventions: ENT consult, home vs. admit to ENT service.
- Posterior epistaxis; stable: ORL consultation, admit to Surgical service.
- Posterior epistaxis; unstable: ORL consultation STAT, admit to SICU.
- All patients going home should get: Oxymetazoline, 3 sprays daily (decreases immediate recurrence) as well as 2 weeks of bacitracin (or petroleum jelly) to the anterior nares twice daily. Role of prophylactic antibiotics is not well established, but bacterial infections such as toxic shock syndrome and sinusitis have been demonstrated in patients primarily receiving

postsurgical packing. Most sources recommend prescribing a short course of cephalexin, amoxicillin/clavulanic acid, and TMP/SMX in patient discharged with nasal packing.

- Dispo Instructions:
  - Return to MD in 2-3 days to get packing removed
  - Avoid heavy lifting, exercise, nose blowing, removing packing material.
- RETURN IF: Nosebleed returns despite packing or, if not packed will not stop with pressure, is a large amount, or returns frequently. Also return if bleeding from other places (urine, stool), feel dizzy, lightheaded, rash, fever, chills, vomiting blood, or any other new or concerning symptoms.

BEWARE...

(!) Always assess for possible posterior epistaxis and elicit key historical features that indicate systemic etiology.

(!) Obtain early ORL consultation for complicated bleeds.

(!) Always manage uncomplicated bleeds with direct pressure and use of topical agents as first line. Using cautery and nasal packing as first line therapy will place patient at increased risk of complications as well as increase hospital and health care costs.

Sources and Further Reading

Schlosser RJ. Epistaxis. *N Engl J Med.* 2009;360:784-9.

Viducich RA, Blanda MP, Gerson LW. Posterior epistaxis: clinical features and acute complications. *Ann Emerg Med.* 1995; 25:592-6.

Pope LER, Hobbs CGL. Epistaxis: an update on current management. *Postgrad Med J.* 2005;81:309-14.

Kucik CJ, Clenney T. Management of Epistaxis. *American Family Physician.* 2005;71(2):305-11.

Leong SCL, Roe RJ, Karkanevatos. No frills management of epistaxis. *Emerg Med J.* 2005;22:470-72.

Krempl GA, Noorilly AD. Use of oxymetazoline in the management of epistaxis. *Ann Otol Rhinol Laryngol.* 1995;104:704-6.

Badran K, Malik TH, Belloso A, Timms MS. Randomized controlled trial comparing Merocel and RapidRhino packing in the management of anterior epistaxis. *Clin Otolaryngol.* 2005;30:333-7.

Gilman C. Focus On: Epistaxis. Available at: https://www.acep.org/Clinical---Practice-Management/Focus-On--Treatment-of-Epistaxis.

Notes

2 ▶ Hematuria

- Hematuria (>5 RBCs/high power field), if transient, is generally a benign etiology. However, in older ages there is an increased risk of malignancy.

- Can be gross or microscopic. Caused by inflammation/injury to kidneys, bladder, ureter, prostate, urethra

- Amount of blood does not correlate with the severity of the etiology

Type of Bleeding	
Bleeding at the beginning of void, that clears	Urethral
Bleeding between voiding that stains clothes	Distal urethral or meatus
Hematuria throughout stream while voiding	Kidney disease
Bleeding at the end of stream/after voiding	Bladder neck, prostatic urethra
Cyclical bleeding	Endometriosis

Urine Color	
Clear (microscopic hematuria)	Stones, kidney disease, UTI
Gross hematuria/clots	Lower urinary tract (post-renal)
Brown/RBC casts/proteinurea	Glomerular disease (renal)

EVALUATION

- **High Yield History**: Is the patient hemodynamically stable?

  — Is the patient obstructed? Passing clots? Adequate urine output? Large post-void residual bladder volume or clots visualized on bedside US?

  — Any risk factors for malignancy: Age >35, smoking history, pelvic radiation, chemical or dye exposure, cyclophosphamide exposure?

  — Any history that points to etiology such as history of stones, renal disease, vasculitis, Afib (embolic syndrome), dehydration/pregnancy/ lymphoma (renal vein thrombosis), hypertension, recent URI, currently menstruating, any dysuria, fever or flank pain? Any blood thinners?

- **Exam**: Should focus on eliciting underlying etiology as well as any bleeding complications

  — Vital signs, examine urine for degree of hematuria or presence of clots. Assess for suprapubic fullness or signs of obstruction.

  — Suprapubic tenderness (cystitis), CVA tenderness (pyelonephritis), hypertension or edema (nephrotic syndrome).

Ddx
UTI
Urologic malignancy
Trauma
Menstruation, endometriosis
Sickle cell
Nephrolithiasis
Renal disease
BPH/prostatitis
Iatrogenic (procedure)
Paroxysmal nocturnal hemaglobinuria
Renal vein thrombosis
Interstitial nephritis
Vasculitis: HSP, Goodpastures, SLE, glomerulonephritis
Medications: NSAIDs, anticoagulation, rifampin

- **Labs**: All patients get a UA with sediment and urine culture as gross blood will make interpreting the UA difficult. Note that positive blood on UA but no RBCs on sediment → rhabdomyolysis; presence of RBC casts → glomerulonephritis.
  — Additional testing based on differential. CBC/coags if concerned about degree of bleeding or on warfarin. BUN/Cr to assess kidney function.
- **Imaging**: Based on differential. An imaging study of the kidneys and collecting system is indicated in patients with unclear cause of hematuria.
  — CT: Abdominal pain and suspect first time stone, or hematuria of unclear cause.
  — Urethrogram: In cases of urogenital trauma.
  — Renal US: In acute renal failure, recurrent nephrolithiasis or pregnancy.
  — Cystoscopy: In hematuria of unclear etiology, persistent or significant bleeding or in cases of blood clots. This can be done as an outpatient based on patient stability.

MANAGEMENT

- In the case of gross hematuria, ensure there are no large clots that could cause an obstruction.
  — If obstructed or large clots visualized within the bladder on bedside ultrasound, perform manual irrigation.
    - Place 20Fr Foley catheter or larger and perform manual irrigation with sterile saline to break up clots.
    - If, after several rounds of manual irrigation, there are no more clots and the urine is light pink, you can remove Foley and treat for underlying etiology.
    - If persistent clots, or if urine continues to be a dark red (signifying persistent bleeding) consult urology and place a 3-way Foley for continuous bladder irrigation. Note: The continuous irrigation helps prevent clotting in persistent bleeding. It is not as efficient at breaking up clots as manual irrigation.
  — If no concern for obstructing clots, treat based on presumed etiology. If unclear etiology patient should follow up with PCP or urologist for urine cytology testing.
  — Urology consult for persistent bleeding, large clots you are unable to break up with manual irrigation, concern for traumatic etiology, or if patient requires continuous bladder irrigation.
- In the case of microscopic hematuria:
  — Cystitis associated with a UTI causing hematuria should be treated with antibiotics for the UTI.
  — Nephrology consults in patients with a glomerular etiology.
- If exam or imaging consistent with a renal stone you should treat this based on size and location (see chapter: nephrolithiasis).

DISPOSITION

- Admit patients with:
  - Significant bleeding (dark red urine or drop in HCT).
  - Persistent bleeding requiring continuous bladder irrigation.
  - Clots that are not cleared with manual irrigation or signs/symptoms of urinary obstruction.
  - Acute renal failure.
  - Hypertensive emergency.
  - Traumatic injuries.
  - Significant comorbidities.
- Discharge patients who:
  - Are hemodynamically stable.
  - Have an identified source of bleeding that is treatable.
  - Can reliably follow discharge instructions and attend outpatient urology/nephrology follow-up
- All patients with hematuria, without a clear etiology, should have cystoscopy (inpatient or outpatient) to detect malignancy.
- All patients with microscopic hematuria or those with hematuria from presumed infection should follow up with their PCP to have repeat urine studies.
- RETURN IF: You become lightheaded, develop chest pain or shortness of breath, are unable to urinate, start passing dark red urine or clots, develop any fevers or chills, or any other new or concerning symptom.

BEWARE...

⚠ Have lower threshold for inpatient workup for patients with a solitary kidney.

⚠ Manual irrigation is not efficient through a smaller Foley catheter, and catheter will become obstructed.

⚠ Ensure that all patients with risk factors for malignancy understand they require close outpatient follow-up for further testing.

Sources

Cohen RA, Brown RS. Clinical practice. Microscopic hematuria. *N Engl J Med.* 2003;348(23):2330-8.

Hicks D, Li CY. Management of macroscopic haematuria in the emergency department. *Emerg Med J.* 2007;24(6):385-90.

3 ▶ Thrombocytopenia

- Platelets < 150,000 (always compare to baseline and compare with other cell lines)
- Surgical and procedural bleeding risk if <50,000. Spontaneous bleeding risk at 10,000-20,000 (not true for ITP)
- Thrombosis risk: HIT, anti-phospholipid syndrome, DIC, TTP/HUS, paroxysmal nocturnal hemoglobinuria

EVALUATION

- **High Yield History**: Recent hospitalization/heparin exposure (HIT), antibiotics (especially vancomycin, PCN and linezolid), AMS/ fever (TTP), infection (DIC), diarrhea, mucosal bleeding, bruising, episodes of epistaxis, recent viral illness/ vaccination, pregnancy (including retained products, abruption, amniotic fluid emboli).

Ddx	
Increased Destruction	**Decreased Production**
TTP/HUS	Myelodysplastic syndrome
HELLP	Liver disease
HIT	HIV
DIC	Malignancies with bone marrow
ITP	involvement
Infection	Sepsis
HIV	Marrow toxic drugs (EtOH,
SLE	chemotherapy)
Drug-induced	

  - Bleeding without systemic symptoms: Drug reaction vs. ITP, HIV, HCV.
  - Bleeding with critical illness: Sepsis, DIC, or bone marrow failure.
- **Exam**: Fever, mucosal bleeding, petechiae, bruising, lymphadenopathy, guaiac, neuro exam (bleeding into CNS), splenomegaly.
- **Labs**: REPEAT THE CBC! BMP, LFTs (liver or renal dysfunction), PT/PTT, +/- LDH, haptoglobin, retic count, fibrinogen, Coombs, sepsis labs, HCG.
- *Getting a peripheral smear is key*. It can confirm true thrombocytopenia (sometimes platelets clump and counts are artificially low) and show signs of microangiopathic hemolytic anemia (seen in HUS/TTP) or schistocytes (DIC). Giant (young) platelets are often seen in platelet destructive processes as the bone marrow tries to compensate. Also, there may be target cells (liver disease).
- Hematology consult if the patient appears sick.

MANAGEMENT

	ITP	TTP	DIC
Etiology	Autoantibodies causing immune-mediated platelet destruction	Inhibition of the enzyme ADAMS13 leading to platelet aggregation	Widespread activation of the coagulation cascade generally in the setting of critical illness
Signs/ Symptoms	Muscosal bleeding most common, splenomegaly	Thrombocytopenia, microangiopathic anemia, neurologic symptoms, fever and renal failure	Laboratory diagnosis (see DIC chapter) ↓platelets and fibrinogen ↑ Elevated PT
Treatment	Steroids, IVIG, or anti-D Immunoglobulin. Avoid NSAIDs.	FFP and plasma exchange	If severe bleeding transfuse appropriate blood products. If clotting start heparin.

- Per primary pathology. If likely HIT, stop heparin. If ITP, steroids and IVIG (if sick). If TTP stat hematology consult for plasma exchange.

Indications for transfusion:

- A "6-pack" of platelets is pooled from 6 donors, thus higher risk of transfusion reactions than other blood products. Should raise platelets by 30,000.
    - <20,000 with any bleeding or with any concurrent coagulation disorder/infection.
    - <50,000 with major bleeding or high risk bleeding: surgery or trauma.
- ITP transfuse only for any life-threatening bleed (space occupying bleed such as ICH or non-compressible such as GI/GU bleed). Anti-platelet antibodies that cause the disease will inactivate the transfused platelets as well. These patients often respond to steroids and hematology consult is indicated.
- Consider DDAVP if bleeding and platelets are non-functional (ie, uremia).
- TTP: Only if life-threatening hemorrhage, as even transfused platelets will aggregate and worsen clinical picture.

DISPOSITION

- Based on primary pathology
- Admit if new thrombocytopenia, bleeding concern, TTP, or DIC. Discharge if otherwise well, chronic thrombocytopenia, or ITP.
- RETURN IF: You experience persistent bleeding, any worsening bruising, severe headaches, head trauma, or any other new or concerning symptoms.

BEWARE...

⚠ Do not transfuse patients with ITP or TTP unless absolutely necessary.

Source

Vanderschueren S, De weerdt A, Malbrain M, et al. Thrombocytopenia and prognosis in intensive care. *Crit Care Med.* 2000;28(6):1871-6.

4 ▶ Disseminated Intravascular Coagulation (DIC)

- Disseminated intravascular coagulation (DIC) is unbalanced clotting and/or bleeding due to fibrin deposition and microangiopathic hemolytic anemia that can occur in any sick patient: severe sepsis, burn, trauma, shock, obstetrical complications, malignancy, TBI, liver disease, envenomation, heat stroke, transfusion, or drug reactions.

- Suspect in patients with end organ damage and inappropriate bleeding/ clotting on exam,

- In acute DIC, the clotting factors are consumed faster than they can be replaced →bleeding is the predominant feature,

- In chronic DIC, the body is able to replace clotting factors →thrombosis predominates,

Ddx
TTP/HUS
HIT
ITP
Liver disease
Anticoagulants
Factor deficiencies

EVALUATION

- **High Yield History**: Patients who develop DIC are generally acutely ill with another underlying disease such as sepsis, trauma, malignancy, head injury, recent surgery, or pregnancy complication. Also a risk with blood transfusions.
    - Bleeding, shortness of breath, chest pain, abdominal pain, confusion.
    - This is a clinical and lab diagnosis and should be suspected in sick patients with any bleeding or thrombotic event.
- Symptoms are the result of bleeding or thrombotic complications or end-organ hypoperfusion. This can be difficult to distinguish from symptoms of their underlying etiology.
- **Exam**: Vital signs (tachycardia, hypotension, tachypnea, or hypoxia).
    - Signs or symptoms of bleeding and thrombosis (arterial or venous):
        - Melena, hematochezia, hematemesis, abdominal pain/distention, epistaxis, hemoptysis, pulmonary edema, hematuria, or oliguria.
        - Skin exam for petechiae, purpura, jaundice, gangrene, cool extremities, or oozing from IV sites.
        - AMS, confusion, focal neurologic deficit.
- **Diagnostics**: Again, this is a clinical and laboratory diagnosis; must consider any lab abnormality in the clinical context.
    - Labs: CBC, Peripheral smear (schistocytes), d-dimer, fibrinogen, haptoglobin, coags (PT, PTT and INR), BMP, UA, and urine HCG.
    - Imaging: Use to evaluate for underlying etiology (eg, CXR for pneumonia).
- **ISTH Diagnostic Scoring System for DIC**: If the patient has an underlying disorder known to be associated with overt DIC
    - Order global coagulation tests (PT, platelet count, fibrinogen, ddimer, haptoglobin)
    - Score the test results:
        - Platelet count (>100K = 0, 50-100K = 1, <50K = 2)
        - Elevated d-dimer, haptoglobin (no increase = 0, moderate increase = 2, strong increase = 3)

- Prolonged PT (<3 s = 0, >3 but <6 s = 1, >6 s = 2)
- Fibrinogen level (>100 mg/l = 0, <100 mg/l = 1)
— **Calculate score**:
  - ≥5 compatible with overt DIC and <5 suggestive for non-overt DIC: repeat score daily

DIC Labs	
Test	**Finding**
Peripheral Smear	Low platelets, schistocytes, RBC fragments
Platelet Count	<100K
PT	Prolonged
PTT	Prolonged
Thrombin Time	Prolonged
Fibrinogen level	Reduced
Fibrin degradation products (D-dimer, haptoglobin)	Elevated
Serum Cr and UA	May be abnormal

- Combination of abnormal fibrinogen and d-dimer: 91% sensitivity and 94% specificity for DIC.
- Differentiate from TTP-HUS: Usually coags are normal in TTP-HUS.

MANAGEMENT

- 40-80% mortality! Key to management is ABCs, supportive care, and treating the underlying cause.
- If severe: **Transfuse**
  — FFP for prolonged coagulation and bleeding.
  — Cryoprecipate (I, V, VIII) for fibrinogen <100 despite FFP.
  — Platelets if <50K and bleeding, if <20K and not bleeding.
  — pRBCs as needed for anemia.
- **Start therapeutic heparin** if large vessel thrombosis or dominant clotting picture, though its use is controversial.
- Consult hematology, blood bank, and others as needed based on etiology.

DISPOSITION

- This is a complication of other concerning illnesses therefore most patients will go to the OR (to treat inciting event) or the ICU.

BEWARE...

⚠ This is a clinical AND laboratory diagnosis, maintain a high index of suspicion and send labs early

Sources

Taylor FB, Toh CH, Hoots WK, Wada H, Levi M. Towards definition, clinical and laboratory criteria, and a scoring system for disseminated intravascular coagulation. *Thromb Haemost.* 2001;86(5):1327-30.

Levi M, Toh CH, Thachil J, Watson HG. Guidelines for the diagnosis and management of disseminated intravascular coagulation. British Committee for Standards in Haematology. *Br J Haematol.* 2009;145(1):24-33.

George JN, Gilcher RO, Smith JW, Chandler L, Duvall D, Ellis C. Thrombotic thrombocytopenic purpura-hemolytic uremic syndrome: diagnosis and management. *J Clin Apher.* 1998;13(3):120-5.

Notes

5 ▶ Gastrointestinal Bleed

These patients have a variety of presentations and a very different morbidity and mortality based on location and etiology of bleed. Though the history and physical, as well as the management, center on the distinction between upper and lower GIB, this is not always immediately clear.

First decision points:

Stable vs. unstable→ABCs and resuscitate; transfuse blood products if indicated.

Upper vs. lower →Use your history and physical to determine if upper or lower GIB if able. This is based on the patient's risk factors, exam findings, and stool appearance.

Ddx
Epistaxis
Oropharyngeal bleed
Vaginal bleed
Ingestion and emesis of red liquid
Beets (turn stool red)
Iron supplements
Bismuth containing medications

EVALUATION

- **High Yield History**: Any hematemesis or coffee ground emesis? Ask color and description of stool as well as frequency of vomiting or diarrhea. Determine any coagulopathies, anticoagulation medications, or antiplatelet agents. History and location of prior GIB or any recent abdominal surgeries. Assess for symptoms of hypovolemia or anemia (ie, chest pain or shortness of breath).
  - **UGIB**: History of epigastric pain, H.pylori infection or recent NSAID or glucocorticoid use to suggest PUD or gastritis? Retching prior to hematemesis to suggest Mallory-Weiss tear? Surgical history such as gastric bypass or Whipple to suggest bleeding from an anastomosis? Any known or risk factors for variceal bleeding, namely history of hepatitis or EtOH abuse?
  - **LGIB:** Last colonoscopy, presence of diverticular disease, or colorectal cancer? Any fevers or abdominal pain? Also assess for weight loss, fatigue, obstructive symptoms, or other signs/symptoms of malignancy.

UPPER GIB	LOWER GIB
Proximal to Ligament of Treitz	**Distal to Ligament of Treitz**
Age <50 Hematemesis or coffee ground emesis Report or presence of melena BUN/Cre>30	Hematochezia Bright red blood per rectum History of diverticulosis
Peptic ulcer: (approx. 50% of UGIB) Esophageal ulcer: (highest mortality) Mallory-Weiss tear Varices Malignancy	Diverticulosis- most common Malignancy Colitis IBD Angiodysplasia Brisk UGIB Hemorrhoid

- **Exam**: VS (Use caution in the elderly or patients on beta blockers.)
  - General: Adequate perfusion? (Mental status, BCR, skin temp?) Stigmata of liver disease? Presence of bruising or petechiae to suggest bleeding diathesis?
    - Abdominal exam:
    - UGIB + epigastric (+/- RUQ) tenderness → PUD (LGIB often painless)
    - UGIB + peritoneal signs → STAT surgical consult (perforated or ischemic bowel)
  - Rectal Exam: Stool color and consistency. Anoscopy may identify bleeding hemorrhoids (these patients can usually be discharged home).
    - **Melena**: Black, tarry stool, generally UGIB or distal small bowel with slow transit
    - **Hematochezia**: (maroon=R and transverse colon; red=left colon and rectum) May also signify brisk UGIB
    - Brown, formed stool covered in BRB suggests hemorrhoids.
- **Diagnostics**
  - **Labs**: BMP (BUN/Cr>30 can be seen in UGIB), CBC, PT/PTT, type and screen. Consider LFTs, EKG, and cardiac enzymes. Sepsis labs if critically ill.
  - **Imaging**: Based on patient stability and suspected location of bleed.
    - Upright CXR: To assess for free air from perforation in the setting of severe abdominal pain or peritonitis.
    - EGD: If concerned for UGIB → early EGD (within 24hrs) if unstable or concern for variceal bleed.
    - Colonoscopy: Inpt vs. outpt based on HD stability.
    - Arteriography: Useful in localizing source of a brisk LGIB. May be done as traditional catheter directed (allows intervention for hemostasis) or as CTA (localization only).

MANAGEMENT

- ABCs and resuscitate. Intubate as indicated for airway protection. Place at least 2 large-bore IVs (18g) and administer IVF. Administer blood products if indicated.
- **Massive GI bleed**: Start massive transfusion protocol (1:1:1 of packed RBCs, platelets and FFP) if indicated. An exsanguinating patient necessitates both an emergent *GI and surgery* consult. Finally, consider placement of Sengstaken-Blakemore tube or Minnesota tube in exsanguinating variceal bleed if EGD not immediately available.
- For all bleeds, make NPO and consider starting bowel prep for stable lower GI bleeds.
- Consider NGT prior to intubation if large amount of UGIB (NOTE: NGT is not considered to be a necessary treatment except in this case).A negative aspirate does not rule out UGIB.
- **Upper GIB**: Will require EGD generally within 24hrs. Urgency of consult and EGD depends on patient stability.
- **Lower GIB**: If stable will need a non-emergent GI consult for inpatient or outpatient colonoscopy. If hemodynamically unstable or severe abdominal pain emergent surgical consult as well as GI consult.

- Medical Therapies
    - **All patients**: Reverse coagulopathies if safe to do so (caution in high risk patient such as mechanical valves).
        - FFP for patients with coagulopathy (INR>1.5), and if giving massive transfusion (liver failure pts). NOTE: for pts on warfarin, pts taking Xarelto or Eliquis, Kcentra (4 factor PCC) may help reverse coagulopathy. Kcentra does NOT work for pts on Pradaxa.
        - Consider platelet transfusion if platelets <50,000, or if taking aspirin or clopidogrel.
        - Vitamin K if on warfarin, 5-10mg (IV or PO based on INR, indication for anticoagulation and severity of bleed.
        - Blood transfusion if hemodynamically unstable or has signs or symptoms of ischemia.
    - **Non-variceal upper GI bleed**
        - Consider IV PPI, no effect on mortality but decreases ulcer severity seen at time of EGD.
    - **Variceal upper GI bleed**
        - Octreotide 50mcg bolus IV->50mcg/hr drip for splanchnic vasoconstriction.
        - Abx: Ceftriaxone, ampicillin/sulbactam, or quinolone. Antibiotic prophylaxis in cirrhotic patients with UGIB shown to reduce mortality.
- Consult GI to obtain early intervention for any hemodynamically significant or large volume bleed.
- Consult surgery for massive bleed, suspicion of bowel ischemia, or if evidence of perforation.

DISPOSITION

- Medical floor vs. ICU depending on stability and comorbidities.
- If exam reveals bleeding from rectal source (hemorrhoids or anal fissure) and workup reassuring, can discharge home.
- Low-risk patients (young, HD stable, guaiac negative, no hematemesis while in ED, stable HCT, no comorbid illnesses) can be discharged home if close follow-up can be arranged. Consider observation status and 6hr repeat HCT.
- RETURN IF: You experience any lightheadedness, dizziness, chest pain, shortness of breath, persistent black tarry stools, bright red blood per rectum, blood in your vomit, any severe abdominal pain, or any other new or concerning symptoms.

BEWARE...

- ⚠ Transfuse cautiously (if symptomatic or unstable; don't use Hgb level only).
- ⚠ Consider occult GIB in differential of patients with nonspecific complaints (weak and dizzy, etc.).
- ⚠ Bismuth will turn stool black and tarry but will not be guaiac positive; iron sometimes causes dark green/black or brown stool to be guaiac positive.
- ⚠ Ask about recent meals, specifically history of red food/drink; a patient's report of hematemesis may just be red juice.
- ⚠ Epistaxis can lead to swallowed blood → nausea → hematemesis but no GI source.
- ⚠ Differentiate hemoptysis from hematemesis and hematuria or vaginal bleeding from hematochezia.

Sources

Capell MS, Friedel D. Initial management of acute upper gastrointestinal bleeding: from initial evaluation up to gastrointestinal endoscopy. *Med Clin N Am.* 2008;92:491-509

Villanueva C, Colomo A, Bosch A, et al. Transfusion strategies for acute upper gastrointestinal bleeding. *N Engl J Med.* 2013;368(1):11-21.

Zuccaro G. Management of the adult patient with acute lower gastrointestinal bleeding. American College of Gastroenterology. Practice Parameters Committee. *Am J Gastroenterol.* 1998;93:1202-8

Notes

6 ▶ Sickle-Cell Disease

- Inherited disease resulting from a mutation in the beta-globin gene (Hgb B)
- Complaints occur from vascular occlusion and thus issues can arise wherever blood flows, making the nature of the complaints extremely variable.
- Episodes can be triggered by infection, cold, physical or emotional stress; often have no clear identifying cause.
- Patients themselves are the best guide, and will tell you how the current episode compares to prior ones.
- Two phenotypes: **Vaso-occlusive type**: Higher Hgb, presents with pain, more likely to present to the ED.

Hemolytic type: Lower Hgb, less pain, more pulmonary HTN, more leg ulcers and high risk of sudden death.

Acute Complications
Common:
Vaso-occlusive crisis
Infection/sepsis
Stroke
Cholelithiasis
Priapism
Less Common:
Hemolytic crisis
Acute coronary syndrome
Splenic sequestration
Osteomyelitis
Renal infarction
Splenic infarction
Mesenteric ischemia

TYPES OF SICKLE-CELL DISEASE

- HbSS: Most severe form. Patient has inherited 2 sickle-cell genes, one from each parent.
- HbSC: Usually a milder form. Patient has inherited 1 sickle-cell gene and 1 for the abnormal hemoglobin "C".
- HbS beta thalassemia: Usually a milder form. Patient has inherited 1 sickle-cell gene and 1 for beta thalassemia.
- Sickle-cell trait (HbAS): Usually asymptomatic. Patient has inherited 1 sickle-cell gene and 1 normal "A" gene ("gene carrier").

EVALUATION

- **High Yield History:** Goal is to understand the severity of the disease, any prior complications, and current pain management.
  - Past complications of SCD: Acute chest, CVA, avascular necrosis, splenic sequestration, priapism, cholecystitis, and any history of cholecystectomy or splenectomy.
  - Pain management: Are they on hydroxyurea to prevent acute pain crises, what is the frequency of pain crises and home pain regimen?
  - History of chronic transfusions? Baseline hemoglobin level? Any scheduled exchange transfusions?
  - History behind their presentation today:
    - For pain crises: Location and severity of the pain? What was tried at home? What usually works for them in the ED?
    - For other complaints: Focused history for potential disease complications. Any exposure to illness? Evaluate for conditions not related to SCD.
- **Exam**: VS to assess for fever, tachycardia, tachypnea or hypotension.
  - HEENT: New scleral icterus? Most patients are anemic and will have conjunctival pallor.
  - Pulmonary: Rhonchi or asymmetric breath sounds suggest PNA or acute chest.

- Abdominal: RUQ tenderness (cholecystitis), LUQ (splenic sequestration or infarction) diffuse pain (mesenteric ischemia).
- MSK: Joint pain or swelling (avascular necrosis), bony tenderness (osteomyelitis).
- Thorough exam for source of fever.
- **Diagnostics**
  - Labs: CBC, reticulocyte count helps evaluate anemia relative to patient's baseline HCT).
    - Consider type and screen early if transfusion may be necessary.
    - *Reticulocyte count low* or 0 suggestive of transient red cell aplasia (caused by parvovirus). *Reticulocyte count increased* suggestive of splenic sequestration palpate for splenomegaly).
    - Increased LDH, LFTs, and indirect bilirubin suggestive of hemolytic crisis.
  - EKG: Higher risk of ischemia in SCD pt of any age with chest complaints.
  - Imaging: CXR to assess for acute chest syndrome.

MANAGEMENT

- IV and monitor. Oxygen only if respiratory distress or hypoxic (<92%). Note: Giving 02 to non-hypoxic patients can reduce circulating levels of erythropoietin and may cause bone marrow hypoplasia.
- **Approach to Vaso-Occlusive Pain Crisis**
  - Treat the pain immediately (see chart). Follow "emergency rescue plans" if pt has one. Note: HR and BP may not be elevated during a pain crisis.
  - Provide analgesia early and reassess Q15-30 minutes until pain is controlled. Early and aggressive pain control is most effective and can result in less overall pain medication given.
  - Provide bolus IVF if hypovolemic (sepsis, diarrhea, vomiting). Once euvolemic give D5 ½ NS @ 1-1.5x maintenance rate. Excess IVF may cause lung atelectasis, which is a known risk factor for the development of Acute Chest Syndrome.

Analgesia Strategy for Adults		
Medication	**Dosing**	**Comment**
Dilaudid	1-2 mg IV push Q15min until pain controlled	Use cardiac monitor. Less pruritus.
Morphine	8-12mg IV push Q15min until pain controlled	Use cardiac monitor
Acetaminophen	650mg-1,000mg PO Q6hrs	Adjuvant therapy
NSAIDS(ibuprofen/ ketorolac)	Ibuprofen 600-800mg PO or Ketorolac 30mg IV q6hrs	Only short course use given renal side effects. Use only after rehydrated.
Diphenhydramine	25mg PO Q6hrs	Useful for pruritus. Avoid IV/IM use.

- **Acute Chest Syndrome** (should ALWAYS be considered in any SCD patient who presents with respiratory symptoms)
  — Life-threatening condition, clinically indistinguishable from pneumonia but will not respond to ABX.
  — Definition (must have 2 of the following): Chest pain, fever >38.5°C (101.3°F), infiltrate on imaging, respiratory symptoms, or hypoxemia.
  — Differential: PNA, fat embolism from bone marrow, pulmonary infarction, PE, acute coronary syndrome, pneumothorax, pleurisy.
  — **Treatment**
    ▪ Mildly ill: Initiate initiate antibiotics for CAP (3rd generation cephalosporin + macrolide to cover *Chlamydia pneumoniae* and *streptococcus pneumoniae*), pain control, and consider transfusion of 1u PRBCs.
    ▪ Moderately or severely ill: Immediately call hematology consult for emergent exchange transfusion and start antibiotics and pain control. Exchange transfusion removes HgS and transfuses PRBCs. If unavailable, transfuse PRBCs.
- **Stroke**
  — Children with SCD have 300-fold increased risk. Most commonly <10yo and >29yo.
  — Mechanism in children is likely from abnormal cell adhesion, intravascular sickling, and abnormal smooth muscle tone.
  — Mechanism in adults is likely from same thromboembolic mechanisms that cause stroke in the general population.
  — **Treatment**: Adults are recommended to receive conventional therapy, tPA. In children thrombolysis is contraindicated, and treatment for acute stroke or TIA is exchange transfusion.
- **Fever**
  — Functional asplenia (from auto-infarction) increases risk of infection with encapsulated organisms.
  — Increased risk of bacteremia, meningitis, septic arthritis, and osteomyelitis (especially in the spine).
  — If unclear source obtain: CBC, blood cx, urine Cx, throat Cx, CXR, UA, LP (if toxic appearing), subperiosteal fluid aspiration and culture (for bone pain), arthrocentesis for acute arthritis.
- **Anemia**
  — Remember: Chronically anemic – always compare to baseline HCT.
  — Other non-hemorrhagic causes of anemia more frequently seen in SCD (decreased RBC production, and increased RBC destruction):
  — **Splenic Sequestration** (normal LDH, elevated reticulocyte count)
    ▪ Usually pediatric diagnosis (have not yet auto infarcted spleen) but can occur in adults. Exam: Splenomegaly.
    ▪ Onset is usually rapid and progressive. Patient is literally bleeding to death into the spleen.
    ▪ Treatment is immediate transfusion of 2u PRBCs. Begin trending HCT.

- Disposition is to ICU because following remobilization of blood from spleen there can be a hyperviscosity syndrome and increased risk of stroke, vaso-occlusive crisis, and Acute Chest Syndrome due to the elevated HCT from post-transfusions.

— **Hemolytic Crisis** (↑ LDH, ↑ reticulocyte count, ↑ indirect bili)
- More indolent in onset.
- Treatment: If symptomatic anemia, then transfuse PRBCs.

— **Transient Red Cell Aplasia** (normal LDH, decreased reticulocyte count)
- Caused by infection with parvovirus B19 → decreased production of RBCs for 5-7 days (SCD pts have abnormally high rate of RBC turnover at baseline).
- Symptoms: Signs of anemia (pallor, fatigue, dyspnea on exertion, chest pain) and recent infection (cough, fever, rash).
- Treatment: IVIG (call hematology consult), PRBC transfusion, and isolation from pregnant patients and health care workers (maternal infection can cause fetal hydrops).

- **Hyphema**
  — **Ophthalmologic emergency** in patients with SCD or Sickle-Cell trait
  — Associated with development of acute narrow-angle glaucoma and frequent re-bleeding into the hyphema.
  — Evaluation should include visual acuity, visual field testing, slit-lamp examination, and intraocular pressure measurement.
  — **Always** obtain an emergent ophthalmologic consult. Consider consultation for any direct eye trauma, even without hyphema.
  — Treatment: HOB elevated 30°. Topical timolol (1st line), topical brimonidine or apraclonidine (2nd line), topical dorzolamide (3rd line).
  — Do not treat with mannitol (can promote sickling) or glycerin (increases serum osmolality), acetazolamide (lowers serum pH), or topical epinephrine (may promote anterior chamber deoxygenation).

- **Priapism**
  — Incidence may be as high as 89% by age 20. Can result in impotence and fibrosis. Etiology is vaso-occlusion.
  — Treatment (see chapter): If <2hrs: analgesics, IV fluids. If >2hrs: 1st line- local intracavernosal aspiration and injection with 1:1,000,000 solution of epinephrine in saline. 2nd line- exchange transfusion and epidural anesthesia. Urology consult.

DISPOSITION

- Contact the patient's hematologist; collaborative discharge plans have the best chance of success. They know their patients well and can help with suggestions for pain control and disposition.
- Many patients require admission for pain control.
- May discharge if: adequate pain control (po opioids, etc.) and no complicating factors.
- RETURN IF: High fevers, chest pain, shortness of breath, pain not controlled by home medications, or any other new or concerning symptom.

BEWARE...

- ⚠ Sickle cell presents variably, so keep a broad differential.
- ⚠ If not similar to prior crises, suspect other pathology(ies).
- ⚠ **Do not** rely on vital signs to determine severity of pain.
- ⚠ Most common complaints are painful episodes that can occur anywhere.
- ⚠ Leading cause of death is Acute Chest Syndrome.
- ⚠ **Do not** over-transfuse. Patients are chronically anemic (check baseline HCT) and have many antibodies from past transfusions.

Sources

Glassberg J. Evidence-based Management of Sickle Cell in the Emergency Department. *Emergency Medicine Practice.* August 2011:13(8)

Brousseau DC, Owens PL, Mosso AL, et al. Acute care utilization and rehospitalizations for sickle cell disease. *JAMA.* 2010;303(13):1288-94.

Tanabe P, Artz N, Mark Courtney D, et al. Adult emergency department patients with sickle cell pain crisis: a learning collaborative model to improve analgesic management. *Acad Emerg Med.* 2010;17(4):399-407.

Notes

Section V.
Chest Pain

1 ▶ Chest Pain Quick Guide

- ALWAYS: ABCs, IV access, place on telemetry and pulse oximetry, with supplemental oxygen if hypoxic (Sp02<93%). Obtain early EKG.
- Can't-miss diagnoses in the first 2 minutes:

  — ACS → dyspnea, diaphoresis, nausea, vomiting, tachycardia, murmur, hypoxia

  — Aortic dissection → aortic insufficiency murmur, unequal pulses, back pain, neurological findings

  — Pericardial tamponade → dyspnea, muffled heart sounds, pulsus paradoxus, elevated JVP, +JVD

  — Pulmonary embolus → dyspnea, hypoxia, swollen extremity, loud P2, pleurisy

  — Tension pneumothorax → absent breath sounds, absent chest rise, tracheal shift, +JVD, hypotension

  — Esophageal rupture → crepitus, fever, recent vomiting (usually prior to onset of pain)

Other Ddx
Valvular heart disease
Pericarditis/myocarditis
GERD/PUD
Esophageal spasm
Esophagitis
Pulmonary HTN
Pleuritis
Musculoskeletal
Herpes zoster
Psychogenic

EVALUATION

- **High Yield History:** Length of symptoms, palliative and provoking factors (exertional, positional or pleuritic). What was the patient was doing at time of onset? Associated symptoms, especially any shortness of breath, palpitations, lightheadedness, diaphoresis, nausea, or vomiting. Any radiation of pain. History of CAD or angina. Any PE risk factors. PMH, meds (Plavix, ASA, nitroglycerin, anticoagulation).

- **Exam:** VS! Cardiac, pulmonary, and neurologic exam (key: new murmurs, signs of volume overload, focal breath sounds), abdominal tenderness to suggest biliary pathology or esophagitis as etiology of pain, check bilateral pulses and lower extremities for signs of DVT.

- **Initial Workup:** Almost all patients get an EKG and CXR. Also consider a bedside US for cardiac and pulmonary source. Then consider CBC, BMP, LFTs, lipase, troponin, d-dimer, and BNP based on risk factors and likely diagnosis.

7 CAN'T-MISS CHEST PAINS LABS

Imaging, Prognosis Scores

1. **ACS** → Serial EKGs, troponin
2. **Aortic Dissection** → CXR, bedside US, CT chest w/ contrast, D-dimer, Type A vs. B, creatinine if concerned for renal extension
3. **Pericardial Tamponade** → Bedside US, CXR, EKG, consider CT if concerned for effusion due to a retrograde aortic dissection
4. **Pulmonary Embolus** → D-dimer, lower extremity US, CTA chest for PE, V/Q scan, EKG, Wells' score, PERC score
5. **Tension Pneumothorax** → CXR, bedside US
6. **Esophageal Rupture** → CXR, CT chest, esophagram
7. **Pneumonia** → CXR, blood cultures (if appropriate), SIRS criteria (WBC, temp, RR, HR), PORT score, CURB-65

Treatment

1. **ACS** → PCI vs. thrombolysis, ASA, morphine, nitroglycerin (*except in inferior and R sided MI), heparin, antiplatelet therapy
2. **Aortic Dissection** → BP control, HR control, avoid ASA and blood thinners, obtain surgical (Type A) or cardiology (Type B) consult
3. **Pericardial Tamponade** → IVF to maintain preload, pericardiocentesis
4. **Pulmonary Embolus** → Heparin (bolus + drip), systemic thrombolysis, IR catheter directed thrombolysis, vascular vs. surgical consult for thrombectomy (rare)
5. **Tension Pneumothorax** → Needle decompression (14G) in 2nd or 3rd intercostal space in midclavicular line or 4th or 5th intercostal space in midaxillary line. Chest tube (pigtail vs. standard).
6. **Esophageal Rupture** → Antibiotics, surgical consult
7. **Pneumonia** → Antibiotics (CAP vs. HAP vs. VAP), respiratory support

BEWARE...

- (!) Compare all EKGs to older ones if available.
- (!) Not all patients refer to chest pain as "pain." Also ask about any pressure, discomfort, etc.
- (!) Young patients can have ACS. Always ask about concerning family history in young patients with ACS.

Sources

Zane RD, Kosowsky JM, et al. Pocket Emergency Medicine. 2nd ed. Philadelphia, PA: Lippincott Williams & Wilkins; 2011.

Ma OJ, Cline D, Tintinalli J, et al. Emergency Medicine Manual. 6th ed. New York, NY: McGraw-Hill Professional; 2003.

Marx J, Hockberger R, Walls R. Rosen's Emergency Medicine: Concepts & Clinical Practice. 5th ed. Maryland Heights, MO: Mosby; 2002.

Hans L, Mawji Y. The ABCs of Emergency Medicine. 12th edition. Toronto, Canada: University of Toronto; 2012.

Medscape News & Perspective. New York, NY: http://emedicine.medscape.com.

2 ▶ EKG Quick Guide

- 1 small box = 1mm = 0.04 seconds (40ms), 1 large box (five small boxes) = 0.20 seconds (200ms)
- Rate=60/(R-R interval)
  OR
  — 1 big box = 300 beats/min (0.2 sec)
  — 2 big boxes = 150 beats/min (0.4 sec)
  — 3 big boxes = 100 beats/min (0.6 sec)
  — 4 big boxes = 75 beats/min (0.8 sec)
  — 5 big boxes = 60 beats/min (1.0 sec)

"SinusRhythmLabels" by Agateller (Anthony Atkielski) Licensed under Public Domain via Commons

Take a systematic approach with attention to possible underlying disease processes. **Questions to answer on all EKGs:**

- **Rate:** Fast or slow?
- **Rhythm:** Is it regular or irregular? Is it sinus?
  Are there P-waves before every QRS and a QRS after every P-wave?
- **QRS:** Is it wide or narrow?
- **Axis?** Normal, left, right, and extreme axis deviation?
- **Intervals:** PR (prolonged?), ST segments (elevated or depressed?), QT (long or short?)
- **Ischemia:** T waves inversions, hyperacute T waves, ST segment changes
- **Assess for ST elevation or depression!**

RATE

- Slow or fast heart rates can compromise cardiac output.
- Adults: Tachycardia >100bpm, bradycardia <60bpm
- Not all rate changes are abnormal (eg, young, fit male may normally be bradycardic).

RHYTHM

- What is the pattern of QRS waveform? **Regular, Irregularly irregular, Regularly irregular.**
  Quickly compare or measure intervals, from one QRS complex to the next, not PR. (Normal PR interval = < 0.20 sec = 5 small boxes)

- **Regular:** Most often sinus, but consider other cardiac pacemakers, particularly when associated with tachycardia. Other possibilities include:
  — First-degree heart block (increased PR)
  — Atrial tachycardia
  — Atrioventricular reciprocating tachycardia (AVRT)
  — AV nodal reentrant tachycardia (AVNRT)
  — Atrial flutter
  — Junctional tachycardia
  — Ventricular tachycardia (assess for AV dissociation, extreme right axis, QRS>0.14)
  — Third-degree heart block (complete heart block) often includes QRS complexes that appear regular and is defined by dissociation (no relationship) between P-waves and QRS complexes. **This is a very unstable rhythm, and emergent cardiology consult is appropriate.**

- **Irregularly irregular:** Most commonly atrial fibrillation. Also consider multifocal atrial tachycardia (MFAT→ HR >100 with P-waves with 3 distinct morphologies) particularly in the setting of pulmonary disease or stimulatory medicines such as theophylline.

- **Regularly irregular:** Often produced by a second-degree heart block
  — Mobitz Type I (Wenckebach): Progressive lengthening of PR, (with associated shortening of R-R) until QRS dropped. Pattern then recurs.
  — Mobitz Type II: Stable prolonged PR interval with intermittent blocked conduction (dropped QRS)
  — Heart block occurring during non-tachycardic sinus rhythm suggests AV nodal dysfunction, which could be intrinsic due to chronic disease or acute ischemia (often inferior STEMI), or due to external dysfunction such as medications, toxins, or excessive vagal tone.
  — Also consider triggered premature atrial or ventricular beats in repeating pattern such as bigeminy or trigeminy.

- **For patients with palpitations or syncope, assess for patterns associated with potentially causative syndromes including:**
  — Wolff-Parkinson-White (delta wave, short PR segment)
  — Brugada (saddle-back appearing ST segment in precordial lead, usually V1 or V2 caused by sodium channel defect)
  — Arrhythmogenic RV Dysplasia (ARVD): epsilon wave in V2 is pathognomonic

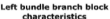

Left bundle branch block characteristics

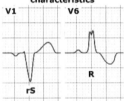

Right bundle branch block characteristics

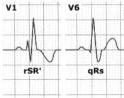

"Left and right bundle branch block ECG characteristics" by A. Rad at English Wikipedia. Transferred from en.wikipedia to Commons. Licensed under CC BY-SA 3.0 via Commons

— Long QT Syndrome (normal QTc in men <440 msecs, women <460 msecs)
- LVH/aortic stenosis (crescendo/decrescendo murmur)
- HOCM (athlete with syncope, murmur that increases with valsalva and decreases with increased preload)
- Tricyclic OD (tachycardia, wide QRS, and increased terminal R wave in aVR)

QRS COMPLEX

- Width: Bundle branch blocks (QRS >0.12 secs or >3 small boxes)
- **Heart Blocks ('William Morrow')**
  - **Left: WiLLiaM → SRS (W) in V1, RSR (M) in V6**
  - **Right: MoRRoW → RSR (M) in V1, SRS (W) in V6**
- Height corresponds to Voltage: (Elevated→hypertrophy, Decreased→pericardial fluid, COPD)
- **Left Ventricular Hypertrophy Criteria (Sokolow-Lyon):**
  - S wave in V1 PLUS R wave in V5 or V6 > 35mm OR
  - R wave in aVL ≥ 11mm
- **Right Ventricular Hypertrophy Criteria** (if present think pulmonary HTN, mitral valve stenosis, PE)
  - Right axis deviation (see chart)
  - Large R wave in V1 (> S wave in V1)
  - V1, V2 inverted T waves suggests RV strain

AXIS

- Consider both QRS and P wave axis.
- P waves that are not positive in leads I and aVF, (0-90 degree axis), or in lead V1 raise concern for an ectopic pacemaker.
- QRS deflections that are primarily negative in leads I and aVF (180-270 degree axis) are more likely to be ventricular in origin

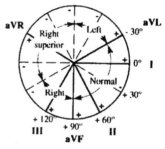

Source: PresentMed

QRS Deflection			Axis
Lead I	**Lead II**	**Lead III**	
Positive	Positive	Positive or Negative	Normal
Positive	Negative	Negative	Left Axis Deviation
Negative	Positive or Negative	Positive	Right Axis Deviation

INTERVALS

- QRS: 0.08-0.12 sec (2-3 small boxes)
- PR: 0.12-0.20 seconds (3-5 small boxes)
  — Long: consider AV block;
  — Short: consider WPW
- QT
  — Check the computed corrected QT interval (QTc) for prolongation. Prolonged QTc above approximately 460-480 milliseconds progressively raises the risk of Torsades de Pointes, a specific form of polymorphic ventricular tachycardia.
  — The QT interval varies inversely with serum Ca levels (see chart).
  — Quick estimate of QT length: If QT interval is less than half the distance of the preceding R to R interval (in sinus rhythm) then the QT length can be considered within normal limits.

ISCHEMIA

- STEMI
  — Evidence of ST elevation in a geographic pattern, and the possibility of associated reciprocal ST depression.
  — If present, are there ischemic symptoms? Is there an old ECG to compare? If new, this requires immediate action.
  — If LBBB present, then use **Sgarbossa criteria**:
    - ST elevation ≥ 1mm CONCORDANT (ie, ST elevation in same direction as deflection of QRS) with QRS→ score 5
    - ST elevation ≥ 5mm where DISCORDANT (ie, ST elevation in direction opposite QRS deflection) with the QRS→ score 2
    - ST depression ≥ 1mm in leads V1, V2, or V3 → score 3
    - A score of ≥3 has sensitivity of 20% and specificity of 90%.
  — **NOTE: Criteria is specific and not sensitive; therefore, you cannot rule out MI when Sgarbossa criteria are absent.**
- NSTEMI
  — Assess for evidence of acute ischemia including symmetric inverted T waves (if deep inversion in the septal leads V2,V3 consider Wellen's Sign which is suggestive of LAD artery stenosis), or ST depression. Prior MI is suggested by pathologic Q waves (see ACS section for territories).

OTHER

- ST segment abnormalities
  — **ST elevation not due to MI:** Pericarditis, benign early repolarization, LV aneurysm, left ventricular hypertrophy, left bundle branch block, WPW, Brugada, hyperkalemia, hypothermia, PE (rare), intracranial hemorrhage (rare)

— **ST depression:** Ischemia, subendocardial or posterior MI (V1, V2), digoxin – check the T wave morphology. Symmetric and diffusely peaked T-waves raise concern for hyperkalemia. Peaked T-waves in anatomical distribution raise concern for hyoperacute T-waves in the setting of MI.

- Disease-specific
  - Pulmonary embolism: EKG findings of S1Q3T3 (not sensitive or specific)
  - Digoxin: Scooping ST, short QT, inverted T
  - Pericarditis: Diffuse ST segment elevation and PR depression
  - Electrolyte abnormalities
    - HyperK: Flattened P, wide QRS, peaked T (late finding is Sine wave)
    - HypoK: Flattened T, U wave
    - HyperCa: Short QT
    - HypoCa: Long QT

BEWARE...

⚠ Always compare to an old EKG.

⚠ If administering a medication for rate or rhythm control, always check an EKG after each intervention.

Sources

Link MS. Evaluation and initial treatment of supraventricular tachycardia. *N Engl J Med.* 2012;367:1438-1448.

Marx J, Hockberger R, Walls R. Rosen's Emergency Medicine: Concepts & Clinical Practice. 5th ed. Maryland Heights, MO: Mosby; 2002.

Notes

3 ▶ Acute Coronary Syndrome (ACS)

Acute Coronary Syndrome (ACS): An acute mismatch of myocardial oxygen supply and demand leading to ischemia and infarction. It is the result of unstable coronary artery plaque rupture → platelet aggregation → clot → obstructed blood flow to myocardium.

- Represents a spectrum of conditions including:

  — **Unstable angina:** Transient obstruction characterized by concerning history with or without ECG changes but without cardiac enzyme elevations.

  — **NSTEMI:** Subendocardial ischemia characterized by concerning EKG changes (ST depression) or history and elevation of cardiac enzymes.

  — **STEMI:** Transmural ischemia characterized by elevated cardiac enzymes and >1mm ST elevations (see chart)

ACS Ddx
Etiologies that can cause ST changes and trop leaks:
• Coronary disease
— Spasm: Prinzmetal's angina, cocaine
— Dissection: Spontaneous coronary, Retrograde from aortic dissection.
— Vasculitis: Kawasaki's, Takayasu, SLE, RA
— Embolism: Endocarditits
• Type II MI: Demand ischemia in setting of fixed lesion
• Myocarditis
Cardiac Contusion

EVALUATION

- **High Yield History**

  — Chest discomfort? If YES- Assess location, character, intensity, onset, duration, radiation, and aggravating/alleviating factors. **NOTE: ACS does not always present with chest discomfort.

  — Atypical symptoms more common in elderly, diabetic, and female pts. May lack chest pain but have pain in jaw, arm, back, epigastrium, or throat. Also consider "non-pain presentations" with dyspnea or syncope as the only presenting symptoms.

  — Associated symptoms? Dyspnea, nausea, vomiting, weakness, diaphoresis, palpitations, AMS, syncope/pre-syncope

  — Past cardiac history? Previous MI, CABG, PCI, abnormal stress test, abnormal ECG, abnormal Echo

  — Risk factors for ACS: Age, DM, HTN, HLD, smoker, cocaine use (helpful in predicting atherosclerosis and long-term complications).

  — Family history of early MI or sudden death? If so, at what ages? Especially important if patient is <40 years old.

- Assess for aortic dissection: Tearing or ripping pain, maximal intensity of pain at onset, radiation to back or legs, neurologic symptoms. If any of these exist, consider further evaluation for aortic dissection prior to administration of any anticoagulant.

- **Exam:** ABCs and VS

- — Evidence of cardiogenic shock: Tachycardia, hypotension, oliguria, cool/clammy/pale skin and extremities
- — Evidence of heart failure: Elevated JVP, presence of JVD, pulmonary congestion
- — Signs of other diagnoses such as unequal breath sounds, unequal pulses, RUQ tenderness, asymmetric lower extremity swelling
- **Diagnostics**
  - — **EKG:** Should be part of the initial set of vital signs (within the first 10min) → see section
  - — **Cardiac biomarkers**
    - ▪ Cardiac troponins (T and I levels will begin to increase as early as 3hrs following onset of symptoms; at 6hrs these have sensitivity and specificity >95%).
    - ▪ Can consider a 3hr rule-out with cardiac markers if a low-risk patient.
    - ▪ Usually you will need to obtain 2 sets of troponins (3-6hrs apart) to trend unless your suspicion of ACS is very low.
    - ▪ CK-MB levels are useful if trying to evaluate a reinfarction in a patient with an MI in the past 1-2 weeks.
  - — Labs: Consider also CBC, BMP, LFTs (to evaluate for biliary process mimicking chest pain). Consider in appropriate patients, BNP or D-Dimer.
  - — CXR: To assess for pneumonia, pneumothorax or widened mediastinum suggesting aortic dissection.

ECG

- For all patients, compare to previous ECGs and ask EMS for their telemetry strips.
- In high-risk patients, those with persistent pain, and those with changing symptoms obtain serial EKGs (Q15min or with any change in symptoms).
- **STEMI definition:** ST segment elevation of 1mm in 2 anatomically contiguous leads other than V2-V3 or 2mm STE in V2-V3 or new LBBB in the setting of clinical presentation concerning for ACS.
- **UA/NSTEMI:** ST segment depressions, deep T wave inversions, or possibly no ECG changes. NSTEMI defined by elevated cardiac biomarkers due to myocyte damage.

I Lateral	aVR Basal Septum	V1 Septal	V4 Anterior
II Inferior	aVL Lateral	V2 Septal	V5 Lateral
III Inferior	aVF Inferior	V3 Anterior	V6 Lateral

- **Lead Anatomy:** (location of infarct)
  - — Anterior: V1-V4 (LAD)
  - — Apical: V5-V6 (Left circumflex vs. distal RCA vs. LAD)
  - — Lateral: I, aVL (left circumflex)
  - — Inferior: II, III, aVF (proximal RCA) in most or left circumflex artery)

— Posterior: ST depression in V1-V3 (this represents reciprocal change for ST elevation that would be seen on posterior leads). Get posterior leads → V7-V9 mirrors V1-V3 (RCA and LCx)

— RV: STD V1-V3; Get right-sided leads and look for STE in V4R (RCA [STE in III>II; no STE in I or aVL] or LCx)

- **Sgarbossa criteria** (rules for defining STEMI in the setting of a pre-existing LBBB)

— Concordant STE ≥1 mm in any lead (i.e. ST elevation in same direction as deflection of QRS) – score 5

— Discordant STE ≥5 mm in any lead (i.e. ST elevation in direction opposite QRS deflection) – score 2

— ST segment depression ≥1 in any lead from V1 to V3 – score 3.

— *A score of ≥3 has sensitivity of 20% and specificity of 90%

EKG FINDINGS AND RISK STRATIFICATION OF ACS

Low Risk	Intermediate Risk	High Risk
TW flattening/TW inversion (<1mm) in non-anatomical leads; normal EKG	Old Q waves, STD (<1mm) or T wave inversions (>1mm) in ≥2 anatomic leads, LV hypertrophy with strain, change from baseline EKG	STE >1mm or new STD (>1mm) in ≥2 anatomic leads, T wave inversions in anatomic leads, hyperacute T waves, new LBBB

MANAGEMENT

- ABCs, IV access, place on telemetry and pulse oximetry, and obtain EKG within 10 min. Consider serial ECGs q15-20 min or with changes in symptoms.

- Principals of management: To reduce pain, reduce demand on heart and thus further infarct, and to prevent further thrombus formation.

- **Dual Antiplatelet Therapy**

— *Aspirin* 324mg (non-enteric coated), chewed

- Can give PR if not able to take PO. Use clopidogrel if **true** aspirin allergy.

- **DO NOT GIVE IF AORTIC DISSECTION IS CONSIDERED.**

— Discuss with Cardiology which of the following medications should be administered to complete "Dual antiplatelet therapy":

- **ADP receptor blockade**:

- Prasugrel 60mg

- Ticagrelor 180mg. Decreased incidence of post-MI complication and death but increased bleeding complications. Shorter half-life, may be beneficial in those high-risk patients going for CABG.

- Clopidogrel 300mg x 1 (conservative treatment) or 600mg x 1 for early invasive (PCI within 48hrs). If given as dual platelet needs to wait 5-7days for CABG if necessary. Requires metabolism in the liver to become activated

- **GP IIb/IIIa Inhibitors** (eptifibatide, abciximab, tirofiban) usually given in cath lab if indicated. No benefit giving prior to PCI and increased risk of bleeding
- **Nitroglycerin** (sublingual 0.4mg Q5min prn x3) IF chest discomfort
  — DO NOT GIVE if evidence of inferior MI with RV extension (RV is pre-load dependent and nitro decreases preload) or if patient uses phosphodiesterase inhibitors or if patient has severe aortic stenosis.
  — If you accidentally give in an inferior MI, hang IVF normal saline to provide increased volume to augment preload. No mortality benefit so if concerned about pre-load better to avoid.
  — For NSTEMI patient, can also start nitroglcerin drip (10mcg/min and titrate up as BP tolerates) if needed to achieve pain-free state.
- **Morphine** (2-4mg IV) can be given q15min prn discomfort, anxiety, air hunger
- **Statin:** Atorvastatin 80mg if not already on a statin. Ideal if given prior to PCI but can be started within 24hrs.
- **Beta Blocker:** If no signs of heart failure, hemodynamic compromise, bradycardia, severe reactive airway disease, or cocaine use.
  — Decreases recurrent ischemia, progression of MI and incidence of arrhythmias.
  — Benefit can be achieved as long as given within 24hrs; **therefore, you do not need to administer in the ED**.
  — Can lead to cardiogenic shock in high risk patients such as those who are already hypotensive.
- **Anticoagulant Treatment**
  — UFH 60U/kg bolus with 12U/kg/hr drip titrated to PTT 1.5-2x control (50-70s) **Can reverse with protamine 20mg/min IV (exact dose dependent upon dose and timing of heparin). If no weight on pt and average size, 4000u bolus, 800u/hr drip to start.
  — LMWH (considered if conservative approach AND CrCl >30): Dalteparin (Fragmin) 120U/kg SubQ BID or Enoxaparin (Lovenox) 1 mg/kg SubQ BID

RISK STRATIFICATION

- Assumes diagnosis of ACS and directs conservative vs. invasive treatment
- TIMI score for UA/NSTEMI - consists of 7 independent predictors of outcome
  — Age >65
  — $\geq$ 3 risk factors for CAD (HTN, HL, DM, current smoker, family history of CAD)
  — Prior coronary stenosis $\geq$ 50% (from previous angiography)
  — Aspirin use in past 7 days
  — $\geq$ 2 angina episodes on past 24hrs
  — ST deviation $\geq$ 0.5 mm
  — Elevated cardiac biomarkers
- For patients with UA/NSTEMI, a TIMI score $\geq$3 places them in an intermediate/high risk group that benefits from early invasive therapy- IIb/IIIa and cardiac catheterization < 24hrs from onset of chest pain.

STEMI Algorithm	NSTEMI Algorithm
• **Reperfusion** — PCI (activate Cath Team) within 90 minutes of arrival. — If PCI not available within 90-120 minutes from arrival to ED then you should consider thrombolysis (alteplase- tPA) if symptoms have been present for <12hrs and the patient has no contraindications. If in community, consider transfer to PCI center if patient can receive PCI within 90-120 min. • **Dual Antiplatelet therapy** — Aspirin 325mg PLUS (speak with cardiology): — ADP receptor blocker- see chart above (only if low risk of bleeding) OR GP IIb/IIIa inhibitor: usually given in cath lab • **Anticoagulant therapy** — Unfractionated Heparin -bolus 60units/kg (max 4000u) followed by drip of 12units/kg/hr (max 1000 u/hr). Goal PTT 50-70 sec. — **Can reverse with protamine 20mg/min IV • **Statin:** Atorvastatin 80mg PO (if not already on statin)	• **Antiplatelet therapy** — Aspirin 325mg PO or PR *Discuss dual antiplatelet therapy with cardiology team. • **Unfractionated heparin** — Bolus 60units/kg (max 4000u) followed by drip of 12units/kg/hr (max 1000 u/hr). Goal PTT 50-70 sec. — OR (If conservative treatment): — LWMH • Dalteparin:120 u/kg SQ inj. (maximum dose: 10,000 int. units) every 12hrs. • Enoxaparin: 30mg IV bolus PLUS 1mg/kg SQ (if age >75 then NO IV bolus). • AVOID in patients with renal failure • **Statin:** Atorvastatin 80mg PO (if not already on statin) • Decrease myocardial O_2 demand by optimizing afterload (BP) and heart rate • **Risk stratify** — IF (+) trop, intermediate/high risk EKG, TIMI ≥3, evidence of CHF, EF<40%, history of PCI or CABG or recurrent ischemic symptoms THEN early invasive strategy within 48hrs. — IF (-) trop, non-diagnostic EKG, age <70, TIMI <2, normal EF will need to rule out UA with stress test. **Can arrange with output providers within 72hrs if all low risk features present.

Test	Sens (%)	Spec (%)	Pros	Cons
ETT with EKG	60	75	Functional capacity; no radiation; low cost	Limited sensitivity
Pharmacologic	60	75	Similar to ETT but for patients who cannot walk/exercise sufficiently for a treadmill	Radiation; Drugs can precipitate bradycardia/ bronchospasm/ tachyarrythmia
SPECT/PET	85	90	Localization; LV function; can use if low exercise tolerance or EKG abnormal at baseline.	Radiation; cost

Echo	85	95	Localization (i.e.- wall motion abnormalities); LV/valve function; no radiation	Operator error; cost
Cardiac CT	95	85	Decreases ED Length of stay, 2+ year "warranty period" for major cardiac adverse event	Cost, radiation, incidental findings

COMPLICATIONS OF ACS

- Conduction disturbances→ bradycardia, AV nodal block, tachyarrhythmias (ventricular and SVTs)
  — You need to treat AV node dysfunction and bradycardia if they are leading to HD compromise
  — Sinus bradycardia:
    - If 1st degree **or** 2nd degree, then should respond to **atropine** (0.5mg IV Q3-5min prn)
    - If unresponsive to atropine, consider **dopamine** (2-10 mcg/kg/min IV)
    - 3rd degree heart block may require transcutaneous pacing while preparing to start transvenous pacing
  — Malignant ventricular arrhythmias (VF/VT): **SHOCK or CARDIOVERT!**
    - If shock refractory VF/VT, then give **amiodarone 300 mg.**
    - If **stable** wide complex tachycardia, then give **amiodarone 150mg IV over 10 min then start 1mg/min IV x 6hrs.**
  — Atrial Fibrillation: BAD in ACS because it ↑ myocardial O2 demand and ischemia as well as loss of atrial kick
    - **If unstable, then cardiovert** to restore sinus rhythm.
    - If stable, then attempt rate control with beta-blockers or calcium channel blockers; may also consider **amiodarone** for rhythm control..
- Hemodynamic disturbances → Resulting from both left and right ventricle dysfunction
  — LV pump failure and cardiogenic shock
  — Treatment focuses on adjustment of preload and afterload to decrease burden on ischemic ventricle
  — NIPPV can decrease acute pulmonary edema but also decreases preload
  — For hypertensive and normotensive patients, **low dose IV nitroglycerin drip** (start at 10mcg/min) can reduce preload and afterload.
  — Inotropes and vasopressors can be used to maintain systemic and coronary artery perfusion. **1st line is norepinephrine** (start at 0.1-0.5/mcg/kg/min). Consider **dopamine** (2-10 mcg/kg/min IV) if bradycardic (know that dopamine is associated with increased risk of arrhythmias)
- Mechanical complications → Ventricular free wall rupture and ventricular septal rupture (rare, requires surgical repair), acute mitral regurgitation due to rupture of chordae tendinae (treat by promoting forward flow with reduction of afterload using IV nitroglycerin or sodium nitroprusside and surgical consultation)

Disposition:

- **STEMI:** Emergent cardiology consult (the clock is ticking), will likely go for PCI and then cardiac ICU or cardiac floor/step-down unit.

- **NSTEMI:** Calculate TIMI score. Medicine vs. cardiac unit (will vary depending on hospital and practice environment).

- **Chest pain concerning for ACS but low risk features:** These are the patients who often require the most thought. Many will warrant a hospital admission or ED observation unit admission (if available) for serial troponins with stress test (guidelines state that all patients who undergo a rule-out for MI should have provocative testing within 72hrs). Dispo will be guided by serial EKGs, trending cardiac biomarkers, performing risk stratification (TIMI score), and clinical judgment.

BEWARE...

⚠ STEs can also be caused by: pericarditis, benign early repolarization, LV aneurysm, LVH, LBBB, WPW, Brugada Syndrome (Coved or Saddleback STE in V_1), hyperkalemia.

⚠ Wellen's syndrome: Deeply inverted T waves or biphasic nondiagnostic EKG → Check posterior and right-sided leads. LCx can be electrically silent.

Sources

Giugliano RP, White JA, Bode C, et al. Early versus delayed, provisional eptifibatide in acute coronary syndromes. *N Engl J Med.* 2009;360(21):2176-90.

Théroux P, Ouimet H, Mccans J, et al. Aspirin, heparin, or both to treat acute unstable angina. *N Engl J Med.* 1988;319(17):1105-11.

O'gara PT, Kushner FG, Ascheim DD, et al. 2013 ACCF/AHA guideline for the management of ST-elevation myocardial infarction: a report of the American College of Cardiology Foundation/American Heart Association Task Force on Practice Guidelines. *J Am Coll Cardiol.* 2013;61(4):e78-140

Wang K, Asinger RW, Marriott HJ. ST-segment elevation in conditions other than acute myocardial infarction. *N Engl J Med.* 2003;349(22):2128-35.

Anderson JL, Adams CD, Antman EM, et al. ACC/AHA 2007 guidelines for the management of patients with unstable angina/non-ST-Elevation myocardial infarction: a report of the American College of Cardiology/American Heart Association Task Force on Practice Guidelines (Writing Committee to Revise the 2002 Guidelines for the Management of Patients With Unstable Angina/Non-ST-Elevation Myocardial Infarction) developed in collaboration with the American College of Emergency Physicians, the Society for Cardiovascular Angiography and Interventions, and the Society of Thoracic Surgeons endorsed by the American Association of Cardiovascular and Pulmonary Rehabilitation and the Society for Academic Emergency Medicine. *J Am Coll Cardiol.* 2007;50(7):e1-e157.

Willoughby SR. Complications of acute coronary syndromes. *EB Medicine EM Crit Care.* 2011 Dec;1(4).

Wright RS, et al. 2011 ACCF/AHA focused update of the guidelines for the management of patients with unstable angina/non-ST elevation myocardial infarction. *J Am Coll Cardiol.* 2011;57(19):1920-1959.

4 ▶ Atrial Fibrillation/Flutter

ATRIAL FIBRILLATION (AF)

- Definition: Supraventricular tachyarrhythmia with uncoordinated atrial activation and consequently ineffective atrial contraction. Atrial rates range from 350-600 but conducted ventricular beats and heart rate varies and can range 70-160bpm.

- EKG: Irregular R-R intervals (when AV conduction present), absence of distinct P waves, irregular atrial activity

Ddx
MAT
Atrial Tachycardia
SVT
Sinus Tachycardia
Atrial Tachycardia

- Classification
  - Paroxysmal: Terminates spontaneously or with intervention within 7 days of onset; may recur with variable frequency
  - Persistent: Continuous Afib that is sustained >7 days
  - Permanent: Not attributed to pathophysiology change but rather decision of patient and clinician to cease further attempts to restore and/or maintain sinus rhythm
  - Atrial fibrillation with rapid ventricular response (Afib with RVR)

ATRIAL FLUTTER

- Typical: Re-entrant atrial tachycardia (loops up the atrial septum, down lateral atrial wall, through cavotricuspid isthmus)
  - Counterclockwise flutter: more common, negative "saw tooth" flutter waves in II, III, aVF, and positive deflection in V1
  - Clockwise (i.e. reverse): less common, positive flutter waves in inferior leads, and negative deflection in V1
  - EKG: Atrial rate is typically 240-350bpm. Monomorphic. No isoelectric baseline. Often even-numbered conduction (2:1, 4:1)
- In general, flutter is often persistent and requires electrical cardioversion or ablation for termination.

EVALUATION

- **High Yield History:** Presence/timing of symptoms. Are they symptomatic? When was the onset of symptoms? Are they anticoagulated?
  - Acute precipitants (infection, electrolyte abnormalities, EtOH, drugs, thyrotoxicosis, MI, myocarditis, PE, pulmonary disease, hypoxia, sympathomimetics or medication noncompliance)
  - Associated symptoms such as dizziness, syncope, chest pain, shortness of breath, palpitations, altered mental status.
  - Risk factors such as HTN, DM, CHF, obstructive sleep apnea, CAD, and prior MI.
  - Watch out for symptoms of angina, end-organ hypoperfusion, symptomatic hypotension.

- **Exam:** VS (assess for tachycardia and for hypotension) and then focus on findings that would guide you to what precipitated the arrhythmia.
  - Signs of volume overload such as elevated JVP, crackles, or lower extremity edema
  - Murmurs, asymmetric lower extremity edema, neuro exam (to assess for cardioembolic ischemia)
- EKG: No P waves, irregularly irregular in atrial fibrillation. Aflutter will have sawtooth pattern in inferior leads and typically have regular QRS intervals though may still be irregular with variable conduction.
- CXR: Evaluate parenchyma, vascularity, pulmonary edema
- Labs: CBC, BMP, cardiac markers. Depending on context, consider LFTs, TSH, tox screen, HCG, BNP, digoxin level, theophylline level, d-dimer, INR.

MANAGEMENT

- **Emergent Stabilization of Critically Ill Patients**
  - IV access. Give IVF bolus if intravascularly deplete. Concurrently evaluate for shock etiology such as MI, infection, and hemorrhage. Initiate revascularization, early sepsis intervention, transfusion, and vasoactive agents, as indicated

CHA2DS2-VASC	
CHF	1
HTN	1
Age ≥75 y	2
DM	1
Stroke/TIA/TE	2
Vascular disease	1
Age 65-74 y	1
Sex (Female gender)	1

  - Remember that the patient may be hypotensive from Afib with RVR **or** may be in persistent Afib but current tachycardia due to another physiologic reaction.
  - If there is no other identifiable cause for shock or hypotension, use synchronized **DCCV at 150J (biphasic)**. A-flutter typically requires lower energy (100-120J). Increase energy in stepwise fashion if not successful.
  - Consider procedural sedation and adjunctive anti-arrhythmic drugs (e.g. amiodarone).
- **Urgent Stabilization**
  - Rate control agents may cause further hypotension, but may be necessary.
  - **Consider push-dose phenylephrine** (goal DBP >60) prior to a slow amiodarone or diltiazem infusion.
  - Consider calcium as pretreatment inopressor.
- **Management of Stable Patients:** Essentially rate and rhythm control as well as antithrombotic therapy
- Overall, rate control rather than rhythm control has not been shown to have any inferior outcomes (symptoms, CV mortality, CVA risk). However, those studies largely looked at patients >60yrs old, persistent AF, structural heart disease, and able to tolerate symptoms. Younger, elderly, and very symptomatic are underrepresented.
- **Rate Control**
  - Rate control in Afib without pre-excitation: IV beta-blocker or calcium channel blocker.
  - Use beta-blockers, calcium channel blockers, and digoxin cautiously in high-degree AV block.

— Magnesium 2mg IV can be an adjunct in achieving rate control.

Common Rate Control Agents			
Class	**Medication**	**IV dose**	**PO dose**
Beta-blocker	Metoprolol	2.5-5mg bolus over 2 min (up to 3 doses)	25-100mg Q6-8hrs
Non-dihydropyridine Ca²⁺ channel blockers	Diltiazem	0.25mg/kg over 2 min, repeat 0.35mg/kg after 15min prn; if needed, infusion at 5-15mg/hr	30-120mg Q6hrs
	Verapamil	2.5-5mg over 2 min, repeat 5-10mg after 15-30min prn, up to 20-30mg	30-120mg Q6hrs
Cardiac glycoside	Digoxin	0.25mg Q2hrs up to 1.5mg in 24h or 0.5-1.5mg: give ½ initially, then give ¼ dose Q6-8h x2 additional doses	Can alternatively load PO; maintenance 0.0625-0.375mg QD or QOD
Class III antiarrhythmic	Amiodarone	150mg over 10min, then 1mg/min x6h followed by 0.5mg/min x18hrs; re-bolus 150mg prn up to daily max 2.1gm	Can alternatively load PO; 1.2-1.8g/d in 2-3 divided doses until 10gm, then 100-200mg/d maintenance

- **Rhythm Control**
  - Long-term Afib management may employ attempts to restore and maintain sinus rhythm, including cardioversion, antiarrhythmic, and ablation in the setting of appropriate anticoagulation and rate control.
  - Elective cardioversion may be done for new-onset Afib or unacceptable symptoms from persistent Afib.
  - Patients with Afib clearly of <48h duration can perform cardioversion without TEE. Ideally if not already anticoagulated, anticoagulation would be given prior to procedure and continue for one month.
  - Use CHA2DS2-VASc risk score to guide decision on whether to initiate long-term systemic anticoagulation.
  - For Afib of >48h duration: Oral anticoagulation with warfarin (INR 2-3) for at least 3 weeks prior and 4 weeks after cardioversion. Alternative strategy is TEE to assess for LA/appendage thrombus.
  - DCCV is the most effective method to restore sinus rhythm. Chemical cardioversion is most likely effective when initiated within 7 days of Afib onset.
  - Antiarrhythmic drugs: Flecainide, propafenone, ibutilide, amiodarone, dofetilide, procainamide, sotalol, dronedarone. Limitations based on cardiovascular disease and should be initiated under the care of an EP physician.

- **Antithrombotic Therapy**
  - Selection of antithrombotic therapy should be based on shared decision-making around the absolute and RRs of stroke and bleeding
  - For non-valvular Afib, use the CHA2DS2-VASc score to assess stroke risk (improved risk stratification among low risk patients)

- — Compare to bleeding risk with anticoagulation such as with HAS-BLED score
- — Oral anticoagulation:
  - **Warfarin** (vitamin K antagonist): 1st choice for a score of 2 or greater, target INR 2-3
  - **Dabigatran** (direct thrombin inhibitor): for nonvalvular Afib; usually150mg BID
  - **Rivaroxaban** (direct factor Xa inhibitor): for nonvalvular AFfib; 20mg QD (15mg for CrCl 30-49mL/min)

DISPOSITION

- Admit: If you are unable to control the patient's heart rate in the ED or the patient had complications (tachymyopathy, cardioembolic event, or acute CHF exacerbation).
- Consider discharge for patients who are otherwise well, are rate controlled, and appropriately anticoagulated. If cardioverted in the ED, patients should be monitored for several hours prior to discharge. All patients should follow up with their PCP within 1-2 wks, or sooner for INR checks.
- RETURN IF: You experience palpitations, chest pain, shortness of breath, dizziness, you pass out, any focal weakness, or changes in vision.

BEWARE...

(!) Treat the underlying precipitant (give missed home med, replete electrolytes, give antibiotics, etc.) or you will have difficult time controlling rate.

Sources

Oishi ML, Xing S. Atrial fibrillation: management strategies in the emergency department. *Emerg Med Pract.* 2013;15(2):1-26.

January CT, Wann LS, Alpert JS, et al. 2014 AHA/ACC/HRS Guideline for the Management of Patients With Atrial Fibrillation: Executive Summary: A Report of the American College of Cardiology/American Heart Association Task Force on Practice Guidelines and the Heart Rhythm Society. *Circulation.* 2014.

Notes

5 ▶ Tachydysrhythmias

- Heart rate >100bmp. It can originate from the atria, AV node, or the ventricles.
- Stable vs. Unstable → If unstable rule out sinus tachycardia and then DCCV!
- Wide vs. Narrow complex → Assume all wide complex rhythms are ventricular tachycardia (VT). This is safer than misidentifying the rhythm and failing to treat VT.

EVALUATION

- **High Yield History:** Palpitations, lightheadedness, dizziness, weakness, fatigue, chest pain, shortness of breath, history of syncope, or abnormal bleeding
  — Past medical history of CAD, CHF, prior arrhythmias and their treatment, hypertension, EtOH, or drug use. Any risk factors for electrolyte imbalance such as diuretics, diet, or infection
  — Medications: Specifically any antiarrhythmic, nodal agents, beta-agonists or blockers, anticoagulation. Any missed doses. Any QTc prolonging medications
- **Exam:** Full set of vital signs, mental status, and any signs of hypoperfusion, volume status and assess for any precipitants
- **EKG:** Obtain as soon as possible. Look for rate, rhythm, and signs of ischemia. Narrow or wide complex? Regular or irregular?
  — Examine baseline EKG for any signs of ischemia, prolonged QTc, or delta waves.
  — Look for P-waves and attempt to determine if they are regular, similar morphology and always followed by a QRS.
  — Any concordance (QRS complex in anterior leads all in same direction), fusion beats, or capture beats→ suggestive of VT

Ddx of Sinus tachycardia
Hypovolemia /hemorrhage
Infection/Sepsis/Fever
Anxiety/ Pain
Hypoxia
Intoxication or withdrawal
Hyperthyroid
PE
Tamponade
Anemia
Beta blocker or Calcium channel blocker withdrawal

Ddx of Tachycardia
Sinus tachycardia
Atrial tachycardia
AVNRT/ AVRT
Junctional tachycardia
Atrial fibrillation
Atrial flutter
MAT
Ventricular tachycardia
Torsades de pointes
Ventricular fibrillation
Pacemaker mediated tachycardia

- **Diagnostics:**
  — Labs: CBC, BMP, Mg, Ca^{2+}, consider serum and urine tox, TSH, D-dimer, digoxin level, UA if concerned for infection, troponin if concerned for ischemia induced arrhythmia. Note that with many tachydysrhythmias, troponin will be elevated due to rate-related demand ischemia.
  — CXR: To assess for infection or volume overload.
  — Bedside US: Conduct after pt stabilized to assess volume status, pericardial effusion, and gross systolic function.
  — Consider further diagnostic imaging based on history such as CTA chest to rule out PE or CT abdomen to rule out hemorrhage if suggested by history.

MANAGEMENT

- Initial steps: Check pulse, ABCs, IV, oxygen, monitor, defibrillator pads (ideally placed anterior-posterior), telemetry/EKG
- If becomes unstable → ACLS. Treat the patient, not the rhythm.

Narrow Complex Tachycardia			
Regular Rhythm		**Irregular Rhythm**	
AVNRT	AV nodal reentrant tacharida (AVNRT)– A re-entry ciruit within the AV node. One limb of the ciruit is usually described as the fast limb and the other the slow limb base on their conduction speeds. Circuit usually set off by a premature atrial contractions in the setting of stress, alcohol, or caffeine intake. Abrupt onset and termination of this rhythm. Treat as SVT with vagal maneuvers, adenosine, or other nodal blocker	MAT	Subset of atrial tachycardia. EKG is characterized by three different P-wave morphologies with varying intervals. **Causes** include hypoxemia, pulmonary disease, electrolyte imbalance (replete Mg and K), methylxanthane, beta-agonists, and dig toxicity. Treat underlying cause and if in RVR, give nodal blockers such a diltiazem or metoprolol.
Focal Atrial Tachycardia	A regular atrial rhythm as a constant rate but comes from a non-sinus focus above AV node. On EKG the QRS complex preceded by a non-sinus P wave. Many etiologies, treat by fixing underlying cause, and consider rate control.	Afib with RVR	Disorganized atrial electrical impulses that are conducted through the AV node at variable rates. On EKG is "irregularly irregular" with no clear P-waves. See chapter.
AVRT	AV reentry tachycardia (AVRT) – A re-entry pathway involving the SA node and an accessory pathway. Majority are "orthodromic" with antegrade conduction down AV node and retrograde through the pathway. Treat with nodal blockade "Antidromic" AVRT (ex WPW) has antegrade conduction down accessory pathway and retrograde up the AV node. EKG with wide QRS complexes. **DO NOT** give nodal blockade.	AFlutter with variable block	A macro reentrant tachycardia with rapid, regular atrial depolarization but variable AV nodal conduction. EKG with classic sawtooth P-waves in inferior leads and may show variable 2:1, 3:1 and 4:1 blocks. Adenosine can be used to slow rythtm enough to see flutter waves.
A Flutter with 2:1 block	A macro reentrant tachycardia with rapid, regular atrial depolarization at rates of 300 bpm. EKG with classic sawtooth P-waves in inferior leads. Classically 2:1 AV conduction ratio and fixed ventricular rate at 150bpm		

- **Narrow Complex Tachycardia**
  - **Sinus tachycardia**: Treat the underlying etiology with IVF, pain control, antibiotics etc. This is usually compensatory mechanism therefore rate control is not helpful. However, do give beta-blockade if due to missed medications or thyroid storm.
  - **SVT**: A tachycardia arising above the AV node. Includes AVRT, AVNRT, and Aflutter with 2:1 or 4:1 block
    - Attempt vagal maneuvers including ice-pack to face, Valsalva, and carotid massage (if no bruits).
    - If recurrent SVT and it is known that patient does not have pre-excitation pathway (i.e. WPW) can give an AV nodal blocker such as diltiazem or metoprolol.
    - Otherwise can give **Adenosine 6mg** IV push. If not effective in 1-2min give 12mg and then another 12mg IV.
      - Adenosine has very short half-life and should be pushed quickly, with flush through proximal IV.
      - Place patient on pads in case s/he develops an arrhythmia or arrest.
      - Have monitor ready to record rhythm strip when patient converts or slows.
      - Give half dose if pushing through central line, heart transplant patients, or patients on carbamazepine.
    - In patients with concern for pre-excitation pathway such as WPW, avoid all nodal agents including adenosine. Consult cards, if unstable cardioversion. If stable consider procainamide.
  - **Atrial Fibrillation/Aflutter**: See chapter. Start with rate control. In appropriate patients consider chemical or electrical cardioversion.
- **Wide Complex Tachycardia (WCT)**: Ventricular origin (VT) or Supraventricular origin (SVT or Afib) with conduction aberrancy. In general, treat as VT until proven otherwise. Place pads, start ACLS, and consult cardiology. Can differentiate between the two based on EKG (presence of extreme R axis, precordial lead concordance, or presence of fusion beats all suggest VT). Presence of multiple risk factors (age, CAD history, structural heart disease, etc.) may suggest VT but is not diagnostic.
  - **Monomorphic VT**: Occurs in patients with structural heart disease, ischemia, and RV outflow tract obstruction.
    - Amiodarone: 150mg IV bolus. Can repeat x1 and then infusion at 1mg/min x6hrs → First line agent
    - Lidocaine: 1-1.5mg/kg (usually 100mg) IV bolus, repeat 0.5-0.75mh/kg bolus Q5-10min up to 3mg/kg and then infusion at 1-4mg/min
    - Procainamide: 20mg/infusion until VT breaks, pt is hypotensive, or QRS prolongs >50%. Avoid in pt with prolonged QTc
  - **Polymorphic VT**: Mainly due to acute ischemia→ Treat as ACS until proven otherwise. Consider amiodarone as previously outlined.
  - **Torsades de pointes**: Polymorphic VT from prolonged QTc
    - Give Mg 2-4mg IV. Avoid amiodarone, which can prolong QTc, and stop all QTc prolonging medications.

- Can attempt overdrive pacing using dopamine or isoproterenol but should be done with cardiology consultation.
  - **Pacemaker mediated tachycardia**: A re-entry tachycardia with the pacemaker firing and then retrograde conduction though the AV node. This is sensed as a P-wave and triggers ventricular pacing → an endless loop of tachycardia at the pacers highest programmed rate.
    - Can attempt nodal blockade to break retrograde conduction.
    - In most cases, place magnet to switch back to DOO mode (no sensing) if dual chamber paced.
  - Other causes of wide complex tachycardia include any atrial or sinus tachycardia with aberrant conduction (ie, a bundle branch block) or pre-excitation. These can be treated the same as their narrow complex counterparts. However, unless it is absolutely clear that the wide complex tachycardia you are seeing is aberrancy, it is safest to assume the rhythm is VT unless proven otherwise.
- Nonsustained VT (**NSVT**) is defined as 3 or more consecutive beats, at rate >120bmp and a duration <30seconds. This can be confused with multiple PVCs but those rates are usually <120bmp. In asymptomatic patients without structural heart disease is not thought to carry increased risk of death. However, it is concerning in patients with history of CAD or RV outflow obstruction.

DISPOSITION

- Admit all patients with ventricular tachycardia, unstable rhythms even if terminated, any patient with a pre-excitation tract with an episode of tachydysrythmia, or any concern for ischemia.
- Polymorphic VT (that is not Torsades) should be evaluated for possible PCI and may be admitted directly to the cath lab versus cardiology.
- Many of these patients will be admitted to a cardiology floor or a cardiology step-down unit. Patients with Afib and Aflutter and can be admitted to the floor with telemetry if they are rate controlled.
- Patients with SVT can generally be discharged home after their rhythm terminates. If there is no concern for pre-excitation, consider discharging with prescription for one time dose of beta-blocker to take at home if they feel their symptoms return.
- Patients with palpitations that have resolved and are not caught on monitor should be admitted to telemetry for monitoring if symptomatic or have significant comorbidties. Otherwise, these patients can be discharged home with PCP follow up for Holter monitor.
- RETURN IF: Palpitations return, you feel lightheaded, dizzy, experience chest pain or shortness of breath, or any other new or concerning symptoms.

BEWARE...

(!) Check pulse to determine how many beats are actually being perfused. HR may be 140bpm but only 70bpm beats may be perfused.

(!) Adenosine has a very short half-life. Give through an IV in the antecubital fossa or more proximal and flush quickly. Warn patients about how uncomfortable they are likely to feel. Many describe it as a roller coaster sensation or that they can feel their heart has stopped.

(!) When giving adenosine always have monitor ready to record a rhythm strip as the rhythm breaks. This will help to determine underlying EKG morphology ifthe heart rate slows but the rhythm does not break.

Sources

Carnell J, Singh. An Evidence-Based Approach to Supraventricular achydysrythimias. *Emerg Med Pract.* April 2008;10(4).

Subramanian NR, Brady WJ. Wide Complex Tahcycardia: Diagnosis and Management in the Emergency Department. *Emerg Med Pract.* 2008;10(6).

Notes

7 ▶ Post-Cardiac Arrest Care

After ROSC is achieved from a medical cardiac arrest, efforts should turn to identifying and treating the etiology of the arrest, preserving neurologic function, managing the resultant cardiovascular dysfunction, and treating any complications from the resuscitation efforts

IMMEDIATE

- Establish definitive airway, complete primary survey, and obtain vital signs.
- Obtain IV and arterial access, ensure that lab work is initiated.
- Obtain 12-lead ECG; if STEMI, initiate reperfusion therapy.
- Obtain collateral information and perform exam to determine etiology of arrest:
  — Use US to assess cardiac function, lung sliding, FAST
- Specific therapy directed at cause of arrest. H's and T's.

H's and T's	
Hypovolemia	Toxins
Hypoxia	Tamponade
Hydrogen (Acidosis)	Tension PTX
Hyperkalemia	Thrombosis (MI)
Hypothermia	Thrombosis (PE)
Hypo/hyperglycemia	Trauma

AIRWAY AND BREATHING

- Avoid excessive ventilation, hypocarbia → cerebral vascular constriction
- Low tidal volume ventilation (6-8 ml/kg), goal $PaCO_2$ of 40–45 mmHg
- Wean FiO_2 as low as possible for goal SaO_2 of 94 – 98% to avoid oxygen toxicity
- Consider waveform capnography
- CXR to confirm endotracheal tube position and evaluate for possible aspiration, pneumonia, or rib fractures after CPR

CIRCULATION

- Administer fluid boluses, vasopressors/inotropes for goal MAP 65–100 mmHg (low flow to brain is very dangerous at this time).
- Continue goal directed hemodynamic optimization using $ScvO_2$ and lactate clearance as resuscitation endpoints.
- Obtain definitive access including central access and place arterial line.
- Consider vasopressors if needed:
  — Epinephrine 0.1-0.5mcg/kg per minute
  — Dopamine 5-10mcg/kg per minute
  — Norepinephrine 0.1-0.5mcg/kg per minute
- Early echocardiography to assess cardiac function
- Consider emergent cardiology consult for intra-aortic balloon pump, ventricular assist device, or ECMO in persistently unstable patients.

DISABILITY (AKA NEUROLOGIC PROTECTION)

- Perform thorough neurologic exam including brainstem reflexes.
- Consider head CT if:
  — Concern for head trauma or intracranial process leading to arrest
  — Lateralizing sign on neurologic exam; should not have asymmetric exam from hypoxic injury alone
- **Initiate Therapeutic Hypothermia** → Can start with cool IVF and ice packs to groin and axilla while in ED
  — **Indications**: Patient does not follow commands or show purposeful movements
  — **Contraindications**: Active non-compressible bleeding (brain or gastrointestinal)
  — Target temperature of 32°C – 34°C if <6hrs of ROSC (though <36 is likely equally effective)
  — Control shivering with sedation and consider neuromuscular blockade if sedation not sufficient
- Glucose control
- Monitor for seizures; if the patient is paralyzed should have EEG to monitor for seizure activity.

BEWARE...

⚠ Do not forget to search for and treat for etiology of arrest after ROSC; failure to do so can lead to another arrest.

⚠ Call family early to obtain collateral information and ensure what you are doing is within the patient's goals of care.

⚠ Treat all patients the same regardless of what you believe will be the neurologic outcome. Even in patients for whom the family will ultimately withdraw care, better care means more time for the family to come to terms with the outcome. It can also mean healthier/viable organs if patient is an organ donor.

Sources

Nielsen N, et al. The TTM Trial Investigators. Targeted Temperature Management at 33°C versus 36°C after Cardiac Arrest. *N Engl J Med*. 2013 Dec 5;369(23):2197-206.

Peberdy MA, Callaway CW, Neumar RW, et al. Post-cardiac arrest care: 2010 American Heart Association guidelines for cardiopulmonary resuscitation and emergency cardiovascular care. *Circulation*. 2010;122:Suppl 3:S768-S786[Erratum, *Circulation* 2011;123(6):e237, 124(15):e403.]

Stub D, Bernard S, Duffy SJ, Kaye DM. Post cardiac arrest syndrome: a review of therapeutic strategies. *Circulation*. 2011 Apr 5;123(13):1428-35.

7 ▶ Aortic Dissection

- Begins with tear in intima → blood into media, separating the intima and adventitia; commonly proximal ascending thoracic aorta

- Diagnostic challenge; time-sensitive (mortality is directly proportional to time of symptoms onset to time of dx and treatment)

- Begins with tear in intima→ blood into media, separating the intima and adventitia; commonly proximal ascending thoracic aorta

- Consider in patients presenting with chest/abdominal/back pain, syncope, focal neurologic deficits, GI bleed

- Death usually from acute aortic regurgitation, major branch-vessel obstruction, pericardial tamponade, aortic rupture

Ddx	
ACS	Peri/myocarditis
Intra-abdominal pathology	Pericardial tamponade
Ischemic bowel	Pneumonia
HTN emergency	GI bleed
Pneumothorax	Esophageal rupture
Pulmonary embolism	Mediastinitis
	Pancreatitis

Types of Aortic Dissection	
Stanford Type A	**Stanford Type B**
<ul><li>All dissections involving the ascending aorta, regardless of site of origin</li><li>Usually require surgical therapy</li><li>More common (68% of dissections)</li><li>Associated with aortic rupture, tamponade, AMI, aortic regurgitation, hemorrhage, stroke</li></ul>	<ul><li>All dissections NOT involving the ascending aorta</li><li>Usually medically managed (BP control) by cardiology or medicine team</li><li>Less common (32% of dissections)</li><li>Usually originates just distal to the left subclavian artery</li><li>Associated with organ/limb ischemia, hemorrhage</li></ul>

EVALUATION

- **High Yield History:** Pain is classically a tearing or ripping sensation in the back or chest that is sudden in onset. It is associated with syncope, diaphoresis, nausea, vomiting, lightheadedness, severe apprehension or focal neurologic signs such as parasthesias. Small number are silent, typically in older patients.

- **Risk factors**: HTN is the most common risk factor. Others include advanced age, aortic valve replacement, bicuspid aortic valve, Marfan's syndrome, Turner's or Ehlers-Danlos syndrome, aortic aneurysm, substance abuse including stimulants, history of TB or syphilis, vasculitis, 3rd trimester of pregnancy, blunt trauma, cardiac surgery or catheterization, tobacco use, and family history.

- **Exam:** Aortic regurgitation (in type A), signs of tamponade (JVD, muffled heart sounds, tachycardia, hypotension), pulse deficits, or unequal BPs in upper/lower extremities, neurologic findings (correspond to location of blood flow interruption).

- **Diagnostics:**
  - Labs: BMP, CBC, cardiac markers, coags, lactate, type and cross 6 units if high suspicion or known diagnosis, consider D-dimer (negative → high negative predictive value)
  - EKG: Not sensitive or specific, can be normal or abnormal, BEWARE: 2-5% patient with ascending dissection have compromise of coronary artery flow and therefore have EKG changes consistent with ACS---usually it is the RCA and hence, an inferior MI.
  - Imaging:
    - CT with IV contrast: high sensitivity and specificity. Identifies intimal flap between true and false lumens.
    - CXR: Not sensitive. May show widened aortic knob or mediastinum, displaced intimal calcification, pleural effusion, left apical pleural cap, indistinct or irregular aortic contour, tracheal or esophageal deviation.
    - US: Not sensitive but is specific if intraluminal aortic flap/dissection visualized. Useful for evaluating for pericardial effusion and tamponade.

MANAGEMENT

- Cardiac monitor; 2 large-bore IVs; bilateral arterial lines
- *GOAL: Rapid control of blood pressure (goal BP systolic 110-120 or MAP 70-80mmHg) and HR (goal 60-80) to* decrease shearing forces and prevent further arterial injury.
- Beta blockers are first-line meds. Can use calcium channel blockers in conjunction with nitrates for patients with contraindications to beta blockade
  - Esmolol (can be used as sole agent): bolus 1 mg/kg, then infusion at 50-200 µg/kg/min (preferred)
  - Labetalol (can be used as sole agent): 20 mg IV bolus and then infusion of 0.5 to 2 mg/min
  - Sodium Nitroprusside: IV infusion 0.3-0.5 µg/kg/min and titrate to maximum 10 µg/kg/min. Requires previous and ongoing beta-blocker or calcium channel blocker to prevent reflex tachycardia (increases wall stress).
- Cocaine-related presentations should NOT be treated with beta blockers; use benzodiazapines, calcium channel blockers, and nitrates.
- If hypotensive evaluate for *pseudohypotension* (falsely decreased BP due to dissection involving brachiocephalic artery) by checking BP in both arms. Then use IV crystalloid and careful use of vasopressors (norepinephrine or phenylephrine) to maintain adequate perfusion.
- Treat pain! This will also help control blood pressure and heart rate.
- Consult cardiothoracic surgery EARLY! Type A dissections are treated surgically while type B dissections are treated medically.
- If patient is unstable DO NOT send to the CT scanner. Consider a cardiology/cardiac anesthesia consult to obtain a bedside TEE.

DISPOSITION

- Type A dissections to the OR.
- Type B admit to the ICU for aggressive blood pressure control.

BEWARE...

(!) If treating an inferior or posterior MI always consider the possibility of proximal dissection into right coronary artery prior to initiating treatment with an anticoagulant or thrombolytic.

(!) Ensure adequate pain control, which will help reduce pain related to tachycardia or hypertension.

(!) Always consider dissection in patients with risk factors and those whose chest pain is associated with back pain or a focal neurologic complaint.

(!) Obtain early cardiothoracic consultation.

Sources

Upadhye S, Schiff K. Acute aortic dissection in the emergency department: diagnostic challenges and evidence-based management. *Emerg Med Clin North Am*. 2012;30(2):307-27, viii.

Woo KM, Schneider JI. High-risk chief complaints I: chest pain – the big three. *Emerg Med Clin North Am*. 2009 Nov;27(4):685-712,x.

Marill KA. Serum D-dimer is a sensitive test for the detection of acute aortic dissection: a pooled meta-analysis. *J Emerg Med*. 2008 May;34(4):367-76.

Marx J, Hockberger R, Walls R. Rosen's Emergency Medicine: Concepts & Clinical Practice. 5th ed. Maryland Heights, MO: Mosby; 2002.

Notes

8 ▶ Pericarditis

- Inflammation of pericardium characterized by granulocytic and lymphocytic infiltration
- **Most common etiologies** (in developed countries): Idiopathic (most cases), viral, post-infarction, neoplasm, or connective tissue disorders

Etiologies				
Infectious	**Collagen Vascular Disease**	**Cardiac**	**Mechanical**	**Miscellaneous**
Viral: Echovirus, coxsackievirus, HIV, hepatitis **Bacterial:** TB Fungal Parasite	RA SLE Scleroderma Sarcoidosis Dermatomyositis Amyloidosis	Post-acute myocardial infarction (Dressler's syndrome)	Trauma Surgery (post-ablation or PVI) Radiation	Idiopathic Uremia Drug-induced Neoplasm Autoimmune

EVALUATION

- **High Yield History:** Chest pain that is sharp, pleuritic, retrosternal, varies with respirations, and generally relieved by sitting forward and worsens with lying down. Can radiate to left shoulder or trapezius.

Ddx
ACS
PE
Aortic dissection
Cardiac tamponade
Pneumothorax
Pneumonia
Cholecystitis
Pancreatitis

- Recent viral infection, fever, myalgias, constitutional symptoms, or any other risk factors (see chart).
  - Can present as isolated shoulder pain. May be associated with epigastric pain, cough, and dyspnea.
- **Exam:** Pericardial friction rub (best heard using diaphragm of stethoscope at LLSB)
- **Diagnostic work-up:** After diagnosis of pericarditis, further workup should be directed at determining etiology.
  - Labs: Consider CBC, BMP (renal function), CRP/ESR (may be used to tailor treatment length), Blood Cx (if febrile/signs of sepsis), PPD, Hepatitis panel, HIV serology, ANA (if indicated for follow up)
  - EKG most reliable tool. Changes often show in sequential stages (EKG changes are typically diffuse but can be anatomic). In the acute setting generally characterized by diffuse ST elevations and PR depressions EXCEPT in aVR/V1 — reciprocal ST depression and PR elevations.
  - ECHO: Can't rule out pericarditis, will be normal unless pericardial effusion. Up to 2/3 of cases will have associated effusion.
  - CXR: To exclude other diagnosis. May reveal an enlarged cardiac silhouette if pericardial effusion is present.
- Ventricular arrhythmia makes diagnosis less likely. Think about myocarditis or other cardiac disease.
- Diagnosis depends on the presence of at least two of the following: typical chest pain, friction rub on exam, stereotypical EKG changes, or presence of pericardial effusion.

MANAGEMENT

- Should focus on treating cause (i.e.- dialysis for uremic pericarditis); otherwise, treatment is symptomatic.
- 1st line: High dose aspirin (750-1000mg Q6-8hrs) or **ibuprofen** (400-800 mg TID) or **indomethacin** (50mg TID) for 2 weeks
  — Consider adding a PPI during treatment in pts with history of PUD, age >65, concurrent use of aspirin, corticosteroids, or anticoagulants
- Alternatives:
  — Colchicine (1-2mg on 1st day then 0.5-1mg/day for 3 months). May cause diarrhea, nausea, vomiting
    - Can be used as an adjunct to NSAID, especially if 1st episode (decreases recurrence)
    - Can be use alone for recurrent pericarditis
  — PO Glucocorticoids (initial dosing 0.25 to 0.50 mg/kg/day of prednisone followed by a slow taper)
    - For use in chronic pericarditis, NSAID contraindicated patients, pericarditis refractory to NSAIDS and colchicine, systemic inflammatory diseases, pregnant patients
    - May be associated with increased rate of recurrence of pericarditis

DISPOSITION

- Depends on clinical appearance and presence of complications, but most patients can be discharged home and will recover within 1-3 weeks.
- Admit patients with concerning associated symptoms such as large effusions, concern for myocarditis, traumatic etiology, or on antiocoagulation.
- RETURN IF: You have worsening chest pain, severe shortness of breath, you pass out, or have any other new or concerning symptoms.

BEWARE...

(!) Thrombolytic treatment is contraindicated ($\uparrow$risk cardiac tamponade).

Sources

Imazio M, Brucato A, Cemin R, et al. A randomized trial of colchicine for acute pericarditis. *N Engl J Med* 2013;369:1522-8.

Maisch B, Seferović PM, Ristić AD, et al. Guidelines on the diagnosis and management of pericardial diseases executive summary: the Task Force on the Diagnosis and Management of Pericardial Diseases of the European Society of Cardiology. *Eur Heart J.* 2004;25:587-610.

LeWinter MM. Clinical practice. Acute pericarditis. *N Engl J Med.* 2014 Dec 18;371(25):2410-6. doi: 10.1056/NEJMcp1404070.

Section VI.
HEENT Complaints

1 ▶ ENT Quick Guide

- ALWAYS: COMPLETE VS and early airway assessment
- Can't-miss diagnoses in first 2 minutes: Epiglottitis, Ludwig's angina, airway foreign body, angioedema, and anaphylaxis
- Viruses cause the majority of pharyngitis. Bacterial infection much less common than viral: group A beta-hemolytic streptococcus is the cause of pharyngitis in 5% of adults.

EVALUATION

- **High Yield History:** Immunocompromised? Severe or repeated infections? Recent antibiotics? Chemotherapy? Radiation? → If yes to any of these then increased risk for fungal colonization (Candida albicans).

- **Exam**: Assess for changes in voice, ability to manage secretions, oropharyngeal swelling, and any stridor. Is the patient febrile?

  — In most cases, if febrile and concern for airway compromise ddx includes epiglottitis, RPA, tracheitis, Ludwig's angina, or lingual abscess. Elderly may not mount a high fever even with infection.

  — In most cases, if afebrile and concern for airway compromise ddx includes foreign body, caustic ingestion, tumor, congenital anomaly, or trauma.

  — Altered phonation or drooling suggests epiglottitis, peritonsillar cellulitis, peritonsillar abscess, or parapharyngeal abscess.

Can't-Miss Diagnoses		
Diagnosis	**Features**	**Treatment**
Epiglottitis	Muffled voice, tripod positioning, fever, tachycardia, stridor, dysphagia, drooling	ENT for OR intubation, IV abx (ceftriaxone and ampicillin/sulbactam), humidified O2, consider IV steroids to decrease edema
Retropharyngeal abscess	Neck pain, muffled voice, fever, dysphagia, odynophagia	Drainage by ENT, IV abx (mixed aerobic and anaerobic coverage), IVF
Peritonsillar abscess	Trismus, muffled voice, , fever, malaise, drooling	Drainage, IV abx (mixed aerobic and anaerobic coverage such as clindamycin)

Trench Mouth (AKA-acute necrotizing ulcerative gingivitis)	Painful, bright red friable gingiva with halitosis. Develop necrosis and/or crater like ulcerations of the gingiva with pseudomembrane formation (grayish film)	Good oral hygiene, salt water rinses, hydrogen peroxide rinses, oral analgesics, viscous lidocaine, dental referral. Untreated or delayed treatment can lead to infection spreading to cheeks, lips, mandible →tissue destruction
Ludwig's Angina	Associated with poor dentition. Exam with edema of the floor of the mouth edema and trismus	IV abx (ampicillin/sulbactam or high dose penicillin and flagyl or clindamycin), emergent ENT consult
Diphtheria	Occurs in non-immunized patients. Characterize by sore throat, pseudomembrane on tonsils/pharynx, swollen neck ("bull neck") and corynebacterium diptheriae on gram stain	Metronidazole, erythromycin, or penicillin G
Suppurative Parotitis	Characterized by tender, erythematous skin over parotid, pus expressed from Stenson's duct, fever and trismus. Risk factors include recent anesthesia, sialolithiasis, dehydration, meds that decrease salivation	Amoxicillin/clavulanate (Augmentin) or ampicillin/sulbactam (Unasyn). Provide sialagogues to optimize salivary flow. Obtain ENT consult

Non-Life Threatening Causes		
Diagnosis	**Features**	**Treatment**
Streptococcal pharyngitis	Symptoms include odynophagia, fever and malaise. CENTOR criteria: fever, tonsillar exudate, tender cervical lymphadenopathy, absence of cough	If 1 CENTOR criteria, no abx. 2-3 criteria then treat if rapid strep is positive. If 4 criteria treat without testing with penicillin x10 days vs. IM penicillin x1
Viral pharyngitis	Sore throat, odynophagia, fever, cervical lymph adenopathy	Supportive care i.e. oral analgesics and salt water gargles
Stomatitis	Prodromal burning or tingling followed by painful ulceration of gingiva, fevers, lymphadenopathy and vesicle formation. Causes: aphthous ulcer, HSV, varicella, coxsackievirus, and chemotherapy	If symptomatic from HSV may use antivirals (i.e. acyclovir if during prodromal phase). For other etiologies treat with analgesia and oral hygiene.
Candida Albicans	Patches of gray or white friable material covering erythematous base	Clotrimazole troches 5x daily, oral ketoconazole, itraconazole, or fluconazole
Sialolithiasis	Pain and swelling of gland, mumps vs. bacteria	Antibiotics, moist heat, sialagogues, massage, hydration
Dental caries	Pain, halitosis, brown discoloration of tooth	Oral analgesics, consider nerve block, dental referral
Dry socket (Post-extraction alveolar osteitis)	Sudden onset of severe pain 2-4 days post-extraction, pain free interval after extraction, foul odor in mouth	Nerve block, oral analgesics, oral abx (eg, penicillin VK 500mg TID)

2 ▶ Ludwig's Angina

- A potentially life-threatening polymicrobial infection of the bilateral submandibular and sublingual spaces most commonly due to an infection of second and third mandibular molar tooth
- Most common cause of death is sudden asphyxiation

Ddx
Dental infection
Deep cervical node suppuration
Peritonsillar and other deep neck space abscess
Parotid and submandibular gland abscess
Angioedema
Submandibular hematoma
Malignancy

EVALUATION

- **High Yield History**: Patients often present with fevers, pain in their throat, jaw, or neck, dysphagia, or changes in their voice.
  - Assess for risk factors including recent dental infections, facial fractures, or other facial trauma.
  - Past medical history for any immunocompromised state.
- **Exam**: Often febrile, tachycardic, and toxic appearing.
  - On exam may have stridor, trismus, voice changes, elevation or protrusion of tongue, elevation and "woody consistency" of floor of the mouth, neck swelling, decreased ROM of the neck, and inability to handle secretions.
  - Note that stridor, tachypnea, dyspnea, drooling, and agitation are highly concerning for impending airway loss.
  - Once this diagnosis is considered, also examine the airway and neck for possible RSI or cricothyroidotomy.
- **Diagnostics**
  - Labs: This is a clinical diagnosis; send labs to exclude other diagnoses or pre-op lab work.
  - CT face/neck is the best imaging study — can identify extent of disease and complications.
  - Soft tissue plain films may show swelling, airway narrowing, subcutaneous gas collections.
  - US can assist with diagnosing abscesses.

MANAGEMENT

- Key to management is to secure the airway and provide early antibiotics.
- **Airway management**: Optimal intubation strategy is fiberoptic guided oral or nasotracheal intubation in the OR with sedation and topical anesthesia. Endotracheal intubation may be difficult due to distorted airway tissues. Cricothyrotomy may be difficult and can spread infection; however, it may be necessary if unable to secure airway.
- **Immediate Antibiotics:** Need to cover hemolytic streptococcus, staph, and bacteroides fragilis.
- Be sure to obtain ENT consult for possible operative intervention/drainage.
- Provide pain control and consider steroids to reduce edema.

Antibiotic Selection	
Immunocompetent Patients	**Immunocompromised Patients**
— Ampicillin/Sulbactam 3gm IV Q6hrs — Penicillin G 2-4 million units Q4-6hrs PLUS metronidazole 500mg IV — Clindamycin 600mg IV Q6-8hrs (if PCN allergy)	— Cefepime 2gm IV Q12h **PLUS** metronidazole 500mg IV Q6h — Imipenem 500mg IV Q6h or meropenem 1gm IV Q8h — Piperacillin-tazobactam 4.5gm IV Q6h
If increased risk of MRSA (eg, IV drugs, DM, nursing home) then add vancomycin 15-20 mg/kg IV q12 **or linezolid 600mg IV q12h	

DISPOSITION

- SICU for airway monitoring and IV abx or to the OR for debridement.
- All of these patients are admitted.

BEWARE...

(!) Recognize the potential for rapid spread of infection.

(!) Be sure to assess and secure the airway early and prepare for a difficult intubation and difficult surgical airway.

(!) Start broad-spectrum IV abx EARLY.

(!) CT imaging requires patient to lay flat and can be unsafe with the evolving airway compromise.

Sources

Hogdon A. Dental and related infections. *Emerg Med Clin North Am*. 2013;31(2):465-480.

Marx J, Hockberger R, Walls R. Rosen's Emergency Medicine: Concepts & Clinical Practice. 5th ed. Maryland Heights, MO: Mosby; 2002.

Notes

3 ▶ Peritonsillar Abscess (PTA)

- Collection of pus located between the capsule of the palatine tonsil and the pharyngeal muscles. Most common deep neck infection; majority of cases are in adolescents and young adults.

- PTA is often preceded by tonsillitis or pharyngitis; it progresses from cellulitis to phlegmon to abscess.

Ddx
Epiglottitis
Retropharyngeal abscess
Retropharyngeal cellulitis
Abscess of parapharyngeal space
Severe tonsillopharyngitis

- PTA usually occurs in the superior pole of the tonsil (but can also occur in the midpoint or inferior pole of the tonsil, or may be dispersed with multiple loculations in the peritonsillar space).

- May compromise the upper airway or spread to the surrounding structures (ie, masseter and pterygoid muscles, carotid sheath).

- Often polymicrobial (most common species are GAS, Staph aureus including MRSA, and respiratory anaerobes like Fusobacteria, Prevotella, Veillonella)

EVALUATION

- **High Yield History:** Paitents often present with severe sore throat (usually unilateral), fever, and "hot potato" (muffled) voice
  - Two-thirds of pts will have trismus (due to irritation and reflex spasm of internal pterygoid muscles).
  - May also have drooling, neck swelling, and ipsilateral ear pain or decreased PO intake due to pain.

- **Exam:** Findings include swollen/fluctuant tonsil with deviation of uvula to opposite side, or fullness or bulging of posterior soft palate near the tonsil with palpable fluctuance
  - Children with peritonsillar cellulitis may have erythematous pharynx and enlarged tonsils with exudate, but less likely to have uvular deviation or trismus.
  - If drooling is present, suggesting concern for epiglottitis, do not be aggressive during examination of oral cavity. Pt may need imaging or examination in OR with controlled airway.

- **Diagnostics**
  - Labs often not necessary, but may be helpful to guide dispo or therapy. Consider CBC and BMP if decreased PO intake.
  - Throat culture for group A strep, gram stain, cultures of abscess fluid if drained (may help guide ABX therapy in immunocompromised patients or those with complications or extension of infection).
  - Indications for imaging: Not needed in straightforward cases, but can help for:
    - Distinguishing cellulitis from abscess (response to a 24hr trial of ABX is an alternative)
    - Looking for spread of infection to parapharyngeal space
    - If exam is inadequate due to trismus

- Exclusion of epiglottitis or retropharyngeal abscess →CT with IV contrast is preferred modality. (PTA will appear as hypodense mass with ring enhancement.)
— Consider lateral neck x-ray to assess for epiglottitis.

MANAGEMENT

- Basic management = (1) Drainage, (2) Antibiotics, (3) Supportive Care
- If pt is anxious, ill-appearing, drooling, or posturing, place on continuous monitoring and prepare for airway intervention if necessary.
- **Drainage** can be via needle aspiration, I&D, or tonsillectomy. Choice of procedure depends on provider experience, age and ability of patient to cooperate, cost, and whether the patient has indications for tonsillectomy (ie, recurrent pharyngitis)
  — **Needle aspiration:** Generally tolerated better than I&D, as it is less invasive and less painful; similar success rates to I&D in randomized control trials. Can usually be done with topical anesthesia. Complications include hemorrhage and aspiration of pus/blood into airway. Pt must be observed after needle aspiration to be sure s/he can tolerate PO abx/ pain meds/fluids. If not admitted, pt should be followed up in 24-36hrs.
  — **I&D:** More painful, with more bleeding than needle aspiration. Complications include aspiration of abscess contents.
  — **Tonsillectomy:** If indicated, can be done immediately during acute infection or as an interval operation.
- **Pearls for Doing the Drainage:**
  — Since visualization of the PTA location can be hard, it may help to use a laryngoscope with a curved blade to provide light and better exposure of the pharynx.
    - Place patient sitting upright and anesthetize area (nebulized lidocaine, 5cc of 2% or 4%, and atomization of additional lidocaine over the tonsil)
    - Insert blade into patient's mouth (just as you would for DL, except they're sitting up) as far posteriorly as tolerated (laryngoscope handle will be below level of pt's mouth, and the curved blade will help to sweep pt's tongue out of the way).
  — Whatever needle you use for aspiration (many providers use a 3.5 inch spinal needle, 18G or 20G), trim the plastic needle sheath so that when replaced, only 1.5 cm of the needle tip is exposed. This prevents you from advancing the needle too far once in the abscess.
  — Using bedside US can allow you to better localize the abscess, but also allows identification of the carotid artery location relative to the PTA, using color Doppler. On intraoral US, the PTA will appear as an echo-free cavity with an irregular border.
- **Antibiotics**: Empiric coverage should include GAS, Staph aureus, and resp. anaerobes
  — **IV:** Unasyn 50mg/kg Q6hrs in children, or 3gm Q6hrs in adults; clindamycin 15mg/kg Q8hrs in children, or 600mg Q6-8hrs in adults. If infection does not respond or is life-threatening, add vancomycin (15mg/kg Q8hrs in kids, 15-20mg/kg Q12hrs in adults with adjustment for trough of 15-20mg).

- **PO:** Should be 14-day course (or completing 14-day course if IV given initially); amoxicillin 45mg/kg Q12hrs in kids, 875mg Q12hrs in adults or clindamycin 15mg/kg Q8hrs in kids, 300-450mg Q6hrs in adults. If empiric therapy for presumed MRSA is used, then clindamycin or linezolid can be used for PO regimen.
- Glucocorticoids: Inconsistent evidence; not routinely recommended (however, the only RCT showed faster symptomatic improvement in patients > 16yo treated with needle aspiration, IV abx, AND glucocorticoids).

DISPOSITION

- Response to Treatment:
  - Success = Symptomatic improvement in sore throat, fever, and/or tonsillar swelling within 24hrs of intervention
  - Failure = Lack of symptomatic improvement or worsening despite 24hrs of antimicrobial therapy (with or without surgical drainage); may occur in patients who have developed complications, are infected with unusual organisms, have incomplete drainage or abscess, or have underlying problems (ie, congenital cyst or tract), and these patients may need imaging or repeat surgical intervention or broadening of abx coverage.
- Complication: Rare but potentially fatal: airway obstruction, aspiration PNA if abscess ruptures into airway, bacteremia, IJ vein thrombosis, jugular vein suppurative thrombophlebitis (Lemierre's syndrome), carotid artery rupture, or mediastinitis. Recurrence of PTA may occur in 10-15% of patients.
- Hospitalization may be needed for adequate hydration and analgesia, especially in younger children. Older patients with uncomplicated PTA may be managed outpatient if well-hydrated and able to take PO medications after drainage procedure.
- Follow up in 24-36hrs if treated as outpatient.
- RETURN IF: You develop shortness of breath, worsening throat/neck pain, trismus, enlarging mass, fever, neck stiffness, or bleeding.

Sources
Afarian H, Lin M. ACEP Tricks of the Trade: Say 'Ah!' – Needle Aspiration of Peritonsillar Abscess. *ACEP News.* May 2008.

Notes

4 ▶ Retropharyngeal Abcess (RPA)

- A deep neck space infection; most common between the ages of 2-4 and may be indistinguishable from uncomplicated pharyngitis early in its course.

- About half of retropharyngeal infections are associated with preceding upper respiratory tract infections; a fourth are related to pharyngeal trauma (ie, penetrating foreign body or dental procedure); another fourth are associated with pharyngitis or vertebral body osteomyelitis.

- RPA is often polymicrobial (GAS, Staph aureus, Fusobacteria, Prevotella).

EVALUATION

Ddx
Epiglottitis
PTA
Croup
Bacterial tracheitis
Uvulitis
Foreign body
Angioedema
Anaphylaxis
Pharyngitis
Neck sprain
Meningitis
C-spine osteomyelitis
Spinal injury
Dystonic reaction

- **High Yield History:** Symptoms include fever, dysphagia, odynophagia, decreased PO intake, and occasionally chest pain if there is mediastinal involvement.

- **Exam:** Patients can present with drooling, torticollis/unwillingness to move or extend neck due to pain, muffled voice or gurgling sound, stridor, neck swelling, or trismus. Tender, anterior cervical lymphadenopathy is frequently present. A neck mass may be palpable if the infection has spread to the lateral pharyngeal space.

  — NOTE: Patient should be examined with suction equipment ready at the bedside in case the abscess ruptures.

  — If visualization is adequate, it may be possible to appreciate midline or unilateral swelling of the posterior pharyngeal wall; mass may be fluctuant.

- **Diagnostics:**

  — Labs: CBC, aerobic/anaerobic blood cultures, standard throat culture, aerobic/anaerobic culture specimens at time of drainage.

  — Imaging: If no signs of airway compromise and the suspicion for RPA is LOW, then lateral neck x-ray may be the initial study.

  - On plain x-ray the prevertebral space may be increased in depth compared to anterior-posterior measurement of adjacent vertebral body (retropharyngeal space considered widened if greater than 7mm at C2 or 14mm at C6 in children).

  - Other signs of retropharyngeal infection on x-ray include loss or reversal of normal cervical lordosis due to muscle spasm/inflammation.

  - If suspicion for RPA is high, then CT with contrast is the preferred study. CT is usually omitted in children with moderate to severe respiratory distress, who usually go to the OR instead for better airway management.

  - CXR should be obtained in pts with suspected retropharyngeal infection, to look for extension (ie, mediastinitis or aspiration PNA).

MANAGEMENT

- Initial therapy depends on severity of respiratory distress and likelihood of having a drainable fluid collection.
  - If concern for airway compromise: Immediate surgical drainage and empiric antibiotic therapy
  - If airway is stable: Management is variable by provider; consider surgical drainage and starting abx versus a trial of abx if abscess is small (< 2 cm area).
- Factors that increase likelihood of having a drainable collection at surgery include: symptoms for more than 2 days, cross-sectional area > 2 cm on CT.
- If pt is early in the clinical course (with a cellulitis or phlegmon in the retropharyngeal space), antibiotics and supportive care may prevent progression and avoid need for surgery.
- Antibiotics: Empiric coverage should include group A strep, Staph aureus, and resp. anaerobes. ***Dosing is given for kids only (as infection most common in ages 2-4.)***
  - **IV:** Unasyn 50mg/kg Q6hrs or clindamycin 20-40 mg/kg/day divided Q6-Q8hrs; if infection does not respond or is life-threatening, add vancomycin (15 mg/kg Q8hrs in children) or linezolid (10 mg/kg Q8hrs for < 12yrs. old, 10 mg/kg Q12hrs in > 12 yrs. old)
  - **PO:** Should be 14-day course (or completing 14-day course if IV given initially). Augmentin 45mg/kg Q12hrs in children or clindamycin 40mg/kg/day divided Q6-Q8hrs in children.
- Supportive care = Maintenance and monitoring of airway, adequate hydration, analgesia, monitoring for complications.

Surgical drainage is usually performed transorally, unless abscess is lateral to neck vessels or involves multiple deep neck space infections.

DISPOSITION

- Hard evidence on management of RPA is lacking. However, in most cases, children with suspected RP infection should be hospitalized and managed with ENT input.
- Complications are largely the same as for PTA. Recurrence may be seen in 1-5% of patients.
- RETURN IF: You develop shortness of breath, worsening throat/neck pain, difficulty opening your mouth, enlarging mass, fever, neck stiffness, bleeding, or any other new or concerning symptoms.

Notes

5 ▶ Dental and Facial Trauma

- Tooth anatomy from external to internal: enamel, dentin, and pulp (central portion with nerves and blood vessels). Area distal to the gum line is crown; proximal is root.

EVALUATION

- **High Yield History:** Generally occurs to due to trauma, therefore it is important to get full trauma history and assess for any other traumatic injuries.
  - Determine if there are any loose teeth, hot or cold intolerance (suggestive of tooth fracture), jaw malocclusion (suggestive of jaw fracture), any facial pain, or epistaxis.
  - Any missing teeth and have they been located (aspiration or intrusion)? In the case of tooth avulsion, determine length of time since the injury (to determine viability of tooth).
- **Exam:** Full trauma exam in addition to focused dental and facial exam.
  - Examine each tooth for fracture, mobility or sensitivity. Account for all missing teeth.
  - Examine soft tissues specifically for any lacerations or imbedded tooth fragments.
  - Assess for jaw malocclusion, midline facial instability or tenderness, nasal septal hematoma, or any other concurrent facial injury.
  - Test each cranial nerve and full motor and sensation of the face.
- **Diagnostics:**
  - Labs not generally indicated.
  - Panorex x-ray: Used to assess all the teeth and the alveolar bone, can also visualize fracture.
  - Maxillary-Facial CT: If concern for facial fractures.
  - CXR: If there are missing teeth that are unaccounted for and there is concern for aspiration.

MANAGEMENT

- Full trauma assessment (see trauma chapter).
- Secure airway as needed and control bleeding.
- Antibiotics for open fractures or patient at risk for subacute endocarditis:
  - Penicillin V: 250-500mg PO Q6hrs
  - Clindamycin (if penicillin allergic): 300mg Q6hrs
- Pain control and tetanus if indicated
- Treatment by injury as listed.

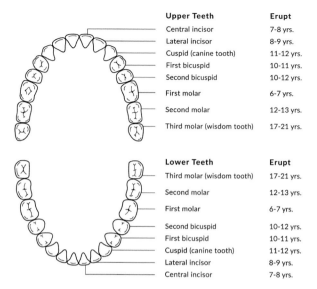

Upper Teeth	Erupt
Central incisor	7-8 yrs.
Lateral incisor	8-9 yrs.
Cuspid (canine tooth)	11-12 yrs.
First bicuspid	10-11 yrs.
Second bicuspid	10-12 yrs.
First molar	6-7 yrs.
Second molar	12-13 yrs.
Third molar (wisdom tooth)	17-21 yrs.

Lower Teeth	Erupt
Third molar (wisdom tooth)	17-21 yrs.
Second molar	12-13 yrs.
First molar	6-7 yrs.
Second bicuspid	10-12 yrs.
First bicuspid	10-11 yrs.
Cuspid (canine tooth)	11-12 yrs.
Lateral incisor	8-9 yrs.
Central incisor	7-8 yrs.

Dental Fracture

- Sorted according to **Ellis Class**
  - Ellis I: Superficial enamel; painless – low risk, can have outpatient dental follow up.
  - Ellis II: Enamel and dentin (yellow at fracture line); sensitive to air, temperature and palpation – risk of infection, should cover (ideally with dental cement) and needs dental follow up in 24-48hrs. Discharge with pain control and advise liquid diet.
  - Ellis III: Involves pulp (pink or reddish), VERY painful (if neurologic bundle severed can be painless) – true dental emergency, need urgent dental consult within 24-48hrs.

Dental Avulsion

- Occurs when tooth is displaced from its socket. The longer the tooth is out the lower the chance of successful re-implantation.
- Management: Only handle by the crown to avoid damaging cells from the periodontal ligament. Rinse debris off gently with normal saline and re-implant. If there will be a delay, soak tooth in normal saline, milk, or (preferably) Hanks Balanced Salt Solution (HBSS).
- Primary teeth in children are never re-implanted (can stunt development of permanent teeth).
- Splint tooth in place and refer for urgent dental follow up (within 24hrs).

Dental Displacement (luxation)

- Sorted according to type
- **Concussion** (mild injury to the periodontal ligament, with some clinical tenderness but no movement of the tooth) and **subluxation** (more significant injury to the periodontal ligament, with clinical tenderness and movement of the tooth, often with bleeding at gum line). Both are non-urgent and can have outpatient dental follow up. Treat pain with NSAIDS and soft diet.
- **Extrusion:** Partial removal of a tooth from its socket. Requires replacing tooth (with firm pressure) to its original position and applying dental splint. Should have close dental follow up (24hrs for permanent splint placement).
- **Lateral luxation:** Lateral displacement of a tooth at an angle, with possible fracture of the alveolar bone. Requires replacing tooth (with firm pressure) to its original position and should be seen by a dentist/oral surgeon for splint placement given likely alveolar bone fracture.
- **Intrusion:** Impaction of a tooth into the alveolar bone, which is also fractured. Often no acute treatment is possible, so should have dental follow up in 24hrs (generally for root canal). This disrupts the blood and nerve supply to the tooth, making it very important that patients follow up.

MAXILLOFACIAL BONE FRACTURES

- Sorted according to Le Fort Classes. These occur with high energy trauma.
  - — Le Fort I (Lower Maxilla): Transverse fracture that separates maxilla from lower pterygoid plate and nasal septum
  - — Le Fort II (Infraorbital Rim): Pyramidal fracture of central maxilla and palate. May be associated with eye, nerve, and vascular injuries.
  - — Le Fort III (Craniofacial Disjunction): Separation of facial skeleton from skull. Fracture extends through frontozygomatic suture lines, orbit, base of nose, ethmoid. May be associated with eye, nerve, and vascular injuries.
- Surgery based on degree of displacement, nasal duct involvement/obstruction (identified by air fluid levels on CT), or CSF leak.
- If surgery not indicated, often send home with prophylactic antibiotics (such as amoxicillin/clavulanate).

DISPOSITION

- Admit if any concerning comorbid conditions, other traumatic injuries, or Le Forte II and III fractures.
- Most patients can be discharged home with close dental or plastic surgery follow up.
- Discharge home with adequate pain control and prophylactic antibiotics if indicated.
- Instruct all patients with dental trauma to follow a diet of soft foods and counsel regarding the possibility of tooth color change, need for root canal, or loss of tooth.
- RETURN IF: You have any severe pain, persistent bleeding, fevers, jaw pain or malocclusion, changes in vision, severe headache, or any other new or concerning symptoms.

BEWARE...

ⓘ Do not be distracted by the dental trauma and miss other traumatic injuries. Do a full trauma assessment.

ⓘ Secure the airway early in anyone with significant injury that may decompensate.

ⓘ Avoid touching the root of an avulsed tooth. You do not want to damage any remaining tissue that is vital to reimplantation success.

ⓘ Account for all missing teeth.

Sources

Zane RD, Kosowsky JM, et al. Pocket Emergency Medicine. 2nd ed. Philadelphia, PA: Lippincott Williams & Wilkins; 2011.

Ma OJ, Cline D, Tintinalli J, et al. Emergency Medicine Manual. 6th ed. New York, NY: McGraw-Hill Professional; 2003.

Marx J, Hockberger R, Walls R. Rosen's Emergency Medicine: Concepts & Clinical Practice. 5th ed. Maryland Heights, MO: Mosby; 2002.

Hans L, Mawji Y. The ABCs of Emergency Medicine. 12th edition. Toronto, Canada: University of Toronto; 2012.

Medscape News & Perspective. New York, NY: http://emedicine.medscape.com.

Notes

6 ▶ Dental Infection

DENTAL INFECTION

- Most often dental carry caused by *Streptococcus mutans*
- Dental caries dissolve enamel and enter the pulp. A track can develop to the root apex and into medullar cavity or maxilla. If untreated this could perforate cortical plates and drain into the superficial tissues or track into deeper fascial planes, causing deep space infection or sinus venous thrombosis.
- If the infection does not drain it develops into a periapical or periodontal abscess.

Ddx
Periapical abscess
Dental caries
Tooth fracture
Aphthous ulcer
Facial cellulitis
Herpes

EVALUATION

- **High Yield History:** Caries often presents with localized pain, edema, and sensitivity to air/temperature. If local infection developed may have fevers; if deeper infection or abscess has formed, may have difficulty swallowing, breathing, or trismus.
- **Exam:** Assess for facial and gingival swelling or fluctuance, tooth tap-tenderness or mobility
  — Necrotizing Ulcerative Gingivitis (trench mouth): Edematous erythematous gingiva with ulcerated, interdental papillae covered with a gray pseudomembrane
  — Periapical abscesses and infections
    ▪ Buccal space infection: cheek edema (infection in posterior teeth/molars)
    ▪ Masticator space infection: trismus (infection of 3rd molar) – can spread to parapharyngeal space
    ▪ Canine space infection: anterior cheek swelling and loss of nasolabial fold (infection of maxillary canine) – can spread to cavernous sinus
- **Diagnostics:**
  — Labs: Generally not indicated unless patient is toxic appearing. Consider CBC, lactate, and cultures.
  — Imaging: Panorex (always requested by dental) is x-ray that can help identify bone involvement; soft tissue x-ray can look for gas and any mass effect, CT for severe infections with concern for deep space involvement.

MANAGEMENT

- Simple dental caries:
  — Antibiotics: Penicillin V 500mg PO Q8hrs or (if PCN allergy) Clindamycin 450mg PO Q8hrs
  — Pain control: Dental infections are painful; offer a dental block depending on which tooth is affected.
- Dental follow up (give a list of dentists!).
  — Necrotizing ulcerative gingivitis:
- Antibiotics, chlorhexidine rinses, pain control, dental follow up.

- — Periapical abscess:
- — I&D area of gingival fluctuance.
- — Provide analgesia with local infiltration of lidocaine.
- — Discharge home with antibiotics, pain control, and dental follow up.

DISPOSITION

- Home with close dental follow up if non-toxic, tolerating POs, and no deep space infection.
- Admit for observation and IV antibiotics if ill appearing, immunocompromised, or unable to handle secretions.
- Admit per ENT if deep space infection for exploration or airway monitoring.
- RETURN IF: Your fevers persist, are unable to tolerate liquids, or have any difficulty breathing or swallowing.

BEWARE...

(!) If the patient also complains of any severe headache or concurrent eye symptoms, consider cavernous sinus thrombosis, which can occur from extension of a dental infection into the cavernous sinus.

Sources

Zane RD, Kosowsky JM, et al. Pocket Emergency Medicine. 2nd ed. Philadelphia, PA: Lippincott Williams & Wilkins; 2011.

Ma OJ, Cline D, Tintinalli J, et al. Emergency Medicine Manual. 6th ed. New York, NY: McGraw-Hill Professional; 2003.

Marx J, Hockberger R, Walls R. Rosen's Emergency Medicine: Concepts & Clinical Practice. 5th ed. Maryland Heights, MO: Mosby; 2002.

Hans L, Mawji Y. The ABCs of Emergency Medicine. 12th edition. Toronto, Canada: University of Toronto; 2012.

Medscape News & Perspective. New York, NY: http://emedicine.medscape.com.

Notes

Section VII.
Eye Complaints

1 ▶ Eye Quick Guide

- ALWAYS: COMPLETE VS including temperature and pulse oximetry, COMPLETE eye exam (see chart), presence or absence for vision loss, and presence or absence of pain.
- Can't-miss diagnoses in first 2 minutes:
  - Caustic injury → Check pH and provide copious irrigation.
  - Acute closed angle glaucoma → Emergent ophthalmology consult, consider timolol (2 drops 0.5%), raise head of the bed 30 degrees.
  - Retrobulbar hematoma (with acute loss of visual acuity, increased IOP, and proptosis) → Lateral canthotomy.
  - Central retinal artery occlusion → Gentle massage though closed lid, nitroglycerin.
  - Globe rupture→ Shield the eye, pain control, antiemetics, antibiotics, and emergent ophthalmology consult.
  - Orbital cellulitis → Broad-spectrum antibiotics.

Eye Exam

Visual acuity (with glasses/contacts if possible, if these are lost you can also use a pinhole to correct)
Visual field
External exam
Extraoccular movements
Pupillary Evaluation
Pressure (tono pen)

EVALUATION

- **High Yield History:**
  - If the patient presents with pain, attempt to characterize the sensation: foreign body sensation (corneal foreign body, abrasion, ulcer), itching (blepharitis, allergic conjunctivitis), burning (irritation of a pterygium, episcleritis, keratoconjunctivitis), dull (increased IOP, sinusitis, temporal arteritis), or sharp (anterior eye pathology – keratitis, uveitis, acute closed angle glaucoma).

Charting the Eye Exam

- Visual Acuity: OD X/X. OS X/X. (or light perception only, no light perception)
- PERL (or afferent pupillary defect)
- Visual Fields: By 4 intact
- Extra Ocular Movements: WNL
- Lids Lashes Lacrimal (LLL): No lesions
- Conjunctiva and Sclera: White and quiet
- Cornea: No fluorescein uptake
- Anterior Chamber: Deep and quiet
- Iris: Round and reactive
- Lens: Clear
- Retina: Sharp disc margins
- Intra Ocular Pressure: 20
  OD: Right Eye, OS: Left Eye

- — Also assess for associated symptoms such as flashing light or falling curtain sensation (retinal detachment), if the patient is immunocompromised or is a contact lens wearer (corneal ulcer, bacterial conjunctivitis), presence of purulent discharge (bacterial conjunctivitis), or any recent eye surgery (uveitis, scleritis, endophthalmitis).
- **Exam**
  - — VVEEPP (see table) including lid inversion and a fundoscopic exam.
  - — Slit lamp exam: Use proparacaine 0.5% for analgesia and fluourosine for staining.
    - ▪ Inspect lids, lashes, conjunctiva, sclera, cornea, anterior chamber, iris, lens.

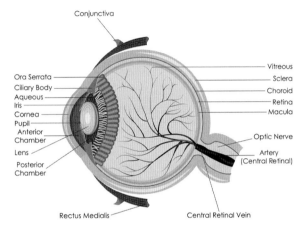

Conjunctiva

Ora Serrata
Ciliary Body
Aqueous
Iris
Cornea
Pupil
Anterior Chamber
Lens
Posterior Chamber

Vitreous
Sclera
Choroid
Retina
Macula

Optic Nerve
Artery (Central Retinal)

Rectus Medialis
Central Retinal Vein

SLIT LAMP

- **Basic procedure: A step-by-step example**

  The basic examination consists of a systematic evaluation of each structure. Master the basic techniques first, and then modify them to suit your individual needs.

  - — Position the patient. Chin in chinrest, forehead against headrest, eyes level with eye level marker. Move the slit lamp table or patient's chair to ensure patient comfort.
  - — Set the ocular head to your specifications. Turn on the power.
  - — Select 1x magnification. Set light source to white light with maximal height and medium width. Set the illumination system to 45 degrees to the temporal side of the eye of interest.
  - — Focus on the outer canthus, adjusting with the joystick (the joystick is what controls focus, not the lenses). Scan across the upper lid, and then back across the lower lid. As you cross the midline, swing the illumination system to the opposite side.
  - — Invert the lids and repeat the procedure.

— Survey the cornea. Focus on any irregularities.

— Set the light width and the aperture to minimum, making a small box or circle of light. Examine the anterior chamber, focusing first in the cornea, the lens, and finally on a point midway between the two. Look for cells and flare. Make sure the room is dark prior to doing this.

— Select the blue filter. Repeat the corneal exam after installation of topical fluorescein.

- **Troubleshooting the slit lamp:**

— **No light:** The reason your light is not coming on is likely that the power is not turned on. Some machines have as many as three switches that all need to be switched on before the light will appear.

— **Poor focus:**

- The slit lamp is a macroscope and sometimes each eyepiece must be focused to your own individual eyes (but try moving the joystick back and forth first).

- The eye pieces were left too close together, or too far apart, and you do not have good binocular vision.

- The joystick is not being properly used to focus in and out.

- The patient does not have his/her forehead up against the headrest.

— **Difficulty aiming light**:

- Make sure the patient's eyes are level with the red line on the frame of the slit lamp. Otherwise you can twirl the joystick all you want, and you will never get the light off the cheek or the forehead.

- Make sure the light source is set "in click."

Red Eye	
Painful	**Painless**
Keratitis, conjunctivitis, episcleritis, scleritis, anterior uveitis, hyphema (can be painful or painless), endopthalmitis, corneal abrasion*, foreign body*, corneal ulcer* (*may only present as pain)	Blepharitis, subconjunctival hemorrhage, hyphemas (can be painless or painful)

Vision Loss	
Painful	**Painless**
Endophthalmitis, acute closed angle glaucoma, optic neuritis	Central retinal artery occlusion, vitreous hemorrhage, central retinal vein occlusion, giant cell arteritis, retinal detachment

TONOMETRY-PEN INSTRUCTIONS

- Use for measurement of the intraocular pressure on tonometry. Normal IOP 10-20mmHg.
- Following instructions are based on use of the Tono-pen:
  - Calibrate Tono-pen or other device based on instructions, and anesthetize the eye with anesthetic drop such as proparacaine.
  - Place patient in seated or supine position and have him/her fix gaze on something.
  - Touch to pen to central cornea lightly and briefly several times. Will hear chirp each time there is a measurement.
  - Machine beeps once for valid readings. Average measurement will appear on LCD.

Sources

Zane RD, Kosowsky JM, et al. Pocket Emergency Medicine. 2nd ed. Philadelphia, PA: Lippincott Williams & Wilkins; 2011.

Ma OJ, Cline D, Tintinalli J, et al. Emergency Medicine Manual. 6th ed. New York, NY: McGraw-Hill Professional; 2003.

Marx J, Hockberger R, Walls R. Rosen's Emergency Medicine: Concepts & Clinical Practice. 5th ed. Maryland Heights, MO: Mosby; 2002.

Hans L, Mawji Y. The ABCs of Emergency Medicine. 12th edition. Toronto, Canada: University of Toronto; 2012.

Medscape News & Perspective. New York, NY: http://emedicine.medscape.com.

Notes

2 ▶ Acute Vision Loss

- Acute vision loss can be the end result of many disease processes, including traumatic injuries, toxic ingestions (methanol), infection (CMV retinitis), cardiovascular (cardioembolic phenomenon), and neurologic (TIA) or a primary ophthalmologic process.

- Diagnosis and management relies on differentiation between a primary ophthalmologic and neurologic etiology.

- The most important initial diagnoses to make and intervene upon are acute angle glaucoma, central retinal artery occlusion, CVA, and chemical burn.

Ddx
Retinal detachment
Central vein occlusion
Retinal artery occlusion
Optic neuritis
Idiopathic intracranial hypertension
Temporal arteritis
Vitreous hemorrhage
Migraine
CVA/ TIA

EVALUATION

- **High Yield Exam:**
  - Primary questions: Is this acute vs. subacute visual loss? Transient (amaurosis fugax) or persistent? Painful or painless? Monocular (pathology anterior to optic chiasm) or binocular (lesion posterior to chiasm), and is there any diplopia?
  - Ask about associated symptoms such as any neurologic deficits (CVA or multiple sclerosis), palpitations, (Afib with embolic disease), headache (glaucoma, giant cell arteritis), any trauma, or systemic symptoms.
  - Have patient describe the pattern and timing of visual loss. Blurry vision vs. complete blackout? Is the entire visual field gone, or are there specific cuts?
  - Past ophthalmic history including baseline eyesight, any surgeries, any history of glaucoma or cataracts, and any eye medications
  - Past medical history for vascular disease, diabetes, malignancy, or any anticoagulant use

- **Exam:** Perform full eye exam (as in Quick Guide) with specific focus on visual acuity, visual fields, and fundoscopic exam
  - Assess for an afferent pupillary defect (slower direct response to light in the affected eye). This suggests unilateral optic nerve pathology.
  - Perform a full neurologic exam, including full cranial nerve exam. Assess for heart murmurs, arrhythmias, carotid bruits, temporal artery tenderness, proximal muscle weakness.

- **Diagnostics:**
  - Labs: Used to assess for comorbidities and risk factors. Specifically, consider ESR (temporal arteritis), coags (vitreous hemorrhage), and more extensive labs if considering neurologic, toxicological, or metabolic etiology.
  - Bedside US can be used to diagnose retinal detachment.
  - Head CT: If concern for hemorrhagic stroke to check for initial screening for edema, hemorrhage, or mass effect from brain mass.
  - CTA/MRI/MRA to assess for ischemic stroke or vertebrobasilar insufficiency

Ophthalmic Etiologies of Painless Loss of Vision			
Diagnosis	**Symptoms**	**Exam/Diagnosis**	**Treatment**
Central retinal artery occlusion ("stroke of the eye")	Sudden, profound, painless monocular vision loss	Visual acuity at presentation is predictive of final visual acuity On fundoscopic exam can see pale fundus and a cherry red macula. Also can see an afferent pupillary defect Diagnose etiology of "stroke of eye"	Emergent ophtho and neuro consult, aspirin and oxygen. Goal is to move embolus to periphery using hyperventilation mannitol, acetazolamide, sublingual nitroglycerin and/or ocular massage
Central retinal vein occlusion	Slow, painless vision loss that may be intermittent and incomplete	"Blood and thunder" appearance on fundoscopic exam due to extensive hemorrhages Can also see disc edema, tortious veins, and/or cotton wool spots	Ophtho consult but here are no clear effective treatments
Retinal detachment	Gradual to sudden onset vision loss, floaters, falling curtain sensation or flashes of lights	Direct ophthalmoscope exam shows pale, detached retina or retinal tears Can be diagnosed with US	Urgent ophtho referral within 24hrs for repair within 1-2 days, Emergent consult if central vision is affected
Vitreous Hemorrhage	Sudden monocular vision loss or decreased acuity (floaters, flashing lights) from bleeding into the vitrea. Can be spontaneous or due to trauma	Vision loss is proportional to amount of blood. Can have afferent pupillary defect, loss of red reflex or inability to visualize fundus	Urgent ophthalmologic consult (within 24hrs) for laser photocoagulation
Temporal Arteritis	Gradual to sudden monocular vision loss associated with headache	Temporal tenderness Elevated ESR Temporal biopsy	High dose steroids (see chapter)

MANAGEMENT

- For presumed neurologic etiology:
  - Obtain appropriate imaging and neurologic consult.
  - For ischemic or hemorrhagic CVA (see chapter).
- Causes of painful vision loss include: Corneal ulcer or burn, acute angle glaucoma, optic iritis, uveitis, and endopthalmitis (see red eye chapter).
- Optic neuritis: Acute monocular vision loss from optic nerve inflammation/demyelination that is associated with multiple sclerosis.
  - Vision loss occurs over hours to days. In many cases is a central scotoma but can be any visual field cut. Loss of color and depth perception most pronounced. Associated with pain on extra ocular movement.
  - Diagnosis: Afferent pupillary defect and/or swollen disc on fundoscopic exam. MRI with gadolinium demonstrates optic nerve inflammation.
  - Early ophthalmology and neurology consult, IV steroids (consider methylprednisone 250mg IV).

DISPOSITION

- Admit anyone with unexplained progressive visual loss, neurologic etiology, or anyone with traumatic etiology.
- Patient with transient vision loss should have a TIA workup.
- Discharge home patients with clear diagnosis, resolution of symptoms or no progression while in the ED, no significant comorbidities, and able to follow up with ophthalmology in next 24-48hrs.
- RETURN IF: Vision loss returns, visual acuity gets worse, any pain with eye movement, any focal neurologic deficits, severe headache, or any other new or concerning symptoms.

BEWARE...

⊘ Always check and document visual acuity on any eye complaint, including both eyes individually.

⊘ Closely search for a neurologic or systemic etiology for any binocular visual complaint.

⊘ Recognize and treat acute angle glaucoma, chemical burns, CVA, and central retinal artery occlusion early.

Source

Graves JS1, Galetta SL. Acute visual loss and other neuro-ophthalmologic emergencies: management. *Neurol Clin.* 2012 Feb;30(1):75-99.

3 ▶ Eye Trauma/Red Eye

- Often benign causes but can be the result of many primary ophthalmologic conditions or systemic illnesses.
- Majority of causes are from conjunctivitis, but the goal in the ED is to exclude life- or vision-threatening illness.

Ddx
Traumatic
Inflammatory
Allergic
Infectious
Other

EVALUATION

- **High Yield History:** Key distinctions to make early: Painful or painless? Any visual changes?
  - Ask about associated symptoms such as pain, foreign body sensation, visual changes (complete loss, blurriness, floaters etc.), photophobia, or any discharge. Also ask about systemic symptoms such as headache, fevers, cough, or rhinorrhea.
  - Determine time of onset, any chemical or allergic exposures, contact use, history of trauma, and any metal work or other potential foreign body exposures.
- **Exam:** Perform full eye exam (see quick guide) including visual acuity, pupillary exam, extra-ocular muscles, lid eversion, slit lamp, and IOP.
  - Assess the pattern of redness: Diffuse redness (conjunctivitis) vs. ciliary flush (keratitis, iritis, or acute angle glaucoma) vs. localized redness (pterygium, foreign body, subconjunctival hemorrhage)
  - If discharge is present, is it purulent or clear?
  - Assess for fluorescein uptake on slit lamp exam (corneal abrasion or ulcer).
- **Diagnostics:** Labs are generally not indicated unless thought to be a systemic etiology. Eye exam and slit lamp are the most useful diagnostic tools. Obtain x-ray or CT (head or facial) if concerned about retained foreign body (metal fragment) or traumatic injury.

MANAGEMENT

- Based on suspected etiology (see below)
- Obtain ophthalmologic consult for anyone with visual loss, increased pressures, acute angle closure glaucoma, iritis, herpes keratitis, episcleritis, corneal ulcer, or any major traumatic injury.
- For all diagnoses, patients should stop wearing their contacts until follow up with ophthalmology.
- Eye patches are not indicated for pain, only to protect open globe injuries.
- Full trauma assessment for any significant eye trauma.

Conjunctivitis

Type	Cause	History	Exam	Treatment	Notes
Viral	Usually adenovirus Can last 2-4 weeks	Initially unilateral then bilateral irritation	Minimal watery discharge, tearing, preauricular LAD	Warm compresses, artificial eye drops for comfort	Very contagious Wash hands, avoid sharing towels
Allergic	Allergies	Seasonal itching/burning Usually unilateral	Clear to thick and stringy discharge	Cool compresses Consider vasoconstrictors such as Vasocon, Naphcon A or cromolyn 4% eye drops as well as antihistamines	Eosinophils can be seen on conjunctival smear
Bacterial	H. flu, Strep, Proteus, Staph, Pseudomonas, Gonorrhea, Chlamydia	Purulent discharge	Purulent discharge	Topical antibiotics (trimethoprim/ polymyxin solution/ointment, ciprofloxacin drops for contact lens wearers). Ophtho follow up in 2-3 days if not improving. PO abx for chlamydia. IM/IV abx for gonorrhea	Complications include corneal ulceration Avoid contact lenses

Glaucoma

Diagnosis	Etiology	History	Exam	Management
Open-angle	Decreased absorption of aqueous humor by trabeculae 90% of glaucoma	Bilateral, gradual onset loss of vision	Increased IOP, increased cup:disc ratio	Outpatient ophtho referral
Acute angle closure glaucoma	Narrow angle between iris and cornea preventing aqueous fluid from reaching trabecular network for absorption	May be precipitated by dark room or dilating eye drops, usually unilateral, painful, decreased vision, photophobia, headache, abdominal pain, and vomiting	Unreactive, mid-dilated pupil, increased cup:disc ratio, IOP>20-30 mm Hg, perilimbal injection, hyperemic conjunctiva, and shallow anterior chamber	Ophtho consult, Timolol, pilocarpine, acetazolamide, mannitol, or glycerin Admission, especially if first episode (see chapter)

Painful Red Eye					
Diagnosis	Cause	History	Exam	Management	Notes
Keratitis	Inflammation of the cornea due to UV, contact lens, infection, dry eye, or drugs	Red eye, painful, irritation	Diffuse corneal breakdown shown as dots in areas of fluorescein staining	Depends on etiology. Artificial tears, antibiotics if infection, cycloplegics if severe	Avoid contact lens
Iritis Anterior uveitis Iridocyclitis	Inflammation of the anterior uveal tract (iris, ciliary body, choroid layer) from TB trauma, syphilis, Reiter's, IBD, ankylosing spondylitis or idiopathic	Painful red eye, consensual photophobia (shine light in the asymptomatic eye, get pain in the affected eye), decreased vision that is usually unilateral, no discharge	Miotic pupil, keratotic deposits on posterior aspect of cornea, cell and flare. Ciliary flushing, pain relieved with dilation, worsened with light. Dilate to rule out posterior involvement (disc swelling, retinal hemorrhage or exudates)	Depends on etiology. PPD, VRDL Ophtho consult, topical steroids, cycloplegics Consider rheumatology or infectious disease consult if indicated	Complications include glaucoma, retinal detachment, and iris adherence to cornea or lens
Episcleritis	Inflammation of scleral membrane, mostly idiopathic, but can be infectious or autoimmune	Itching, irritation, sudden onset, mild or no pain, and absence of discharge	Normal vision, conjunctival erythema, mobile nodule, episcleral vessels look like rays of sun from iris	Artificial tears, mild steroid eye drops in consultation with ophtho	Benign
Scleritis	Destructive disease of sclera caused by infections, vasculitis, autoimmune disease IBD, or connective tissue disease	Dull orbital pain, lacrimation, photophobic and decreased vision	Injected sclera, blue-red hue. Non-mobile vessels that fail to blanch with phenylephrine drops	Ophtho consult, NSAIDs, systemic steroids, Labs and CXR to assess for etiology	Chronic condition

Diagnosis	Cause	History	Exam	Management	Notes
Herpes	Herpes simplex or Varicella zoster	Redness, vision loss, flashes, floaters, pain and irritation	Hutchinson's sign, corneal dendrites/ disciform pattern edema or pseudodendrites	Optho consult. Acyclovir + Viroptic drops Q2hrs, IV abx if immunocompromised or intraocular). If varicella, Famvir 500 mg BID	
Corneal ulcer	Viral, bacterial (pseudomonas), fungal, traumatic, contact lens, topical steroid use, rheumatoid arthritis	Erythema of eyelid and conjunctiva, mucopurulent discharge, foreign body sensation, blurry vision, pain, and photophobia	Slit lamp exam with fluorescein uptake. Also corneal erythema, ciliary injection and purulent discharge (obtain culture)	Optho consult if severe or in line of sight or organism unclear. Gentamicin or ciprofloxacin eye drops for bacterial infection Avoid topical steroids Cycloplegics for pain	Complications: perforation, scarring, vision loss, glaucoma, and cataracts

Cellulitis		
Diagnosis	**Signs/Symptoms**	**Treatment**
Preseptal/periorbital (patient is well-appearing)	Infection anterior to orbital septum Normal vision, extraoccular movements intact. Inflamed, edematous, warm and tender eyelids	Augmentin 875mg PO BID x 10days or Clindamycin 450mg PO TID x 5days Warm compresses Consider admission and/or CT orbit if uncertain
Postseptal/ orbital (looks ill/ uncomfortable)	Pain on eye movement, decreased vision and proptosis	CT orbit Admission Antibiotics (Vancomycin AND Unasyn) Surgical drainage

Traumatic Red Eye			
Injuries	**Presentation**	**Diagnosis**	**Treatment**
Corneal foreign body/ Abrasions	Irritation, pain worse with blinking Conjunctival injection Sometime will report foreign body exposure	Tetracaine drops Fluorescein, slit lamp shows darker green under cobalt blue Consider imaging for possibility of intraocular injury	Anesthetize with tetracaine drop and remove metallic foreign body with 25g needle held parallel to cornea Erythromycin topical ointment and close ophtho follow up
Chemical burns	Painfully, blurry vision, blepharospasm, photophobia More severe with alkali burns due to liquefactive necrosis. Mace and tear gas burns are self-limited.	Irrigation with NS until pH~7.4 and recheck Q30mins Slit lamp exam to assess for corneal damage	Ophtho consult Tetracaine drops and cycloplegics for pain Erythromycin topical ointment
Ruptured globe	Periorbital trauma, decreased visual acuity, hyphema, irregular shaped pupil, lens opacity, and severe subconjunctival hemorrhage	Decreased anterior chamber depth Seidel test (fluorescein leakage into the anterior chamber) Do not measure IOP CT orbit	Ophtho consult Eye shield, antibiotics to prevent endophthalmitis, antiemetics, analgesia, leave foreign body alone Sinus precautions: no nose blowing, no straws, and sneeze with closed mouth
Blow out fracture	Blunt trauma to orbit with fracture of orbital floor. Eyelid edema, ecchymosis, diplopia, vertical gaze palsy, and injury to infraorbital nerve	Cranial nerve III, IV, and VI exam CT orbit **Entrapment**: inferior rectus muscle prolapses.	No immediate intervention unless there is entrapment →consult facial surgery Close ophtho follow up for consideration of surgery
Traumatic iritis	Photophobia, blurry vision, and consensual photophobia	See iritis	Prednisolone to prevent synechiae formation (when the iris adheres to the cornea)
Retro-orbital hematoma	Pain, nausea, diplopia, decreased vision, globe displacement, and proptosis	Increased IOP, compromised extra ocular movements, and afferent pupillary deficit	Lateral canthotomy/inferior catholysis
Hyphema	Blood in anterior chamber	Careful exam to rule out other eye injuries	Cycloplegics (cyclopentolate 0.5%) Admission to monitor for rebleeding (often in 3-5 days after injury) or close follow up

- **Medications:** Lubricating eye drops are available over the counter. Steroid drops should only be used with ophtho consult.
  - Antibiotics for bacterial conjunctivitis, corneal abrasions/ulcers, or infectious keratitis. Contact wearers need pseudomonas coverage.
    - For non-contact lens wearers, Erythromycin 0.5% ointment Q3-6hrs, polytrim drops 4x/day.
      - Corneal ulcer: Ciprofloxacin 0.3% 1-2 drops Q1-2hrs, ofloxacin 0.3% 1-2 drops Q1-2hrs or polytrim drops 4x/day.
    - For contact lens wearers: Tobramycin, ofloxacin or ciprofloxacin for both abrasions or ulcers.
  - Cycloplegics for pain control in iritis or keratitis: i.e. atropine 1% 1-2 drops prn or tropicamide 0.5% 1-2 drops prn

DISPOSITION

- Admission indicated for first-time acute angle closure glaucoma, open globe injuries, retrobulbar hematoma, or large corneal ulcers.
- Many patients can be discharged home with close (1-2 day) ophthalmology follow up.
- RETURN IF: Any visual changes, severe pain, worsening symptoms, symptoms not improving, or any other concerning symptoms.

BEWARE...

- ⚠ Always obtain a full eye exam, especially visual acuity and slit lamp exam.
- ⚠ Do not obtain an intraocular pressure if there is concern for globe rupture.
- ⚠ Lateral canthotomy/inferior cantholysis is an uncommon but vision-saving procedure. All ED providers should be familiar with the technique.

Sources

Mahmood AR, Narang AT. Diagnosis and management of the acute red eye. *Emerg Med Clin North Am.* 2008;26(1):35-55, vi.

Zane RD, Kosowsky JM, et al. Pocket Emergency Medicine. 2nd ed. Philadelphia, PA: Lippincott Williams & Wilkins; 2011.

Ma OJ, Cline D, Tintinalli J, et al. Emergency Medicine Manual. 6th ed. New York, NY: McGraw-Hill Professional; 2003.

Marx J, Hockberger R, Walls R. Rosen's Emergency Medicine: Concepts & Clinical Practice. 5th ed. Maryland Heights, MO: Mosby; 2002.

Hans L, Mawji Y. The ABCs of Emergency Medicine. 12th edition. Toronto, Canada: University of Toronto; 2012.

Medscape News & Perspective. New York, NY: http://emedicine.medscape.com.

4 ▶ Acute Angle Glaucoma

- Optic neuropathy caused by increased intraocular pressure (IOP) from narrowing or closure of the anterior angle channel occluding the flow of aqueous humor from the anterior chamber

- Classic presentation is a patient who presents with sudden onset of painful vision loss upon entering a bright room after spending time in a dark environment (i.e. the movie theater).

Ddx
Conjunctivitis
Temporal arteritis
Retinal detachment
Iritis or Uveitis
Corneal abrasion
Ocular Migraine

EVALUATION

- **High Yield History:** The rapid onset of IOP results in abrupt onset severe eye pain, decreased visual acuity with blurred vision and halos, frontal headache (may be chief complaint), nausea, and vomiting
  — Risk factors include farsightedness, female sex, age >50yo, and family history
  — Medication precipitants include midriatics, anticholinergics, sympathomimetics, topiramate, TCA, antipsychotics, antihistamines. May also be precipitated by rapid change in ambient light and emotional triggers.

- **Exam:** Common findings include conjunctival injection with ciliary flush, cloudy cornea, mid-dilated sluggish/fixed pupil, decreased visual acuity, and elevated IOP (rises rapidly, but anything > 20 is diagnostic, particularly if only in affected side).
  — Perform full eye exam including visual acuity, tonometry, and slit lamp exam.

- **Diagnostics:** This diagnosis is made by history and measurement of IOP. Normal IOP 10-20mmHg.
  — Calibrate Tono-pen or other device based on instructions, and anesthetize the eye with anesthetic drop such as proparacaine.
  — Place patient in seated or supine position and have him/her fix gaze on something.
  — Touch to pen to central cornea lightly and briefly several times. Will hear chirp each time there is a measurement.
  — Machine beeps once for valid readings. Average measurement will appear on LCD.

MANAGEMENT

- This is an ophthalmologic emergency! Goal is to reduce the intraocular pressure as quickly as possible.
- Immediate ophthalmologic consultation and treatment with topical medications
- If visual acuity is markedly reduced use both topical and IV therapies.
- IOP<50 without significant loss of visual acuity can start with topical only. Topical beta-blockers are first-line agents.
- Treat until pressure decreases and pain resolves. If no resolution of symptoms with medications, will need laser iridotomy with ophthalmology.

Topical		
Medication	**Mechanism of Action**	**Dose**
Timolol 0.5% top	Beta-blocker, decreases aqueous humor production	1 drop Q30min
Apraclonidine 1% top	Alpha2-agonist, decreases aqueous humor production	1 drop x 1
Pilocarpine 1-2% top	Constricts pupil and moves iris away, opening up channel	1 drop Q15min x 2
Prednisolone acetate 1% top	Corticosteroid, reduces inflammation	1 drop Q15min x 4
Systemic		
Mannitol	Hyperosmotic agent, decreased aqueous humor	1-3 mg/kg IV over 45 min
Acetazolamide	Inhibits aqueous humor secretion	250-500 mg IV

DISPOSITION

- Most patients will be admitted for observation, especially those with severe pain, those who received IV medications, and those who do not have complete resolution of their symptoms or elevated pressures.

- Consider discharge home with close (<24hrs) ophthalmology follow up for patients with initial minor presentation and complete resolution of symptoms.

- Majority of patients will ultimately require peripheral laser iridotomy to prevent recurrence.

- RETURN IF: You develop any changes in vision, severe pain, and headaches or have any lightheadedness/pass-out (side effects of topical medications). Avoid any antihistamines or decongestants.

BEWARE...

(!) This is a true ophthalmologic emergency. Always consider measuring IOP in patients presenting with an acute onset headache.

Section IX.
Environmental
Complaints

1 ▶ Toxicology Quick Guide

- ALWAYS: IV, O2, Monitor, COMPLETE VS, EKG (arrhythmias or specific patterns consistent with toxic ingestion), point-of-care glucose, airway equipment nearby if needed.
- Can't-miss diagnoses: Acetaminophen, TCA, calcium channel blockers, aspirin, and lead.

EVALUATION

- **High Yield History:** Determine which drugs were taken and what dose, formulation (i.e. extended release), and total amount. What time did the ingestion occur? Was anything else taken, and what else did the patient have access to? Use family, friends, EMS, and call their pharmacy. Finally, why were they taken: recreationally or as a suicide attempt?

Toxins by Smell	
Garlic	Arsenic, Organophosphates, dimethyl sulfoxide (DMSO)
Bitter almonds	Cyanide
Pears	Chloral hydrate
Gasoline	Hydrocarbons
Fruity	Isopropanol,paraldehyde, chloroform, nitrates, nitriles, alcoholic ketoacidosis
Wintergreen	Methyl salicylates, methanol
Rotten eggs	Hydrogen sulfide, disulfiram, N-acetylcysteine (NAC)
Ammonia	Ammonia
Vinegar	Acetic acid, hydrofluoric acid
Mothballs	Napthalene, camphor
Pepper	o-chlorobenzylidene, (tear gas)

- **Vital Signs:**
  - **Bradycardia** (clonidine, calcium channel blocker, beta blocker, digoxin, opiates)
  - **Tachycardia** (anticholinergics, antihistamines, amphetamine, theophylline and sympathomimetics)
  - **Hypotension** (clonidine, calcium channel blocker, beta blocker, opioids, ethanol, sedative hypnotics)

- **Hypertension**: (sympathomimetics, anticholinergics)
- **Hyperthermia**: (anticholinergics, sympathomimetics, salicylates, NMS, serotonin syndrome)
- **Hypothermia**: (opiates, ethanol, oral hypoglycemic)
- **Exam:** Assess for level of consciousness, skin flushing, diaphoresis, and any pathognomonic odors.
  - Full neurologic exam to assess for cerebellar signs, reflexes, and tone
  - Eye exam for pupil reactivity and size, disconjugate gaze, and any nystagmus (note if horizontal or vertical)
  - Any signs of track marks or nose bleeds to suggest means of ingestion
- **Initial Workup:**
  - Labs: These patients can be unreliable historians. Have low threshold to obtain lab data including CBC, BMP, Ca^{2+}, Mg, LFTs, coags, lactate, VBG, serum osmolarity, acetaminophen and aspirin level, UA, HCG. Though they are usually of low utility, consider also serum and urine tox to screen for co-ingestions. For specific exposures consider drug levels such as digoxin.
  - EKG: An EKG should be obtained early! Assess for interval changes (widened QRS or prolonged QTc), specific morphology changes (digoxin or TCA), AV nodal blockage (calcium channel blockers or beta blockers)
  - Imaging: Iron, other heavy metals, some extended release formulations can be seen on x-ray

Toxidromes		
Category	**Agents**	**Exam**
Anticholinergic	Antihistamines, atropine, TCAs, antispasmotics, antipsychotics	Hot as a hare (hyperthermia), red as a beet (flushed skin), dry as a bone (NO diaphoresis), blind as a bat (mydriasis), mad as a hatter (delirium). Can also see tachycardia, hypertension, ataxia, and urinary retention.
Cholinergic	Organophosphates, pesticides, nerve agents	SLUDGEM: Salivation, lacrimation, urination, diarrhea, diaphoresis, GI upset, emesis, miosis. Also bronchorrhea, bradycardia, respiratory failure, and seizures
Sympathomimetic	Cocaine, amphetamines	Psychomotor agitation, diaphoresis, mydriasis, piloerrection, tachycardia, hypertension, hyperthermia, seizures
Sedative hypnotic	Benzos, barbiturates, GHB	Confusion, delirium, somnolence, diplopia, hallucinations, nystagmus, apnea, ataxia
Opioid	Heroin, methadone, oxycodone	Miosis, hypoventilation, bradycardia, hypotension, somnolence
Serotonin syndrome	SSRIs and MAOIs	AMS (agitation or stupor), hyperthermia, hypertension or hypotension, tachycardia or bradycardia, skin flushing, diaphoresis, mydriasis, myoclonus, nystagmus, hyperreflexia
Neuroleptic Malignant syndrome (NMS)	Antipsychotics (haldolperidol, promethazine), levodopa, metoclopramide	AMS (agitation or stupor), hyperthermia, hypertension or hypotension, tachycardia or bradycardia, skin flushing, diaphoresis, mydriasis, bradykinesia, and extrapyramidal rigidity

DECONTAMINATION

- **External:** First, protect yourself and other staff. Must remove any source of persistent exposure: remove patient's clothes and provide copious irrigation with water or NS if skin, eye, or mucus membranes were exposed. Irrigate and check pH frequently.

- **Internal:** There is little evidence for bowel decontamination. If going to use, the patient must be fully awake or intubated with NGT in place.

  — Activated charcoal: Potentially useful for certain ingestions if given within one hour of ingestion. Dosed as 1gm/kg or 10:1 ratio of charcoal to poison. Not useful for: lithium, iron, alcohols, lead, hydrocarbons, or caustics. Can cause nausea, vomiting, and pneumonitis if aspirated.

  — Cathartics: Used in conjunction with activated charcoal to increase GI transit time and decreased absorption. Should not be given without activated charcoal. No clear benefit but possible harm; infrequently used.

  — Whole bowel irrigation: Used for toxins that are not absorbed by charcoal (ie, lithium, iron, alcohols, lead, hydrocarbons, or caustics). Can place NGT and give polyethylene glycol until stool is clear. Do not use in patents with ileus or obstruction.

Antidotes	
Acetaminophen	N-acetylcysteine (NAC)
Anticholinergics	Physostigmine
Arsenic	Dimercaprol/ BAL
Beta blockers	Glucagon, high-dose euglycemic therapy
Benzodiazepine	Flumazenil
Calcium channel blocker	Calcium, high-dose euglycemic therapy
Cholinergics	Pralidoxime (2-PAM) and atropine
Copper	Penicillamine
Cyanide	Thiosulfate, hydrocobalamin
Digoxin	Digoxin specific immune Fab fragments
Ehylene glycol	Fomepizole
Glypizide	Glucose, octreotide
Heparin	Protamine
Hydrofluoric acid	Calcium
Iron	Deferoxamine
Isoniazid	Pyridoxime
Lead	Dimercaprol
Lidocaine	Sodium bicarbonate, intralipid
Magnesium	Calcium
MAOIs or SSRI	Cyproheptadine or Bezos for serotonin syndrome
Methemoglobinemia	Methylene blue
Methotrexate	Folic acid, leucovorin
Mercury	Dimercaprol (BAL), EDTA or DMSA
Opiods	Naloxone
TCA	Sodium bicarbonate
Warfarin	Vitamin K

- **Indications for hemodialysis:** Potentially useful for agents that have a large volume of distribution or are protein bound i.e. lithium, methanol, ethylene glycol, or salicylates.

BEWARE...

- ⚠ Toxidromes are most useful in the setting of a single drug overdose, but the clinical picture may be clouded in the setting of polyingestion.
- ⚠ The presence of sweating is what differentiations sympathomimetics and anticholinergic.
- ⚠ If multiple patients present with similar toxidromes, or if seen in patients during a mass causality incident, always consider chemical attack.
- ⚠ Always consider causes of altered mental status in the setting of vital signs abnormalities.
- ⚠ Always consider concurrent tox ingestion in patients presenting with a traumatic suicide attempt.

Source

Flomenbaum N, et al. Goldfrank's Toxicology Emergencies (8th edition). McGraw-Hill Professional. 2006.

Notes

2 ▶ Acetaminophen Toxicity

PHARMACOKINETICS/MECHANISM OF TOXICITY

- Rapidly and completely absorbed from GI tract (peak serum levels within 4 hrs in immediate release, slower with co-ingestions like anticholinergics or opioids as in some sources of acetaminophen)
- Elimination half-life is 4hrs in therapeutic doses.
- Normal metabolism: Majority sulfated or glucuronidated, small amount oxidized via cytochrome P450 system into a toxic, highly reactive, electrophilic intermediate, N-acetyl-p-benzoquinoneimine (NAPQI) which is then detoxified by glutathione.
- Overdose: Normal metabolism saturated and more acetaminophen is shunted down the P450 pathway.
- Once 70% of glutathione has been depleted, NAPQI reacts with local cells, causing irreversible injury and hepatocellular necrosis.
- Can lead to hepatic toxicity, renal toxicity, spontaneous abortion, and fetal death in pregnancy.

Sources of Acetaminophen
Tylenol
Paracetamol
Panadol
Liquiprin
Excedrin ES
Lorcet
Norco
NyQuil
Percocet
Vicodin
Unisom Dual Relief
Sominex 2
Tylenol #3,
Vicks Formula 44-D
and MANY more…

EVALUATION

- "Stages" of acetaminophen poisoning are outdated and rarely referred to clinically.

  — Early (<24 hrs) after acute ingestion: Nausea, vomiting, diaphoresis, pallor, lethargy, and malaise. Many pts are asymptomatic in this phase.

  — 24 to 72 hrs: This is when pts become "sick." Transaminitis, prothrombin time, and bilirubin levels rise. Of patients that develop hepatic injury, >50% will demonstrate aminotransferase elevation within 24 hrs, and ALL have elevations by 36 hrs. On exam may have RUQ pain and tenderness.

  — 72 to 96 hrs: "Live or die"– Systemic symptoms re-appear with jaundice, encephalopathy, severe transaminitis, synthetic function defects, hyperbilirubinemia, and cardiomyopathy. Acute renal failure occurs in 25-50%. Patients who reach this state may require emergent liver transplant. Death most commonly from cerebral edema, hemorrhage, ARDS, sepsis, and multisystem organ failure.

  — >96 hrs: Recovery if the patient survives. Begins at 4 days and takes up to 3 months, usually 7-14 days.

- **Diagnostics:**

  — Labs: POC glucose, BMP, LFTs, coags. HCG, serum. and urine tox. Consider pH, lactate, phos for risk-stratification.

    ▪ Obtain a 4-hour post-acute-ingestion level and use the modified Rumack-Matthews nomogram to determine need for treatment. Patients with a serum acetaminophen level >150mcg/mL at 4hrs are at risk for liver injury.

- In patients without timing of ingestion, it is safest to assume the initial serum level is the 4hr level.
- Repeat level in 4 hrs if extended release prep or delayed ingestion.
— Nomogram is NOT useful in chronic/repeated/multiple ingestions. Also limited usefulness if ingestions involve sustained-release acetaminophen or combos with opioids or anticholinergics, which may slow intestinal motility/absorption.
— EKG: As part of general toxicology work up
— Head CT: If patient presents with AMS and suspect trauma or late-stage cerebral edema

MANAGEMENT

- If safe to do so, administer activated charcoal in first 2-4hrs after ingestion for GI decontamination.
- N-acetylcysteine (NAC) is antidote. It replenishes hepatic glutathione allowing for detoxification of NAPQI.
- Best if given within 8 hrs, but never delay treatment if suspect potentially toxic ingestion!
  — Start ASAP in "late-presenters." Dosing can be done over different time periods and can be given PO or IV. Sample regimen:
  — IV 150mg/kg over 1 hour, then infuse 12.5mg/kg/hr x 4 hrs, then 6.25 mg/kg/hr x 16 hrs
- PO 140mg/kg x1, then 70mg/kg q4h x 17 doses
- Note that the IV formulation can result in an anaphylactoid reaction. The oral formulation is associated with nausea and vomiting.
- If this was a suicide attempt, also look for and treat any coingestions and consult psychiatry.

DISPOSITION

- All patients with suspected acetaminophen overdose should be admitted.

BEWARE...

ⓘ When in doubt, start NAC Remember: 150 is the magic number with acetaminophen poisoning: 150 mg/kg = potentially toxic ingestion, 150 mcg/mL at 4 hrs potentially toxic level, 150 mg/kg = loading dose of IV NAC

Source

An Evidence-Based Approach to Acetaminophen (Paracetamol, APAP) Overdose. *Emergency Medicine Practice*. Sept 2010;12(9).

Notes

3 ▶ Salicylate Toxicity

PHARMACOKINETICS

- Notorious for erratic absorption and metabolism, so DO NOT be falsely reassured by time from ingestion or quantitative serum level (half life in non-toxic ingestions is 2-5 hrs).

- Absorbed from stomach/small intestine and eliminated by hepatic metabolism (and renal metabolism during overdose)

- Acute ingestion of 150mg/kg is toxic; severe intoxication likely after >300mg/kg.

Sources of salicylates
Aspirin (acetylsalicylic acid, ASA),
Topical keratolytics (salicylic acid)
Topical analgesics (methyl salicylate)
Oil of wintergreen (methyl salicylate)
Certain antacids (bismuth subsalicylate)
Yew bark and other herbal medications

MECHANISM OF TOXICITY

- CNS stimulation:
    - Stimulation of respiratory center leads to hyperventilation and respiratory alkalosis.
    - Stimulation of chemoreceptor trigger zone causes nausea and vomiting.
    - Tinnitus
- Interference with cellular metabolism (Krebs cycle, oxidative phosphorylation)
    - Metabolic acidosis
    - Hyperthermia
- Inhibition of cyclooxygenase (decreases synthesis of prostaglandins, prostacyclin, and thromboxanes) leads to:
    - Platelet dysfunction
    - Gastric mucosal injury
- Cerebral and pulmonary edemas (by mechanisms unknown) are the deadly effects of salicylates.

EVALUATION

- **High Yield History/Exam:** Patients can present with an acute or chronic toxicity. If acute always attempt to determine exact quantity taken, through collateral information or pill bottles, and assess for possible coingestions.
    - Acute: Signs and symptoms include nausea, vomiting, hyperpnea, tinnitus, and lethargy
        - Mixed acid base disturbance (respiratory alkalosis and metabolic acidosis) may result in normal-ish pH
        - If severe: hyperthermia, pulmonary edema, hypoglycemia, seizure, coma, death
    - Chronic: Signs and symptoms include confusion, dehydration, acidosis, cerebral and pulmonary edema
        - Think of the elderly/demented patient who is chronically taking aspirin for pain for their CAD.
        - There is usually no clear history of ingestion but suspect in any patient who is on aspirin-containing prescribed or over-the-counter medications.

- **Diagnostics**
  - Labs: Check a full panel including FSGS, BMP, coags, ABG, HCG, and urine tox. Do not be reassured by a normal Anion Gap, as chloride levels are falsely elevated in severe toxicity.
  - Salicylate levels:
    - 10 to 30 mg/dL is therapeutic, >40 mg/dL is toxic, >100 mg/dL is severe (NOTE: Different labs use different units, so convert if necessary.)
    - Single levels are NEVER sufficient in salicylate poisoning due to 1) erratic pharmacokinetics, 2) potential for bezoar formation, 3) rapid diffusion between blood and CSF.
    - We don't really *care* about the serum level; it is a *proxy* for the CSF level (harder to obtain).
  - EKG: As part of toxicology evaluation and to assess for coingestions.

MANAGEMENT

- Airway: Sedation and frequent vomiting often put the airway in danger; however, be aware that intubation is high risk for these patients.
  - Patients need to hyperventilate to blow off CO_2 to maintain pH. ACMT suggests giving a bolus of IV sodium bicarbonate when intubating "in a sufficient quantity to maintain a blood pH of 7.45-7.50 during intubation;" however, there is no evidence to support this maneuver.
- Circulation: These patients universally present severely hypovolemic (4-6L dry) due to vomiting, hyperventilation, sodium loss, hyperthermia, and diaphoresis.
  - Hypovolemia impairs elimination of salicylate due to decreased renal and hepatic circulation.
  - An ideal indication for bedside ultrasound! Evaluate that IVC!
  - Place a Foley for UOP monitoring.
- Alkalinize *the blood* (the urine is a secondary bonus).
  - Alkalemic blood pH limits an increase in CNS salicylate concentration, so aim for pH of 7.5 or higher.
  - 2 amps/100meq $NaHCO_3$, followed by D5W with 150meq $NaHCO_3$/L at 200-250 mL/hr titrate to goal pH
- Decontamination and elimination:
  - Charcoal: Data from human volunteers and animal models suggest this improves salicylate clearance, but no evidence suggests this action improves clinical outcome (charcoal never part of standard of care, always weigh with risk of aspiration).
  - Hemodialysis indications: Serum level >100mg/dL (1000 mg/L at MGH), acidosis refractory to bicarb or limited by volume overload, pulmonary or cerebral edema, seizure, coma, AMS, or other signs of severe poisoning (consult renal early; you never know when patient may crash)

- Monitoring
  — Salicylate levels, ABG, K levels required every 2hrs until patient consistently improving.
  — Beware the decreasing salicylate level! Small decreases in blood pH can lead to large shifts of drug into CNS, so a decreasing level is only good if mental status is improving at the same time.
  — IV potassium repletion is critical to avoid paradoxical aciduria.

DISPOSITION

- All patients with true salicylate toxicity should be admitted.

Source
Pearlman BL, Gambhir R. Salicylate intoxication: a clinical review. *Postgrad Med.* 2009;121(4):162-8.

Notes

4 ▶ Digoxin Toxicity

PHARMACOKINETICS/MECHANISM OF TOXICITY

- Digoxin inhibits Na/K ATPase pump in cardiac cells increasing inotropy and automaticity while decreasing the depolarization period. This results in a slower SA/AV conduction and increased vagal tone. Commonly used for Afib, a-flutter, atrial tachycardia, and CHF.
- Patients can develop hyperkalemia with acute ingestions and hypokalemia with chronic toxicity leading to life-threatening arrhythmias.
- Digoxin has a large volume of distribution and half-life of approximately 15-20hrs. It is renally cleared.

EVALUATION

- **High Yield History:** Symptoms include visual disturbances (yellow vision/halos are specific but not sensitive), vague symptoms (weakness, weight loss, fatigue, nausea, vomiting, abdominal pain), and neuropsychiatric symptoms (hallucinations, confusion, seizures, delirium).
  - Acute toxicity – Cardiac symptoms predominate
  - Chronic toxicity – Noncardiac symptoms predominate
  - Determine amount taken (>10mg is fatal), timing (serum level should be measured at least 6hrs after ingestion), and if ingestion was intentional.
  - Obtain full review of symptoms and past medical history. Renal failure and infection can increase serum levels and result in toxicity. Medications such as verapamil, quinidine, amlodipine, amiodarone can increase levels.

Ddx
Beta blocker/Calcium channel blocker toxicity
Nicotine
Antipsychotic
MI
Herbal Supplements
CHF
Antihistamine
CHF
TCA
Myo/pericarditis
Clonidine
TCA
Electrolyte abnormality
Thyroid disturbance

- **Exam:** Patients can present with tachycardia or bradycardia, hypotension, and altered mental status.

- **Diagnostics:**
  - Labs: BMP, Ca/Mg/Phos. Hypokalemia and hypomagnesemia can sensitize myocardium.
  - Acute: Digoxin level 6hr post-ingestion. Chronic: Digoxin level immediately. Although therapeutic at 0.5 – 2.0; pts can be toxic in normal range.
  - EKG and continuous monitor! Watch for high-grade AV block, refractory VT, VF, and hyperkalemia.
    - 4 typical **EKG findings**: T-wave changes; short QT; scooping of ST ("hockey stick");↑U-wave amplitude
    - Can cause virtually any arrhythmia, but PVCs most common.

MANAGEMENT

- Continuous telemetry

- GI decontamination can be considered with charcoal for acute ingestions within 1-2 hrs. (rarely done)

- Medication:

    — Digoxin immune FAB: Acute: 10 vials (a repeat 10-vial dose if necessary); chronic: 1-2 vials (repeat if needed).

    Indications for Digifab / Digibind

    - AMS attributed to dig tox
    - Ingestion of >10 mg of dig
    - Acute OD with serum steady-state level >10 ng/mL
    - Chronic toxicity with serum SS level >6 ng/mL
    - K > 5.5 with acute OD
    - Hemodynamic instability
    - Life-threatening brady/tachy dysrhythmias
    - Toxicity with nondig cardioactive steroids (i.e. plant or animal)

    - Effect within 30-120min.

    - A single vial binds 0.5 mg of digoxin. Above is empiric treatment. If known amount, calculate # of vials needed.

    - Lab test measures total digoxin, including amount bound to Fab. Further therapy should rely on clinical status and not serum levels, which are no longer useful. Note that Fab is renally excreted.

    — Atropine (0.5-1 mg) for bradydysrhythmias.

    — Magnesium for VT/VF (while awaiting digoxin immune FAB!)

    — Beware of pacing and cardioversion, which can cause VT/VF due to cardiac cell irritation.

    — Theoretically should avoid Ca^{2+} administration for hyperkalemia (impaired intracellular K pumping so cells are hypercalcemic).

DISPOSITION

- Admit to a step-down unit, ICU, or cardiac care unit.

BEWARE...

(!) Administer DigiFab early in unstable patient.

(!) Look for subtle signs of chronic toxicity.

Source

Palatnick W, Jelic T. Emergency Department Management of Calcium-Chanel Blocker, Beta Blocker, and Digoxin Toxicity. *Emergency Medicine Practice*. 2014;16:2.

Notes

5 ▶ Opioid Overdose

PHARMACOKINETICS/MECHANISM OF TOXICITY

- All opioids undergo hepatic metabolism and renal elimination.
- Stimulation of opioid receptors results in sedation and respiratory depression.

Routes of Administration	Findings in Overdose	Findings in Withdrawal
Oral: Ask EMS about pills **Parenteral**: Track marks? **Nasal** **Rectal** **Buccal**: Look under tongue **Pulmonary** **Transdermal**: Look for fentanyl patches	Respiratory depression Miosis Stupor Absent or hypoactive bowel sounds Hypothermia Hepatic injury (due to Tylenol or hypoxemia) Prolonged down time →rhabdomyolysis and/or compartment syndrome	Restlessness/agitation/anxiety Dysphoria/drug craving Mydriasis Nausea/vomiting Diarrhea/abdominal cramps Myalgias Piloerection Yawning Lacrimation/rhinorrhea Diaphoresis

- Meperidine and normeperidine (toxic metabolite) have prolonged half-life in patients with cirrhosis and renal insufficiency and can lead to seizures.

EVALUATION

- **High Yield History:** Determine what opiate caused the overdose (long vs. short half-life) and amount taken. Was there a coingestion of other drugs (i.e. Tylenol in Percocet/Vicodin, alcohol), and was this a suicide attempt?
  - It is important to know if EMS or bystanders gave naloxone. Also, did anyone witness traumatic injury, and any concern for aspiration?
- **Exam:** Common physical findings include hypotension, bradycardia, decreased respiratory rate, hypoxia, and miosis.
  - Look for signs of other ingestions, any signs of trauma, or any complications of IVDU. (ie, cardiac murmurs from endocarditis or abscess)
- **Diagnostics:** If patient endorses opiate use, did not have prolonged down time and no persistent hypoxia, labs are not generally indicated. Otherwise consider CBC, BMP, LFTs, CK, basic serum tox, urine analysis, urine HCG, urine tox, EKG, and CXR is concerned about aspiration.

MANAGEMENT

- **ABCs:** Support ventilation with BVM. Place on end-tidal CO_2 monitor. Use caution when administering supplemental oxygen, as this may lead to normal pulse oximetry but will mask hypoventilation and rising CO_2.
- **Naloxone:** Duration of effect is variable and may last as little as 30mins or up to 2hrs. Therefore, if overdose on long-acting opiate then repeat doses or establish a drip→ Dose drip at two-thirds of the effective initial dose per hour.

- — Do not give naloxone if patient is maintaining adequate ventilation, as it can precipitate withdrawal.
- — Initial adult dose: **0.4mg IV**; initial pediatric dose 0.1mg/kg (max 2mg). If no effect escalate dose Q2-3 minutes until increase in respiratory rate occurs (2mg →4mg→ 10mg→ 15mg)
- — In a code or peri-code situation start with 2mg IV naloxone
- Management of opiate withdrawal:
  - — Clonidine: central alpha$_2$-agonist: suppresses sympathetic hyperactivity and shorten withdrawal duration→**initial dose 0.1mg PO**. You can repeat dose every 30-60 minutes. Hypotension may limit the treatment so monitor BP closely.

Opiate	Half-life (T ½)
Heroin	30 minutes
Morphine	2-3 hrs (PO, IV, IM)
Hydromorphone	2-3 hrs
Oxycodone	2-3 hrs
Meperidine	2-3 hrs
Hydrocodone	3.8-6 hrs
Fentanyl	20 minutes IV, 7 hrs transderm
Methadone	15-60 hrs
Buprenorphine	20-70 hrs

DISPOSITION

- Patients who did not receive naloxone with EMS and can give a reassuring history can usually be discharged without further intervention.
- If naloxone given and monitored for 4-6 hrs and no additional naloxone needed, the patient is back to baseline health, and no concern for intentional self-harm, then they can be discharged.
- If concern for intentional self-harm or other psychiatric condition, then medically clear patient and collaborate with psychiatry.
- Patients requiring 2 or more doses of naloxone in ED or if coingestion that also causes somnolence generally require admission.
- Patients on a naloxone drip due to ingestion of long-acting opioid generally require admission to the ICU.
- RETURN IF: You have any fevers, shortness of breath, severe back pain, focal weakness, or numbness.

BEWARE...

(!) Always consider concurrent acetaminophen overdose in patients with opioid overdose.

Source

Boyer EW. Management of opioid analgesic overdose. *N Engl J Med*. 2012;367:146-155.

Marx J, Hockberger R, Walls R. Rosen's Emergency Medicine: Concepts & Clinical Practice, 7th ed. Maryland Heights, MO: Moslay Elsevier.

6 ▶ Tricyclic Antidepressant Toxicity

PHARMACOKINETICS/MECHANISM OF TOXICITY

- Medications for depression, migraines, obsessive-compulsive disease, panic disorder (most names end in –line, -mine, or –pine, with exception of doxepin)
- Very long elimination half-lives (8 to >50hrs)
  — Highly lipophilic; protein bound with large volume of distribution.
  — Enterohepatic circulation after hepatic metabolism may further prolong effects.
  — Anticholinergic effects may lead to delayed or prolonged absorption from the GI tract.
- Narrow therapeutic indices (less than 10x the therapeutic dose may produce toxicity, 10mg/kg for a potentially life-threatening ingestion)

There are SEVEN mechanisms of TCAs, each with specific clinical effect	
Mechanism	**Effect**
Presynaptic neurotransmitter reuptake inhibition (norepinephrine and serotonin)	Makes you happier (in therapeutic doses)
Na+ Channel influx blockade (AKA Class IA antiarrhythmic)	QRS duration prolonged, (right) bundle branch blockade / Intraventricular conduction delay, dysrhythmias (VT, VF)
Slow K+ Channel efflux blockade	QTc prolongation→ Torsades de Pointes is rare
Muscarinic acetylcholine receptor blockade (aka anticholinergic)	Tachycardia, mydriasis, decreased sweating, hyperthermia, flushing, ileus and urinary retention
Histaminic (H1) blockade	Sedation OR Stimulation
Non-specific Alpha receptor blockade	Hypertension possible, followed by hypotension
GABA receptor blockade	Seizures, status epilepticus

EVALUATION

- **High Yield History and Exam:** Presentation is a variable combination of antimuscarinic, cardiovascular, and/or CNS toxidromes. As with all overdoses attempt to confirm amount taken, which formulation, and any other ingestions.
  — Antimuscarinic:
    - "Mad Hatter Syndrome": Tachycardia, mydriasis, decreased sweating, hyperthermia, flushing, ileus, urinary retention, and delirium
  — Cardiovascular: Sinus tachycardia with prolongation of PR, QRS, and/or QTc
    - Variable intraventricular conduction delay and AV block
    - QRS duration >120msec predicts severe neurologic and cardiovascular effects
    - R' in aVR is a sensitive and specific measure of toxicity
    - VT and VF may occur (and should NOT be treated with Class I antiarrhythmics)
    - Hypotension and pulmonary edema are common

— CNS: Variable delirium (antimuscarinic effect) to obtundation or coma (antihistaminic effects)

- Seizure and status may occur (resulting in brain damage, rhabdomyolysis, hyperthermia, multisystem organ failure, and death)

- **Diagnostics**
  — Clinical diagnosis! (AMS/seizures plus tachycardia and any of above EKG changes)
  — Check full panel of electrolytes, FSBS, CPK, ABG, and CXR.

MANAGEMENT

- Airway/Breathing: Intubate if needed for airway protection
- Circulation
  — Sodium bicarbonate to overcome arrhythmia
    - Bolus 100 mEq for QRS over 100, repeat q5min until QRS narrows (also indicated if R' in avR over 3mm)
    - Once QRS below 100, start drip (150mEq/1L of d5W, infusing at 150/hr) until goal pH 7.45 to 7.55
    - If pH target in range and QRS still prolonged, there is some evidence for benefit of lidocaine (1.5mg/kg)
  — BP support
    - Start with IV fluid – fill the tank to get ready for them to bottom out.
    - May need to add pressors (neosynephrine or norepinephrine preferred to overcome alpha blockade).
    - Consider hypertonic (3%) saline to saturate Na channels.
- Decontamination and Elimination
  — IV intralipid (may sequester lipophilic drug away from heart/brain where it causes the most damage)
    - Central administration preferred
    - 1ml/kg to 1.5ml/kg bolus Q3-5 min to a total of 3ml/kg
    - IV drip started at 0.25ml/kg/min - 0.5ml/kg/min for 1hour (or until max dose of 8ml/kg delivered)
  — Wondering if charcoal will work? No evidence to support it will, but always worth consideration if presents within 1hr of ingestion and airway is secure (Note: Always weigh with risk of aspiration, and remember it is NEVER standard of care).
- Treat seizures with GABA-agonists (benzodiazepines and barbiturates).
  — Consider barbiturate loading and propofol infusion for status epilepticus.
  — If pt is in status epilepticus despite GABA agents, paralyze the patient with a long-acting neuromuscular blocker while continuing treatment to prevent rhabdomyolysis/hyperthermia (remember pt may still be seizing and an EEG will be required).

DISPOSITION

- All patients with confirmed or suspected TCA overdose should be admitted and monitored on telemetry.

BEWARE...

- ⓘ Do NOT give sodium channel blockers: caution with lidocaine (as first line), NO phenytoin loading, etc.
- ⓘ Do NOT give physostigmine for anticholinergic toxidrome; it may cause asystole in TCA overdose.

Notes

7 ▶ Hyperthermia

- Core body temp > 37.5 °C due to failure of thermoregulation (NOT fever due to infection and cytokine activation)
- Presentation ranges from dehydration and electrolyte derangements to multiorgan failure

ETIOLOGIES				
Heat Stroke	Neuroleptic Malignant Syndrome	CNS	Toxic	Metabolic
Non exertional (old people who can't thermoregulate) **Exertional** (young athletes)	Reaction to dopamine blockade – lead pipe rigidity, AMS, choreoathetosis, autonomic disarray	Hypothalamic stroke Cerebral hemorrhage Status epilepticus Encephalitis/ Meningitis/ Brain abscess	Salicylate, Lithium, Anticholinergic, Sympathomimetic agents, Serotonin Syndrome	Thyroid storm Pheochromocytoma

EVALUATION

- **High Yield History:** Presentation varies by etiology and ranges from anhidrosis to profuse sweating and CNS dysfunction ranging from confusion to coma.
  - Patients may complain of headache, nausea, muscle cramp, or syncope.
  - Assess for precipitants: increased physical exertion, lack of access to air conditioning, medication, drug effect, or preceding illness.
  - Risk factors that inhibit heat dissipation include extremes of age, obesity, certain skin conditions, concurrent febrile illness, or heart disease.
- **Exam:** Full VS: Get rectal temp and expect tachycardia, tachypnea, widened pulse pressure, and hypotension.
  - Assess for any toxidrome, including a full neurologic exam and evaluation for muscle rigidity.
- **Diagnostics:**
  - CXR to evaluate for pulmonary edema (common in heat stroke)
  - EKG to evaluate for arrhythmias/conduction disturbances or Heat-related MI
  - Labs: CBC and coags (coagulopathy and DIC), BMP, Mg/Phos/Ca, and CPK (acute renal failure, rhabdomyolysis), liver enzymes (acute liver failure), tox screen
  - Head CT and LP if CNS process is suspected

MANAGEMENT

- Pearls to stabilize the ABCs
  - Treat hypotension with discrete IV boluses of isotonic crystalloid (NOT pressors, which will decrease heat dissipation)
  - Continuous rectal/esophageal monitoring!
  - In case of seizure, follow normal benzo protocol
- Cooling measures: Used in the case of heat stroke, and should be stopped after a temperature of 38 to 39 °C has been achieved.
  - Evaporative cooling most effective, and proven to decrease morbidity and mortality in older patients with classic heat stroke (well-tolerated by the awake patient).
  - Spray patient with lukewarm water and position fans to blow over the skin.
  - Ice baths can be used in the younger/exertional heat stroke patients; however, they complicate monitoring and can increase mortality in the elderly patient with classic heat stroke.
  - Applying ice packs to axillae, neck, and groin is safe but is poorly tolerated by conscious patients.
  - Cooling blankets and cold IV fluids (22° C) may also be used.
- Medications: Most often, none!
  - Antipyretics ineffective in heat stroke
  - Benzos should be used to treat shivering/agitation, and can also be used to treat muscle rigidity in serotonin syndrome. Suppress shivering with diazepam (5 mg IV) or lorazepam (1 to 2 mg IV); chlorpromazine should be avoided (unless neuroleptic malignant syndrome is NOT suspected).
  - In malignant hyperthermia dantrolene can be used (1 mg/kg IV push until symptoms subside, or max dose of 10mg/kg).

DISPOSITION

- Heat stroke, severe metabolic derangement, and a neuromuscular malignant syndrome should be admitted to the ICU.
- Most other patients can be discharged home but consider longer period of monitoring or admission in the elderly, significant electrolyte derangements a sign of AKI.
- RETURN IF: You develop severe headache, changes in vision, stop urinating, have a seizure, pass out, or have any other concerning symptoms.

BEWARE...

(!) Do not confuse febrile illness with heat stroke. Maintain a high index of suspicion for infection.

8 ▶ Hypothermia

- Mild: 35 to 32°C, Moderate: 32 to 28°C, Severe: Below 28°C
- Rectal thermometers may be artificially low if next to cold stool, and esophageal thermometers may be artificially high due to warm tracheal air.
- Patient is not dead until s/he is warm and dead. Longest CPR in survivors: adult 190min, child 6hrs.

Ddx
Hypothyroidism
Adrenal insufficiency
Sepsis
Neuromuscular disease
Malnutrition
Thiamine deficiency
Hypoglycemia

EVALUATION

- **High Yield History:** Assess for etiology including cold exposure, water or snow submersion, medication effect, adrenal insufficiency, or hypoglycemia.
  - If from a submersion, get full report of down time, water temp, initial core temp, and any arrhythmias.
- **Exam:** See table. Also, perform full trauma exam and skin exam for injuries (i.e. frostbite)
- **Diagnostics**
  - Labs: ABG (Metabolic acidosis and/or respiratory alkalosis), BMP (no predictable trends), glucose (initial hyperglycemia, followed by hypoglycemia in severe hypothermia), CBC (↓WBC/platelet from splenic sequestration and ↑ Hgb/HCT from concentration), coags (falsely normal despite pro-coagulopathic state), lipase (risk for pancreatitis)
  - EKG: Prolonged PR/QRS/QT, ST elevations, T wave inversions, or Osborn waves
  - CXR: Aspiration pneumonia, pulmonary edema, vascular congestion

Evaluation			
Organ System Manifestation	**Mild hypothermia → 32-35°C**	**Moderate→ 28-32°C**	**Severe <28°C**
Neurologic	Confusion, slurred speech	Lethargy, hallucinations, unconsciousness	Coma
Cardiovascular	Tachycardia, HTN, Osborn wave	Bradycardia, Hypotension	VF, asystole
Pulmonary	Hyperventilation, bronchorrhea	Hypoventilation	Pulmonary edema, apnea
Renal	Diuresis	More diuresis	Oliguria
Gastrointestinal	Ileus, pancreatitis	Acute hepatic failure	Stress ulcers
Musculoskeletal	Shivering	Decreased/no shivering, global rigidity	Pseudo-rigor mortis
Hematologic	Procoagulation	Procoagulation	Procoagulation

MANAGEMENT

Avoid jostling when possible to avoid risk of inducing cardiac arrhythmia, but this should not get in the way of doing what you have to do.

- Stabilize your ABCs
  - Low threshold for intubation
  - If hypotensive, give warm crystalloid → Dopamine (low-dose 2-5 micrograms/kilogram/minute) if necessary
  - If arrhythmia present, may persist until rewarmed: IGNORE atrial arrhythmias with slow ventricular response
  - Ventricular fibrillation is common: defibrillation typically ineffective below 30 degrees

When to call the code
No ROSC at 32-35C
No ROSC and K>12mmol
No VS and burial time <35min (likely died from other cause)
No VS/burial time >35min and asphyxial death/airway occluded

- Rewarming
  - **Mild hypothermia** → Passive external rewarming: Goal rate: 0.5 to 2°C per hour
    - Remove clothing and cover with blankets/insulation.
    - May not be effective in elderly population given low reserve.
  - **Mod/Severe hypothermia** → Active external rewarming: Goal rate: 2°C per hour
    - Warm blankets, warm baths, or warm humidified air
    - Warm the core before the extremities to avoid core temperature afterdrop (cold, acidemic blood in the extremities is shunted to the heart, causing arrhythmia/hypotension).
  - **Severe hypothermia** → Active internal rewarming
    - Consult cardiac surgery EARLY for cardiopulmonary bypass for cardiac instability, core temp<28C/82F, OR cardiac arrest from hypothermia.
    - Warm IV crystalloid (42°C), peritoneal/pleural 37, irrigation with warm crystalloid if bypass or ECMO are not available

DISPOSITION

- All but the mildest cases in otherwise healthy patients should be admitted, even if to observation status in order to monitor and continue warming.

BEWARE...

- ⓘ For homeless patients with cold exposure, ensure that you do a full exam so you do not miss a hypothermic injury (frostbite), and consult social work to help find warm shelter.
- ⓘ Remember that hypothermia can be seen in sepsis. Not all infected patients are febrile.

Section XI.
Fever

1 ▶ Fever Quick Guide

- ALWAYS: IV, O2, monitor, **COMPLETE** VS, EKG (arrhythmias or specific patterns consistent with toxic ingestion), fingerstick glucose, airway equipment nearby if needed
- Can't miss diagnoses in first 2 minutes:
  — Sepsis→ Early goal directed therapy, IVF and antibiotics
  — Bacterial meningitis →Ceftriaxone 2gm IV + vancomycin 1gm IV
  — Neutropenic fever→ Neutropenic precautions and early antibiotics against gram negatives
  — Neuroleptic malignant syndrome → benzos! Consider dantrolene

Definition: Single temp >101 or temp >100.4° for more than 1hr

- *Not to be confused with hyperthermia = temp >37.5° C
- 35°C=95°F, 36°=96.8°, 37°=98.6°, 38°=100.4°, 39°=102.2°, 40°=104°

Infectious Causes						
Respiratory	**CV**	**GI**	**GU**	**Neuro**	**Skin/Bone**	**Systemic/ Blood**
Pneumonia	Endocarditis	Peritonitis	UTI	Meningitis	Cellulitis	Sepsis/bacteremia
Peritonsillar abscess	Pericarditis	Appendicitis	Pyelonephritis	Cavernous venous	Infected decubitus	Meningococcemia
Retrophyarngeal abscess	Myocarditis	Biliary infection	Perinephric abscess	sinus	ulcer	Parasitic disease (ex. Malaria or
Otitis media	Pericardial effusion	Diverticulitis	Infected renal	thrombosis	Soft tissue	Babesiosis)
Sinusitis		Pancreatic	stone	Encephalitis	abscess	Fungal infections:
Viral phyaryngitis		pseudocyst	Tubo-ovarian	Intracranial	Necrotizing	(Coccidio-
Strep pharyngitis		Necrotizing pancreatitis	abscess	abscess	soft tissue	domycosis)
Bronchitis		Intra-	PID	Spinal	infection	
Influenza		abdominal	Endometritis	epidural	Osteomyelitis	
TB		abscess	Cystitis	abscess	Septic	
Epiglottitis		Colitis	Epididymitis		arthritis	
		Gastroenter-	Prostatitis		Infected	
		itis			hardware	
		Hepatitis			Indwelling	
					line infection	

EVALUATION

- **High Yield History:** Ask about localizing symptoms of source of infection including headache, neck pain or stiffness, cough or congestion, chest pain, nausea, vomiting, diarrhea, abdominal pain, dysuria, back pain, rashes, or indwelling lines or catheters.
  - Assess for immunosuppression risk: Diabetes, steroid use, history of transplant or malignancy, chemotherapy, HIV
  - Social history: Recent travel, exposures (bug or animal bites, needles, food), sexual partners, IVDU, alcohol use, housing situation (homeless, nursing home) work exposures, sick contacts
  - Any recent antibiotic use, previous infection, culture data
  - Full medication review to assess for drug reactions
- **Exam:** Full set of VS. Thorough system-based exam including skin (sacral decubitus ulcers, track marks). Look for any signs of rheumatologic disease (joint pain or swelling, malar rash).
- **Initial Workup:** Consider CBC, BMP, LFTs, lipase, troponin, lactate, UA, UCx, BCx, CXR, EKG, and LP. Then peel off labs that are not indicated for your patient. For example, blood cultures generally only indicated in a systemically ill patient unless screening for endocarditis.
  - Consult the Centers for Disease Control website for potential exposures in the recently returned traveler with fever.

Non-Infectious Causes		
Pulmonary embolism/ infarction	Recent seizure	Drug/medication related fever
Neuroleptic-malignant syndrome	Sickle Cell Disease	Malignancy
	Transplant rejection	Crystal arthropathy (Gout/CPPD)
Malignant hyperthermia	Pancreatitis	Sarcoidosis
Thyroid storm/thyrotoxicosis	Deep Vein Thrombosis	Inflammatory Bowel Disease
Acute adrenal insufficiency	Environmental exposure	Autoimmune disorder
Bood product transfusion reaction		
Toxic ingestion		

Common Infectious Causes of Pediatric Fever		
Age	Bacterial Causes (Unique to age in bold)	Viral Causes
0-28 days	**GBS**, Listeria, E. coli, **C. trachomatis**, N. gonorrhea	HSV, varicella, enteroviruses, RSV, influenza
1-3 months	**H. influenza**, S. pneumoniae, N. meningitides, E. coli	Varicella, enteroviruses, RSV, influenza
3-36 months	S. pneumoniae, N. meningitidis, E. coli	Varicella, enteroviruses, RSV, flu, Mono, roseola, adenovirus, Norwalk, coxsackievirus
≥ 3 years	S. pneumoniae, N. meningitidis, E. coli, **Group A streptococcus**	Varicella, enteroviruses, RSV, flu, Mono, roseola, adenovirus, Norwalk

PEDIATRIC CONSIDERATIONS

- Fever in infants 0-28 days old require complete sepsis workup (CBC, blood culture, UA and urine culture, lumbar puncture), empiric antibiotics, and hospital admission.

  — Ampicillin (100mg/kg/24hrs divided Q6h) **plus** either gentamicin (5mg/kg/24hrs divided Q8h to Q12h) or cefotaxime (150mg/kg/24hrs divided Q8hrs)

  — Avoid ceftriaxone in infants <28 days old due to possibly inducing acute bilirubin encephalopathy.

  — If risk factors for HSV are present (review hospital chart and obtain history) then empiric acyclovir should be administered (60mg/kg/24hrs divided Q8hrs).

Pediatric Fever Criteria and Work Up		
	Philadelphia Criteria	**Boston Criteria**
Age	29-60 days	28-89 days
Temp	≥38.2° C	≥38.0° C
Exam	Well-appearing, no focal site of infection	Well-appearing, no focal site of infection
Lab Values (defines low risk)	WBC count <15K, No bands on differential, UA <10 WBCs, CSF < 8 WBCs, negative Gram stains on UA and CSF, CXR/stool negative (if obtained)	WBC count <20K, CSF <10 WBCs, UA <10 WBCs, CXR negative (if obtained)
High Risk	Admission + IV abx (ampicillin + cefotaxime +/- vancomycin)	Admission + IV abx (ampicillin + cefotaxime +/- vancomycin)
Low Risk	Home, no abx	Home, empiric abx (Ceftriaxone IV or IM 50mg/kg), re-evaluation within 24hrs

Sources

Wing R, Dor MR, McQuilkin PA. Fever in the pediatric patient. *Emerg Med Clin North Am.* 2013;31(4):1073-1096.

Marx J, Hockberger R, Walls R. Rosen's Emergency Medicine: Concepts & Clinical Practice. 7th ed. Maryland Heights, MO: Mosby; 2009.

Notes

2 ▶ Sepsis

Bacteremia: Presence of bacteria in the blood as evidenced by positive blood cultures (present in less than half of patients with septic shock)

Systemic Inflammatory Response Syndrome (SIRS): Having 2 of the following is considered positive (Remember, SIRS is not specific to infection):

- Temperature >100.4°F or <95°F
- RR >20 breaths/min or PaCO$_2$ <32mmHg
- Heart rate >90 beats/min
- WBC >12K or <4K or >10% bands

Sepsis: SIRS with proven OR suspected infection source

Severe sepsis: Sepsis with one or more signs of **organ dysfunction**, hypoperfusion, or hypotension (i.e. metabolic acidosis, acute AMS, oliguria, or respiratory difficulty)

Septic shock: Sepsis with hypotension that is **unresponsive to fluid resuscitation** plus organ dysfunction or perfusion abnormalities

Ddx
MI
Pulmonary Embolus
Acute pancreatitis
Acute adrenal insufficiency
GI hemorrhage/anemia
Trauma
DKA
Thyrotoxicosis
Anaphylaxis
Transfusion reaction
Adverse drug reactions

Acute Respiratory Distress Syndrome (ARDS)*: Must have the following

- Ratio of PaO2 (need ABG) to FiO2 of <300. This ratio also known as P:F ratio. (Example: PaO2 of 150 on 50% O2 results in P:F ratio of 150 / 0.5 = 300).
- Bilateral pulmonary infiltrates on CXR
- No alternate explanation for symptoms (ex: pulmonary edema due to CHF)

EVALUATION

- **High Yield History:** Ask about any recent fevers, headaches, neck stiffness, cough, abdominal pain, vomiting, diarrhea, rashes or dysuria, confusion, or altered mental status (delirium).
  - Obtain an infectious past medical history such as C.diff infection, recurrent UTIs.
  - Assess for immunosuppression: chemotherapy, chronic steroids, neutropenia, splenectomy, neoplasm, renal failure, hepatic failure, HIV, or history of transplant.
  - Determine risk for multidrug resistant organism infection including prior culture data, recent hospitalizations, or nursing home resident.
- **Exam:** Full set of VS for fever, tachypnea, tachycardia, hypotension, or hypoxia
  - Assess for source of infection including abnormal breath sounds, abdominal tenderness, CVA tenderness, sacral decubitus ulcer, or rash.
  - Examine indwelling lines or catheters that could be nidus for infection.
  - In patients who are high risk, urogenital exam to check for PID or Fournier's gangrene.
- **Diagnostics:** Goal is to determine source of infection and assess for end-organ dysfunction.
  - Labs: CBC with differential, BMP, LFTs, **lactate**, VBG or ABG, coags, UA (consider DIC labs if concerned)

- Lactate >4 is indicative of tissue hypo-perfusion and is associated with increased risk of death*
- **Cultures prior to antibiotics:** blood x 2, urine, consider sputum
— EKG: To assess for ischemia or arrhythmia
— Imaging: Based on likely source of infection. Consider CXR, CT head, CT chest, CT abd/pelvis or RUQ US.

MANAGEMENT

- Place on monitor, oxygen, and intubation as needed. Consider placing Foley, central line, and arterial line.
- Five sepsis goals in the ED:
  — **Early identification of presence of sepsis** ("time is tissue" → Limits organ dysfunction and decreases mortality)
  — **Source control** (remove bacteria)- You can remove the Foley but you will have to call surgery to remove gallbladder or IR to drain an intra-abdominal abscess, etc.
  — **Early appropriate antibiotics:** Broad spectrum based on likely pathogen and prior culture data if available
  — **Increase O2 delivery to tissues:** The lactate is elevated because tissues aren't receiving enough O2! Supplemental O2 increases oxygen content, IV fluid increases cardiac output, blood transfusions increase O2 carrying capacity, vasopressors increase MAP, inotropes increase cardiac output
  — **Assess response** to therapy: UOP can be followed with goal is 0.5-1 cc/kg/hr. Lactate can be followed serially, you should recheck at the 3hr and 6hr marks, and ScvO2 can be serially monitored with goal ≥70%.

FLUID RESUSCITATION

- Patients are typically significantly hypovolemic in sepsis (usually at least 2-4L volume down). Goal of IV fluids is to improve volume status, tissue perfusion, and blood pressure. First-line IV fluids are crystalloid such as normal saline or lactated ringers. Randomized control trials have shown no benefit in outcome with albumin, and the cost of albumin is much higher.
  — Administer IVF boluses until you are no longer improving tissue perfusion or blood pressure with each additional bolus.
  — After each bolus, assess for fluid responsiveness to the bolus as well as for pulmonary edema.
  — Patients with sepsis are predisposed to developing noncardiogenic pulmonary edema (ARDS), and you should also be aware if your patient has a history of CHF. If any form of pulmonary edema develops, stop bolusing IVF.
- Methods to assess volume status include:
  — **CVP:** Studies have shown that CVP may not be as reliable as previously believed. Value is obtained from tip of central line catheter. Rivers protocol calls for goal CVP of 8-12. While you should not necessarily use CVP as an endpoint for volume resuscitation, it is a useful additional data point, especially if it is low (i.e. 0) or if it is high (i.e. 20).

— **Blood pressure**: Improvement in MAP (2/3*diastolic BP + 1/3*systolic BP) following a bolus suggests improvement in cardiac output (i.e. fluid responsive). You can also perform a **passive leg raise** at the bedside to provide a transient autotransfusion of 250cc blood and assess BP responsiveness to the "bolus."

— **Bedside Ultrasound**: Using a subxiphoid view with a phased array probe the IVC should be visualized entering the right atrium. If IVC is collapsing during inspiration, this suggests hypovolemia. If IVF is plethoric, this suggests adequate volume resuscitation. This is much more accurate on the extremes of measurements and more accurate when collapsing than when plethoric.

— **Pulse pressure variation**: Requires arterial line and intubated patient in sinus rhythm. Refers to the variation in the radial artery pulse pressure that occurs with each respiration. If variation is present, this suggests a patient who will likely respond to an additional IVF bolus.

ANTIBIOTICS

- Early antibiotics matter in sepsis and should be **targeted towards the suspected source**.
- DO NOT forget to obtain cultures PRIOR to abx, and to think about source control.
- Take a moment to review any previous culture data, as this can help guide abx selection - especially if the patient has a history of multi-drug resistant organisms.
- If source is unknown, an appropriate starting abx regimen includes pipercillan/tazobactam (3.375g IV Q6h) plus vancomycin (1gm IV Q12h with adjustment for low GFR) **or** cefepime (1-2gm IV Q8hrs) plus vancomycin (1gm IV Q12hrs with adjustment for low GFR) plus metronidazole (500mg IV Q8hrs).
- Always start the antibiotic targeted against gram negatives first due to the high morbidity and mortality of GNR bacteremia.

VASOPRESSORS

- AFTER adequate IVF resuscitation, if a goal MAP ≥65 has not been achieved then a vasopressor should be started. If you have a central venous catheter then norepinephrine should be started first.
- If you have a peripheral IV: Phenylephrine can be used; however, it is not the first-line agent and can cause reflex bradycardia and myocardial depression. You can consider using peripheral norepinephrine but **beware** that there are reports of limb ischemia and damage if it extravagates into surrounding tissues.
- Questions to answer if considering to start a second vasopressor agent:
  — Was the patient adequately fluid resuscitated? (Consider giving an additional 1-2L NS IVF)
  — Is the patient hypocalcemic? (Obtain ionized calcium and replete as needed)
  — Is the patient bleeding somewhere? (Perform guaiac, FAST exam)
  — Does the patient need inotropy (ie, dobutamine)? (Perform bedside US to estimate cardiac ejection fraction)
  — Is this an endocrine problem (ie, adrenal insufficiency or hypothyroidism)? (You can empirically give hydrocortisone 50mg IV Q6h and check a TSH level)

- Typical second-line pressors are vasopressin or epinephrine. Epinephrine provides more inotropy than vasopressin and may be more optimal in patients with a decreased cardiac EF.

Typical Vasopressor Doses	
Agent	**Dose Range (no maximum dose if ongoing HD response)**
Norepinephrine-both beta1 and alpha1 agonist	Initial starting dose is 8-12 mcg/min. Weight based dosing = 0.01-3mcg/kg/min. Titrate to desired response. Increases BP and HR.
Epinephrine beta1 > beta2 agonist and alpha 1 agonist (2nd line agent)	Initial starting dose 5-35 mcg/min. Weight based dosing= 0.1-0.5 mcg/kg/min. Titrate to desired response. Increases BP and HR.
Vasopressin: anti-diuretic hormone (2nd line agent)	Fixed dosing at 0.04 units/min. If BP improves, then first titrate down other pressors before discontinuing vasopressin.
Phenylephrine: alpha 1 agonist	Initial starting dose 25-180 mcg/min. Weight based dosing = 0.5 mcg/kg/min. Titrate to desired response. Can cause reflex bradycardia.

*Studies suggest dopamine is inferior to norepinephrine in sepsis and has an increased risk of dysrhythmias. Therefore, dopamine is usually not administered for treatment of sepsis.

DISPOSITION

- If pt is on vasopressors, has significant lab abnormalities, or comorbidities, admit to ICU.
- Many patients can be managed on the medical floor if they receive adequate fluid resuscitation in the ED, source control, and early antibiotics.
- Some pts with infections such as strep pharyngitis or influenza will meet criteria for sepsis based on initial VS. If otherwise healthy, improved with antipyretics, and no concern for other infection, these pts can be discharged home.

BEWARE...

① Think about sepsis in anyone who meets SIRS criteria. Failure to think about sepsis can lead to delayed diagnosis, which is harmful given that early antibiotic administration is essential in the management of sepsis.

① Do not start vasopressors until you have provided adequate IV fluid resuscitation. If severely hypotensive then you can start vasopressors but do not stop IVF (even if you achieve MAP ≥65 with pressors) until euvolemia is achieved.

① Always think about source control and call the appropriate consultant.

① Look at previous culture data. Typical sepsis antibiotics may not be sufficient in someone with recent known infection with resistant organisms (ie, ESBL→It doesn't look good if you administer cefepime to a patient just recently treated with imipenem for a similar infection).

Sources

Singh N, Weingart SD. Current guidelines for the management of severe sepsis and septic shock. *EB Medicine Emerg Med Practice.* April 2013.

Maloney PJ. Sepsis and septic shock. *Emerg Med Clin North Am.* 2013;31(3):583-600.

Reifel Saltzberg JM. Fever and signs of shock: the essential dangerous fever. *Emerg Med Clin North Am.* 2013;31(4)907-926.

Marx J, Hockberger R, Walls R. Rosen's Emergency Medicine: Concepts & Clinical Practice. 7th ed. Maryland Heights, MO: Mosby; 2009.

Notes

3 ▶ Pneumonia

Types of Pneumonia	Definitions
Community Acquired Pneumonia (CAP)	Patients diagnosed with PNA who do not meet criteria for other forms of PNA
Health Care-Associated Pneumonia (HCAP)	PNA that occurs in a non-hospitalized patient with significant health care contact by meeting any of the following criteria: • Residence in nursing home or other long-term care facility • Hospitalization for ≥2 days within the past 90 days • IV therapy (i.e. chemo) within the past 30 days • Attendance at a hospital or hemodialysis clinic within the past 30 days
Hospital-Acquired Pneumonia (HAP)	Also known as nosocomial PNA. Occurs ≥48 hrs after admission and did not appear to be present at time of admission
Ventilator-Associated Pneumonia (VAP)	Form of HAP that develops ≥48 to 72 hrs after endotracheal intubation

EVALUATION

- **High Yield History:** Symptoms include increased cough or sputum production, dyspnea, fever, pleuritic chest pain, and AMS/lethargy in elderly. Abdominal pain and back pain are less common symptoms.

  — Red flag symptoms include hospitalization within past 3 months, nursing home placement, antibiotic use within past 3 months, recent influenza infection, or exposures to birds, bats, rabbits, farm animals, haystacks.

  — Assess for any immunosuppression either by disease process or therapy (i.e. HIV, chemotherapy, transplant).

  — Obtain past medical history with focus presence of COPD, asthma, cystic fibrosis, end-stage renal disease on dialysis, sickle-cell disease, asplenia, alcohol abuse, smoking, IV drug abuse, TB risk factors, or relevant travel.

- **Exam:** Vital signs may be notable for hypoxia, tachypnea, tachycardia, hypotension, or fever.

  — Pulmonary exam for any focal changes in breath sounds, rhonchi, wheezing, or absence of breath sounds

  — Look for other etiologies of fever including rash, abdominal pain, or meningitis

  — Determine volume status and assess for other etiologies of shortness of breath

- **Diagnostics**

  — Labs: To risk stratify and to evaluate for other diagnoses

    ▪ CBC: Assess for leukocytosis, neutropenia, and lymphopenia

    ▪ BMP: Assess renal function (abx choice and dose) and acidosis (sepsis and prognosis). Hyponatremia is seen in Legionella PNA.

Ddx
Pulmonary embolism
CHF
Pneumothorax
Pneumonitis
ACS
COPD or Asthma
Cardiac tamponade
URI
Pericardial effusion
Sarcoidosis
Goodpastures
Malignancy

- Lactate is helpful in patients who meet sepsis criteria (2 out of 4 SIRS and a suspected source). Don't hesitate to obtain and trend!
- Consider trop or BNP if high concern for ACS or CHF. Additional considerations: rapid influenza test, urine legionella antigen.

— **Cultures:** Obtain blood cultures in all patients admitted to ICU. Consider in immunocompromised, sepsis, prosthetic valves. Get BEFORE antibiotics if possible. Consider sputum culture in patients being admitted to the hospital and patients with risk factors for unusual pathogens

— **CXR:** Pay special attention to the heart and diaphragm borders as well as the retrocardiac region.

— **Chest CT:** Consider in patients with serious underlying disease, sepsis, or shock

Etiology Quick Guide

- Most common for CAP: S. pneumoniae, H. influenza, Mycoplasma pneumoniae
- Hospitalized patients: Pseudomonas, Staph
- Nursing home/extended care facility: ↑risk resistant organisms including pseudomonas, Klebsiella, Acinetobacter, MRSA
- MRSA: Causes severe PNA, associated post-influenza infections, cavitations
- Klebsiella: Alcoholics, DM, high antibiotics resistance
- Legionella: Hyponatremia, abd pain, diarrhea
- Viral: Parainfluenza, influenza, CMV, metapneumovirus
- Fungal: Histoplasma, blastomyces, coccidioides (Midwest and SW)
- PCP: HIV/AIDS or malignancy
- Mycobacterium tuberculosis
- Rare: Hantavirus (rodent urine/feces), plague (yersinia pestis–fleas from rodents), tularemia (mammals–rabbits), psittacosis (birds), Q fever (cattle/sheep/cats)

MANAGEMENT

- Management focuses on determining likely organism based on risk factors, exposures, and symptoms. Etiology is rarely identified in the ED; therefore, you need to cover organisms based upon risk factors.
- ABCs: If profoundly hypoxic or not protecting airway, intubate.
  - Provide supplemental oxygen if needed
  - If septic, initiate early goal directed therapy
- Initiate early antibiotics based on presumed etiology (see chart).

Outpatient Therapy		
PNA Classification	**Antibiotics**	**Comments**
Community-acquired PNA (CAP) in previously healthy people	- Azithromycin 500PO x 1 and 250mg PO QD x 4 days, OR - Doxycycline 100mg PO BID x 7 days	Treats common typical and atypical bacterial pathogens
CAP with comorbidities or recent antibiotics	- Levofloxacin 750mg PO QD x 5 days, OR - Cefpodoxine 200mg PO BID + Azithromycin 500mg PO QD x 7 days *If aspiration is suspected, add clindamycin or metronidazole	Can substitute moxifloxacin or gemifloxacin. Augmentin can be substituted for cefpodoxime.

Inpatient Therapy		
PNA Classification	**Antibiotics**	**Comments**
Community-acquired PNA (CAP)	Floor admit: Levofloxacin 750mg PO/IV or ceftriaxone 1gm IV Q12 **PLUS** azithromycin 500mg PO/IV ICU admission: add vancomycin to above	Indications for anaerobic coverage (clindamycin or metronidazole) include lung abscess, necrotizing PNA, post-obstructive PNA
Health Care-Associated PNA (HCAP) Hospital-Acquired PNA (HAP) Ventilator-Associated PNA (VAP)	Cefepime 2gm IV Q12h + levofloxacin 750mg IV QD + vancomycin 1g IV Q12h **If risk of pseudomonas is low** you can hold either cefepime or levofloxacin.	— Can substitute imipenem/zosyn/meropenem for cefepime. — Can substitute vancomycin with linezolid. — If VAP consider Acinetobacter and treat with carbepenem — If ESBL use carbepenem
Presumed PCP PNA	Trimethoprim-sulfamethoxazole 240/1200mg IV Q6h consider steroids	Can substitute pentamidine + ceftriaxone, clindamycin + primaquine or atovaquone + ceftriaxone for sulfa-allergic patients

DISPOSITION

- Admit to the ICU any patients who are intubated, are profoundly hypoxic, in septic shock, or who have significant comorbidities.

- Several decision-making tools exist to help determine which patients to admit or discharge based on their risk stratification. These include CURB-65 or the Pneumonia Severity Index (PSI) (use online calculator).

- Consider discharge home in younger patients (<65yo), stable on room air, otherwise minimal medical comorbidities, reassuring exam and vitals, and ability to fill and take prescribed medication. Discharged patients should have follow up within the next 2-3 days.

- RETURN IF: Persistent fever, worsening shortness of breath or chest pain, unable to fill or take antibiotics, failure of symptoms to improve in next 2-3 days, or have any other new or concerning symptoms.

BEWARE...

(!) Obtain cultures PRIOR to abx administration. However, never delay antibiotics if obtaining cultures is difficult. Patients presenting to the ED with PNA have **better outcomes if treated with antibiotics within 6 hrs.**

(!) **Aspiration**: Systemic corticosteroids for acute aspiration are of no benefit and are not indicated. Although many patients go on to develop PNA after an acute aspiration event, prophylactic antibiotics are controversial and generally not recommended unless signs of acute infection are present.

Source
Lim WS, Van der eerden MM, Laing R, et al. Defining community acquired pneumonia severity on presentation to hospital: an international derivation and validation study. *Thorax.* 2003;58(5):377-82.

Notes

4 ▶ Neutropenic Fever

- This is a medical emergency. Delay in antibiotic therapy has been associated with up to 70% mortality

- Usually chemotherapy induced. Mucosal barrier immune defense breaks down and results in translocation of bacteria

- **Fever:** A single temperature >101 OR a sustained temperature >100.4 for an hour

- **Neutropenia:** ANC (absolute neutrophil count) <500 cells/microL OR <1000 cells/microL with an expected nadir <500 cells/microL in the next 48hrs. ANC= WBC x (% neutrophils + % bands)

Ddx
Pneumonia
Cellulitis
Viral illness
Typhlitis
Cholecysitis
Sinusitis
Transient bacteremia

EVALUATION

- **High Yield History:** It is important to appreciate that neutropenic patients may not demonstrate typical signs and symptoms of infection due to their immunocompromised state — fever may be your only clue.

  — Obtain a complete review of systems to determine affected organ systems and possible infectious source (i.e. headache, photophobia, vomiting, mouth/ throat pain, cough, shortness of breath, chest pain, abdominal pain, diarrhea, hematochezia, melena, dysuria, wounds/ulcers).

  — Does the patient have indwelling lines? (i.e. PICC lines, ports, central lines, Foley) and when were they last accessed?

  — Obtain infectious history, including current antibiotic prophylaxis, past infections, any history of antibiotic resistant organisms.

  — Obtain full oncologic history including what type of cancer, if the patient is on chemotherapy or radiation therapy, and when the last treatment was given.

- **Exam:** (Signs of infection may be subtle given lack of inflammatory response)

  — Examine any port, lines, or indwelling catheters for signs of cellulitis.

  — Check mucosal surfaces (skin, mouth, perineum) for mucositis.

- Do thorough exam for infectious source, including beyond lungs, skin, and abdomen (i.e. look for sinusitis or pharyngitis).

- **DO NOT PERFORM DIGITAL RECTAL EXAM, as this can introduce bacteria into the fragile mucosal surface.**

  — Diagnostics: Have a low threshold to test for any complaint.

  — Labs: CBC with differential, BMP, lactate, LFTs, UA

  — Cultures: Peripheral blood and indwelling line cx, urine cx, sputum cx (bacterial and fungal cx)

  — Imaging: CXR in all patients

    ▪ Head CT and LP if headache or AMS (consider addition of cryptococcal antigen and PCR for HSV or VZV)

- Send stool Cx, C. diff, and consider abdominal CT for typhlitis (necrotizing enterocolitis) or abscess if abdominal discomfort/diarrhea
- Consider CT sinus if any sinusitis symptoms
- Have low threshold for CT chest if respiratory symptoms given increased sensitivity for identifying PNA or other infectious pulmonary process.

MANAGEMENT

- ABCs, IV access, telemetry, and fluid resuscitation
- If patient is septic start early goal directed therapy (see sepsis chapter).
- **Early antibiotics** (within 60min) are essential. A patient's well appearance can be deceptive. The majority of neutropenic fever is from a bacterial source and thus all neutropenic fevers should be treated as if the patient is bacteremic.
  - Goal is to treat the most likely organism and most deadly.
  - If the patient has a likely source of infection, treat broadly for likely organisms (not targeted therapy as in immunocompetent hosts).
  - If no clear source, always cover for gram negative organisms. Do not forget neutropenic dosing and to review past culture data.
  - Do not treat empirically for gram positive bacteria unless the patient has a likely gram positive infection (i.e. line infection), is septic, or has a history of MRSA (see chart).
- Anti-fungal therapy should be added if hemodynamically unstable or concern for fungal infection (typically anti-fungal coverage is not added until fever >4 days while on abx). Appropriate empiric coverage including Amphotericin B, caspofungin, voriconazole, or itraconazole. Consider immediate infectious disease consult.
- IF oral ulcerations are present (HSV vs. Candida) then consider addition of acyclovir and fluconazole.
- The patient's primary oncologist, or their coverage, should be called. They can provide invaluable information about the patient's risk factors, chemotherapy course, and other possible complications.
- As with all bacterial infection, source control is key. Consult surgery or IR as indicated for intraabdominal infections, though effort should be made to avoid surgical intervention if possible given risk of infection and poor wound healing in this patient population.

Gram negative abx	Gram positive abx	Anaerobic abx
— Cefepime 2gm IV Q8hr, OR — Ceftazidime 2g IV Q8hr, OR — Piperacillin/tazobactam 4.5gm IV Q6H **Alternate agents**: Imipenem 500mg IV Q6hr, OR Meropenem 1gm IV Q8hrs **If PCN allergic**: Ciprofloxacin + clindamycin, OR Aztreonam + vancomycin	**Should NOT be empirically given.** Increasing concern now over breeding abx resistant organisms. **Vancomycin should be added if** history of MRSA **or** suspected catheter related infection, skin or soft tissue infection, PNA, signs of sepsis, or HD instability. Dose vancomycin by nomogram -or- Vancomycin 1gm IV Q8hs If history of VRE then linezolid 600mg IV Q6H	If HD unstable, abdominal symptoms, diarrhea, or concern for C. difficile colitis: Metronidazole 500mg IV Q6hrs

DISPOSITION

- Patients who are low risk and hemodynamically stable can be admitted to the oncology or medical floor.

- Patients who are high risk (from the comorbidities or oncologic process) or are septic should be admitted to the ICU.

- A select group of low risk patients (expect short duration of their, neutropenia, no medical comorbidities, good follow up) may qualify for outpatient treatment. However, this decision should always be made in conjunction with the patient's primary oncologist.

- RETURN IF: You have recurrent fevers, develop any focal infectious symptoms such as abdominal pain or rash, are unable to tolerate oral hydration, or have any other new or concerning symptoms.

BEWARE...

⚠ These patients are sick and can decompensate quickly; appreciate that fever may be the only sign of a serious infection.

⚠ Early appropriate antibiotics are imperative! Touch base with nursing staff regarding importance.

⚠ DO NOT forget to look at the differential on the CBC (patient may have 3000 WBC but almost 0 neutrophils).

⚠ Look at past culture data to ensure you are providing adequate antimicrobial coverage.

⚠ Remember that a patient whose ANC is still slightly >500 but expected to drop further in the next 1-2 days should be treated as if s/he is neutropenic.

Sources

McCurdy, Mitarai, Perkins. Oncologic emergencies, part II: Neutropenic fever, tumor lysis syndrome, and hypercalcemia of malignancy. *EB Medicine Emerg Med Practice*. March 2010.

Marx J, Hockberger R, Walls R. Rosen's Emergency Medicine: Concepts & Clinical Practice. 5th ed. Maryland Heights, MO: Mosby; 2002.

5 ▶ Meningitis

- A CNS infection with inflammation of the meninges resulting in fever, nuchal rigidity, altered mental status, and headache.

- **Bacterial meningitis** is a potentially deadly infection with potential lifelong neurologic sequelae. Early identification and treatment are vital.

- **Aseptic meningitis** (aka viral meningitis) cannot easily be distinguished from bacterial meningitis. Most are caused by enteroviruses and many need only symptomatic care.

EVALUATION

- **High Yield History:** Symptoms include headache, nausea, vomiting, fever, nuchal rigidity, and AMS. May also report seizure activity.

  — The **triad of fever, AMS, and neck stiffness** is only 46% sensitive; however, the absence of all three makes the diagnosis of meningitis much less likely.

Ddx
Tox/metabolic
CVS
Encephalitis
Malignancy
Abscess
ICH
Viral meningitis

- **Exam:** VS may be normal, but typically patients will have fever and possible tachycardia.

  — Examine for photophobia, pailledema, altered mental status, and any focal neurologic deficits.

  — Skin exam for meningococcal rash, viral exanthema, or herpetic lesions

  — Classic signs (both low sensitivity):
    - Brudzinski sign: Spontaneous flexion of hip with passive flexion of neck
    - Kernig's sign: With hips flexed 90 degree, resistance of full extension of the knees

- **Labs:** CBC (leukocytosis or leukopenia, thrombocytopenia), BMP (anion gap metabolic acidosis, hyponatremia), blood cultures x 2

  — Obtain a CT prior to LP only if: focal neurologic deficit, papilledema, immunocompromised, history of CNS process (mass, CVA, focal infection, abnormal level of consciousness, GCS <10, new onset seizure)

  — LP (see procedure section for specifics regarding procedure).
    - Obtain opening pressure especially if concerned for cryptococcus.
    - In addition to typical tests consider TB culture, India Ink and fungal cultures, and cryptococcal antigen as indicated.

LP results			
	Normal	**Viral**	**Bacterial**
WBC	<5 /mm3 <1 PMN/mm3	<250 /mm3 (mostly lymphocytic)	500-5000 /mm3 (mostly PMN, however early can be lymphocytic)
Protein	<50mg/dL	50-300 mg/dL	100-500 mg/dL
Glucose	0.6:1 (CSF to serum) 50-80mg/dL	Normal	<0.4:1 ratio <40mg/dL

- Traumatic LP:

— True CSF WBC = measured CSF WBC x [(csf RBC x blood WBC)/blood RBC] or subtract 1 WBC/ 700 RBC

— Subtract 1mg/dL of protein/ 1000 RBC

Gram stain				
Gram + cocci, single	Gram + cocci, pairs	Gram +rods	Gram – cocci, pairs	Gram – rods
Staph	S. pneumo	Listeria	N. meningitidis	E. coli, pseudomonas

Meningitis (microbiology)					
Peds (<1 mo)	Peds (1mo–23mo)	Adult (Community)	Healthcare associated	Viral	Other
Group B strep E. coli Listeria	S. pneumoniae N. meningitidis Group B strep H. influenza E. coli	S. pneumoniae H. influenza N. meningitis Listeria	Staph, Gram –bacilli, Psuedomonoas (risk if ventricular drain or recent neurosurgery)	HIV, HSV, West Nile, VZV, mumps, enteroviruses, lymphocytic choriomeningitis	Mycobacteria, Fungi (cryptococcus), Spirochetes (T pallidum, B. burgdorferi)

MANAGEMENT

- Early administration of antibiotics is key, along with patient isolation.

- If LP is delayed, BC x2 should be obtained before empiric antibiotics.

- Consider dexamethasone (0.15mg/kg IV Q6H x 2-4 days) before or at first dose of antibiotics.

- Treat based on the suspected pathogen (for bacteria this varies by age).

- Antibiotic prophylaxis for confirmed meningococcal meningitis: Should be administered within 24 hrs of index case to those with "close contact" to the patient (ie, 8 hrs of contact, close proximity <3ft, direct oral secretion contact during week prior to illness).

- For adults give ciprofloxacin 500mg PO x 1 dose OR rifampin 600mg PO Q12h x 2 days. For children give IM ceftriaxone or PO azithromycin.

- If HSV meningitis suspected give Acyclovir 30mg/kg Q8hrs IV.

Antibiotics				
Pediatrics <1 month	Pediatrics >1 month	Adults	Health care associated	Other
Ampicillin (50mg/kg QID) **PLUS** Gentamicin (2.5mg/kg IV TID) **PLUS** Cefotaxime (50mg/kg IV QID)	Ampicillin (50mg/kg IV QID) **PLUS** Cefotaxime (100mg/kg IV TID), **OR** Ceftriaxone (50mg/kg IV BID) **PLUS** Vancomycin (15mg/kg IV QID)	Ceftriaxone 2g IV BID **OR** Cefotaxime 2g q4h **PLUS** Vancomycin (15-20mg/kg IV BID) **PLUS** Ampicillin 2g q4h (if >50) to cover listeria	Vancomycin (15-20mg/kg IV BID) **PLUS** Cefepime 2g IV TID **OR** Meropenem 2g IV TID	**HSV:** Acyclovir 10mg/kg IV TID **Cryptococcus:** Amphotericin B 0.7-1mg/kg IV qD and Flucytosine 25mg/kg PO QID **Tuberculosis:** IZD 300mg PO QD, Rifampin 600gm QD, Pyrazinamide 2gm PO QD, and Ethambutol 1.6gm PO qD

DISPOSITION

- Patients with bacterial or fungal meningitis patients are admitted to floor or ICU if obtunded, systemically ill, or significant comorbidities.

- Can discharge patient home if clear case of aseptic meningitis and patient not toxic, not immunocompromised and is able to follow up closely with PCP or has ability to return with any worsening symptoms.

- RETURN IF: You experience persistent symptoms, severe headache, have a seizure, or have any focal numbness or weakness.

Sources

Attia, et. al. The Rational Clinical Examination: Does This Adult Patient Have Acute Meningitis. *JAMA* (1999), 281(2), 175-81

Heckenberg SG, Brouwer MC, Van de beek D. Bacterial meningitis. *Handb Clin Neurol.* 2014;121:1361-75.

Kim KS. Acute bacterial meningitis in infants and children. *Lancet Infect Dis.* 2010;10(1):32-42.

Tunkel AR, Hartman BJ, Kaplan SL, et al. Practice guidelines for the management of bacterial meningitis. *Clin Infect Dis.* 2004;39(9):1267-84.

Van de beek D, De gans J, Tunkel AR, Wijdicks EF. Community-acquired bacterial meningitis in adults. *N Engl J Med.* 2006;354(1):44-53.

Notes

Section X.
Headache

1 ▶ Headache Quick Guide

- ALWAYS: ABC, IV, O2, Monitor, complete VS (fever, HTN, bradycardia), EKG (ST changes in SAH and increased ICP),
- Can't miss diagnoses in first 2 minutes:
  - ICH/Herniation → Hypertonic saline and mannitol
  - Meningitis→ Vancomycin 25mg/kg and ceftriaxone 2gm
  - SAH → BP control and reverse any anticoagulation
  - Epidural hematoma → Emergent evacuation
  - Hemorrhagic stroke→ BP control and reverse any anticoagulation
- Quick differential: BITE ME (Bleed, Infection, Thrombosis, Eye, Mass, Environmental)
- ED can't miss differential (the "10 deadly headaches")

Benign Ddx
Migraine
Tension
Trigeminal neuralgia
Post-LP
Cluster
Dental pain
Exertional
Post-coital headache

EVALUATION

- **High Yield History:** Important questions to ask: Maximal intensity at onset? Activity at onset? Trauma? Fever/immunocompromised? Intensity? Is this consistent with previous headaches? Any oncologic history? Anticoagulation?
- **Exam:** VS! Full neurologic exam (key: level of consciousness, pupils, reflexes), temporal tenderness, eye exam, meningeal signs, rash. Papilledema and optic nerve sheath diameter on US (>5mm and 3mm behind globe) to evaluate for ICP.
- **Initial workup:** Usually limited Most "deadly headaches" get CT and/or LP (including opening pressure, 9-18cm H2O is normal). CBC and blood cultures for meningitis, ESR for suspected temporal arteritis, HCT if anoxic headache suspected.

Diagnosis	Typical Presentation/ History	Initial Workup
Subdural or epidural hematoma	Trauma, can be minor if elderly, intoxicated, or anticoagulated	CT, general trauma exam, and workup
Subarachnoid hemorrhage	Worst headache of life (atypical), maximal intensity at onset, onset with exertion, syncope, vomiting, HTN, polycystic kidney disease	CT (adequate in first 6 hrs), most get CT/LP
Meningitis or encephalitis	Recent ear, nose or throat infection, immunocompromised, + jolt accentuation (pt rotates head horizontally at 2 cycles / sec, + test is worsening of existing headache)	LP, CBC, droplet precautions, antibiotics (low threshold)
Hypertensive emergency	History of HTN, pregnancy, current CVA/ICH, sympathomimetics	Full labs, EKG, UA
Carotid or vertebral dissection	Thrombophilia, OCPs, cancer, rotational head or neck trauma	CT head and neck with IV contrast
Temporal arteritis	Age >50, temporal tenderness, jaw claudication, collagen/vascular disease	ESR, give steroids
Acute angle closure glaucoma	Pain in dark environment, red eye with ciliary flush, poor vision	Tonometry
CO poisoning	Winter, location specific, other people in house with headache	CO level, co-oximetry, high flow oxygen
Central venous thrombosis	Mostly women of child-bearing age, also: OCPs, known thrombophilia/previous clots, malignancy	CTV or MRV
Increased ICP	History of increased ICP/shunt or malignancy. On exam Cushing response, cranial nerve findings (especially III, IV), AMS	CT, shunt series. Only LP if CT neg. Mannitol/hypertonic saline. Call neurosurgery

BEWARE

⚠ Response to conservative treatment does not rule out dangerous headache.

⚠ Exercise caution when making a specific diagnosis for benign headache.

2 ▶ Benign Headache

- Complaint of headache represents between 3-5% of all ED visits. Majority are tension headaches, 30% unknown etiology, 10% migraines, 8% potentially serious causes (i.e. tumor or glaucoma), and 1% are thought to be life-threatening (i.e. SAH).

- Blood vessels and meninges are the sensate areas of the brain (with no sensation in the parenchyma). The scalp, neck muscles, skin, and mucosa of the sinuses can also contribute to headache-like pain. Cranial nerve V is most often responsible for mediating headache pain (although VII, IX, and X are also sometimes implicated), leading to poor localization of pain.

Ddx (Does not include the "ten deadly headaches" from the quick guide)					
Neuro/Vascular	Toxic/metabolic	ENT/Eye	MSK	Allergy/Infection	Misc
Migraine Trigeminal neuralgia Post LP	Chemical ingestion	Temporomandibular joint disease	Cervical strain Tension Cluster	Sinusitis Dental Infection	Effort dependent/post-coital

EVALUATION

- **High Yield History:** Obtain detailed history on timing, onset, palliative, or provoking factors, quality, etc. Focus should be on mental status changes over time and relation to headache, any focal findings, history of trauma, presence of vertigo, or fever.
  - Ask about red flags including history of trauma (SAH, SDH, EDH), sudden onset of pain (thunderclap), "worst headache of life" (SAH), AMS (involvement of brain tissue), history of HIV or immunocompromised (abscess), multiple family members with same symptoms (CO), meningismus (meningitis), vomiting, morning headache or visual disturbance (tumor), and any facial tenderness (temporal arteritis).

- **Exam:** VS often normal. Presence of fever or hypertension are concerning signs.
  - Full physical exam with focus on mental status, focal findings, full neurologic exam, and assessment for tenderness over temporal arteries

- **Diagnostics**
  - Labs: Labs are not indicated for benign headaches. They are indicated only to evaluate for more concerning etiology.
  - Imaging: CT (trauma, AMS, focal neurologic findings, meningismus). Note: For minor trauma see Canadian CT Head Rules to guide your decision to image.

Diagnosis	Diagnostic Features
Tension headache	Frequent exacerbations, no nausea or vomiting, no photo or phonophobia. At least 2 of: non-pulsatile, does not prohibit activity, bilateral location, and not worse with routine physical activity
Migraine HA	More common in women. Patient will often have a migraine history. Can have associated photo/phonophobia and/or nausea and vomiting. At least 2 of: Unilateral, pulsating, moderate to severe pain, and worse with routine physical activity
Cluster HA	Unilateral, associated with any of following: scleral injection, lacrimation, congestion, rhinorrhea, facial sweating, miosis, ptosis, or eyelid edema
Exertional/Sexual HA	Onset with physical/sexual activity

MANAGEMENT

- Low risk if ALL are present: Previous identical headache, normal mental status, normal neck exam (no meningismus), normal vital signs, non-focal neurologic exam, and improvement under observation with treatment.

- If low risk, diagnose as primary (benign) headache and proceed to analgesia. There is little value (and success) in differentiating type of headache in the ED.

- Analgesia (based on underlying etiology): Start with NSAIDS in most cases. Triptans are recommended for acute treatment if previous episodes have not been controlled by simple analgesia.

Treatment Options			
Tier	Mild / Moderate HA	Severe HA or n/v	Cluster HA
1	Ibuprofen 800mg, acetaminophen 1000gm and/or caffeine 200 mg (all PO)	Ketorolac 30mg IV + Prochlorperazine 10mg IV (or Metoclopramide 10mg IV) + IVF	Oxygen 6-10L and sumatriptan 6mg SQ
2	Ketorolac 30mg IV (if ibuprofen not given above) + Prochlorperazine 10mg IV (or Metoclopramide 20mg IV) + IVF	Consider Dexamethasone 20mg IV (NNT 10 for prevention of recurrence)	Add + Prochlorperazine 10mg IV (or Metoclopramide 20mg IV)
3	Consider dexamethasone 20mg IV (number needed to treat is 10 for prevention of recurrence)	Add Sumatriptan 6mg SQ and re-dose Prochlorperazine / Metoclopramide	Consider opiate (last resort)
4	*Pregnant patients: APAP 650 PO and/ or Metoclopramide 20mg PO / IV	Consider opiate (last resort)	

Drug	Contraindications	Side effects
Triptans	HTN, CAD, peripheral vascular disease , arrhythmias, recent MAOI, SSRI or triptan use (Serotonin syndrome)	High rate of relapse, chest pain / tightness, sweating and dizziness
APAP	Liver disease	N/A
Prochlorperazine	Pregnancy, Parkinson's (with Metoclopramide)	Dystonic reaction (treat with Benadryl), QTc prolongation
Ibuprofen	Kidney disease, 3rd trimester	Bleeding

DISPOSITION

- Vast majority of patients with benign headaches can be discharged home.

- Consider admission if post-LP headache or complex migraine.

- Patients should follow up with their PCP to discuss further care or abortive medications.

BEWARE...

① Not adequately working up a pt's headache if it's different from his/herusual.

① Dismissing an older patient with a migraine diagnosis without adequate work up (think temporal arteritis).

① Do not routinely work up patients (ie, expose them to imaging) if this is the same headache they have had in the past – the priority in this case is pain management and outpatient follow up.

① Expecting that the patient will be headache-free at discharge.

① Not realizing that recurrence of pain is common (educate your patient and provide guidance for recurrence).

Sources

Zane RD, Kosowsky JM, et al. Pocket Emergency Medicine. 2nd ed. Philadelphia, PA: Lippincott Williams & Wilkins; 2011.

Ma OJ, Cline D, Tintinalli J, et al. Emergency Medicine Manual. 6th ed. New York, NY: McGraw-Hill Professional; 2003.

Marx J, Hockberger R, Walls R. Rosen's Emergency Medicine: Concepts & Clinical Practice. 5th ed. Maryland Heights, MO: Mosby; 2002.

Hans L, Mawji Y. The ABCs of Emergency Medicine. 12th edition. Toronto, Canada: University of Toronto; 2012.

Medscape News & Perspective. New York, NY: http://emedicine.medscape.com.

Notes

3 ▶ Hemorrhagic Stroke

- Intracranial hemorrhagic (ICH) has a 30-day mortality of up to 50% – many of which occur in the first few days.

- Hemorrhagic stroke can be classified as intraparenchymal, subarachnoid (typically from aneurysm), and intraventricular.

- Etiology most commonly from acute hypertension in the setting of cerebral amyloid angiopathy but also includes vascular malformation, ruptured aneurysm, and malignancy.

- Traumatic ICH such as epidural and subdural hematomas are uniquely managed, and the management strategies in this section do not apply directly.

Ddx
Ischemic stroke
Migraine
Seizure
Intracranial abscess
Malignancy
HTN emergency
Meningitis
Encephalitis
Intoxication
Hypoglycemia

EVALUATION

- **High Yield History:** Presenting symptoms depend on the size and location of the bleed. In general, patients present with a headache and a focal neurologic deficit. Patients may also present with altered mental status, vomiting, decreased consciousness, or seizure activity.

  — In contrast to a SAH these symptoms are not usually "thunderclap" and maximal at onset.

  — Risk factors: HTN (bleed is typically in basal ganglia), Smoking Amyloid angiopathy (typically lobar located), and anticoagulant use,

- **Exam:** Presenting markedly elevated blood pressure and possible decreased level of consciousness

  — Focal neurologic deficits are based on location of the bleed.

  — Symptoms and exam findings may be transient in smaller bleeds.

- **Diagnostics:** Obtain emergent brain imaging. Is ICH suspected? Then a non-contrast head CT should be priority after patient is stabilized.

  — Labs: Obtain CBC, BNP, coags, type, and screen

  — EKG: Various EKG changes can be seen with ICH, including ST segment changes and tall T waves.

  — Head CT: Should be obtained emergently to diagnose ICH and to determine size, if there is surrounding edema, extension into the ventricular system, or signs of midline shift.

  — Contrast MRI/MRA: Can be useful if concern that the bleeding is from a tumor or vascular malformation.

  — CT angiogram can assess for bleeding from an aneurysm, vascular bleed as well as any ongoing bleeding.

MANAGEMENT

- ABCs (if intubation indicated, consider pre-treatment with lidocaine 1mg/kg and fentanyl 100 mcg IV)

- Big picture: Secure airway, obtain STAT head CT, and then prevent further bleeding, seizures, and increased ICP.

- Whom to consult? For large ICH, or patients in whom you are concerned about elevated ICP, the neurosurgical team should be consulted for evaluation/treatment of aneurysm and consideration of EVD placement +/- hematoma drainage. If the ICH is small it may be appropriate to only consult the neurology team.

- **Stop further bleeding:** Immediately reverse any anticoagulation and transfuse platelets if on an antiplatelet agent and control blood pressure to SBP <160mmHg, or even to SBP 140mmHg if safe to do so.

Anticoagulant/Antiplatelet Reversal Options		
Anticoagulant	**Treatment**	**Comments**
Warfarin	• **Vitamin K:** 5-10mg IV over 10min (INR corrected in 6-24 hrs) **plus either:** • **FFP:** 3-6hrs to infuse (INR corrected in ~12hrs) **or** • **Prothrombin-complex concentrate (PCC):** dosing weight based. (INR corrected 15 min after 1 hr infusion) — 3-factor contains factors II, IX, and X — 4-factor contains II, XII, IX, and X	-IV Vitamin K has risk of anaphylaxis -Volume associated with FFP can be prohibitive in patients with heart failure or aortic stenosis -PCCs are expensive and should be limited to life-threatening bleeds -No trials comparing 3 and 4 factors PCC. If giving 3-factor consider supplementing factor IIX with FFP or factor concentrate
Aspirin	Platelet transfusion	Discuss with consulting team. Obtain consent for blood products.
Unfractionated heparin/ LMWH	Protamine sulfate: dose dependent on dose of heparin, route given and time of last dose	Call pharmacy
Dabigatran	No antidote. Half-life 12hrs in patients with normal renal function. One-third protein bound with 60% removed 2-3hrs after hemodialysis	

- **Controlling ICP**
  - Head of the bed elevated to 30 degrees, avoid all hypotonic fluids.
  - If intubated, is the patient adequately sedated? If not, consider additional propofol or midazolam.
  - Is pain controlled? If not consider IV morphine. Pain increases SBP. Avoid NSAIDs.

— Is the blood pressure at goal? If presenting with SBP 150 – 200 then goal SBP should be 140mmHg. If presenting with SBP >200 mmHg then aim to acutely lower SBP ~25% and discuss with consulting team ultimate BP goal.

Blood Pressure agents		
Medication	**Dosage**	**Comments**
Nicardipine (dihydropyridine calcium channel blocker)	Initial rate of 5mg/hr IV. Can increase by 2.5mg Q15min until desired BP or max rate of 15mg/hr. Once goal BP achieved titrate down to 3mg/hr	Most commonly used medication to control BP in ICH. Use cautiously in patients with heart failure who are already taking beta blockers
Labetalol (beta and alpha blocker)	10-20mg IV Q10min (max dose 80mg/dose)	Contraindicated in bradycardia, heart failure, severe COPD. Be cognizant of possible bradycardia if patient is currently taking calcium channel blocker
Hydralazine (vasodilator)	10-20mg IV Q4-6hrs (max dose 40mg/dose)	BP response may be delayed and unpredictable. Typically only for patients with contraindication to labetalol

- **Seizure prophylaxis:** Risk/benefit of prophylactic anti-epileptic drugs is unclear. Typically more often recommended for ICH involving the cortex. Discuss with the consulting team prior to administering unless patient has already had a seizure.
  - Levetiracetam is the typical seizure prophylaxis medication → dose is typically 750-1000mg IV x1
  - Alternate agent is Fosphenytoin → dose is 10-20mg phenytoin equivalent per kg x1

- **Adequate and appropriate IV access?** Ensure adequate IV access for all necessary infusions (sedation, BP control, anticoagulation reversal, etc.). If inadequate peripheral IV access then consider a central line.
  - Prior to placing central line discuss with consulting team regarding location (often internal jugular central lines are avoided given increased ICP if thrombosis, and operative approach may necessitate central line on specific side of the body).
  - If elevated SBP then place arterial line → Again, discuss which side of the body the consulting team prefers as this can assist patient care in the OR (ie, anesthesia not having to climb under the table for ABGs).

- **Additional or scheduled repeat imaging studies**
  - For any significant worsening neurologic status.
  - If there is suspicion for an arteriovenous malformation, aneurysm, or other vascular abnormality often a CTA head/neck is obtained.
  - Often a repeat non-contrast head CT is obtained 6 hrs after the initial non-contrast head CT to assess for hematoma enlargement. If patient was transferred from outside facility take note of when the initial CT was performed as the 6 hour repeat head CT may already be due.

- Next steps if the patient starts to show signs of herniation? If clinical evidence of transtentorial herniation (dilated pupil and pupil down-and-out) immediately notify neurosurgery to discuss use of mannitol or hypertonic saline as well as ICP monitoring.

Ddx
Necrotizing soft tissue infection
Hypothermia
Rhabdomyolysis
Muscle inflammation / myositis
DVT
Acute limb ischemia

  — Mannitol dose is 1gram/kg IV infusion with goal serum osmolality of 300-310 (side effects include hypovolemia from diuresis)

  — Hypertonic saline dose is typically 30mL of 23.4% saline over 20mins. Requires infusion through a central line (3% saline does not).

  — Cerebral Perfusion Pressure (CPP) = MAP – ICP. Goal CPP is 50-70 mmHg

  — Hyperventilation had an effective but short-lived effect and should be the last measure used and as a bridge to get to the OR.

- **Does the patient have an advance directive or pre-specified code status?** Given the morbidity and mortality associated with hemorrhagic stroke it is prudent to speak with the patient or family member, contact PCP, or examine the chart to assess code status and goals of care.

DISPOSITION

- Likely admit to neurosurgical or neurology team.
- Many patients will be admitted to the ICU. Even if they seem clinically well many will need aggressive nursing care including frequent neurologic checks and strict blood pressure control. Also patients with a high-risk bleed (patients on anticoagulation, or bleeds in certain areas of the brain) will also need ICU level care.
- Some patients, especially those who have had stable repeat imaging, can be admitted to the floor.

BEWARE...

(!) Neurologic deficits may not be present in hemorrhagic stroke.

(!) Be cautious in attributing a sudden onset or different quality than normal HA to a benign cause.

(!) All patients on warfarin who receive FFP for reversal should also receive vitamin K to achieve sustained reversal.

Sources

Broderick J, et al. Guidelines for the management of spontaneous intracerebral hemorrhage in adults: 2007 update. *Stroke.* 2007;38(6):2001-2023.

Caceres JA, Goldstein JN. Intracranial hemorrhage. *Emerg Med Clin North Am.* 2012;30(3):771-794.

Marx J, Hockberger R, Walls R. Rosen's Emergency Medicine: Concepts & Clinical Practice. 5th ed. Maryland Heights, MO: Mosby; 2002.

4 ▶ Subarachnoid Hemorrhage

- Subarachnoid hemorrhage (SAH) can be spontaneous or traumatic.
- Most spontaneous SAH is from an aneurysmal bleed, usually berry aneurysms that occur at the bifurcation of two arteries. They can also be secondary to vascular malformations, mycotic aneurysms (from endocarditis), or malignancy.
- Some patients may have a "sentinel bleed," which is a classic SAH headache that self-resolves and is not associated with other symptoms. It is just as important to diagnose these in order to prevent possible catastrophic SAH later.

Ddx
Migraine
Malignancy
Intracranial abscess
HTN emergency
Cerebral venous sinus thrombosis
Vertebral dissection
Carotid dissection
Seizure
Ischemic stroke
Hemorrhagic stroke
Meningitis
Subdural or epidural hematoma

EVALUATION

- **High Yield History:** Classic history is a sudden onset headache ("thunderclap") that is worst of life, peaks within seconds to minutes, and is maximal at onset. Also associated with vomiting, altered mental status, syncope, seizures, focal neurologic deficits, and neck pain/stiffness from meningeal irritation. Can occur after sexual intercourse or heavy lifting but most often occurs spontaneously.

    — Assess for risk factors including family history, Ehlers-Danlos syndrome, polycystic kidney disease, hypertension, smoking, or sympathomimetic drug use.

    — If SAH is the result of trauma, obtain full trauma history. Traumatic SAH is usually much more benign and the etiology and treatment are markedly differently than an aneurysmal SAH. An isolated traumatic SAH with a normal neurologic exam, no other serious trauma and in a patient who is not anticoagulated may possibly be discharged.

- **Exam:** May be notable for elevated blood pressure, focal neurologic deficits, neck stiffness, and photophobia. In severe cases patients can have AMS and become unresponsive.

    — Perform full trauma survey if the result of blunt injury to head.

- **Diagnostics**

    — **Non-contrast head CT** is **nearly** 100% sensitive if performed within 6 hrs of symptom onset. However, this sensitivity decreases if the head CT is not performed within 6 hrs of symptom onset or if the SAH is minor. Therefore, if there is a strong suspicion of SAH in the setting of a negative initial head CT, then a lumbar puncture must be performed.

    — **Lumbar puncture findings:** Elevated opening pressure and elevated RBC count that does not decrease from tube 1 to tube 4 (less reliable than xanthochromia)

      - **Xanthochromia:** Is present from 2 hrs (and up to 2 weeks) after onset of SAH. Caused by by-products of hemoglobin degradation and is HIGHLY suggestive of SAH. This can be diagnosed at the bedside (then confirmed by the laboratory) by the presence of a pink or yellow tint in the vial of CSF compared to a vial of plain water when compared against a white sheet of paper

- — Labs: CBC, BMP, coags and type and screen. Of note troponin can be elevated in about a quarter of these patients
- — EKG: may mimic ischemic changes
- — **Brain CT Angiogram:** Once the presence of subarachnoid blood is noted on head CT or LP, goal is to determine sources of bleed, not indicated in traumatic bleed. This can detect even small aneurysms, persistent bleeding and can help with planning any future coiling or aneurysmal clipping

MANAGEMENT

- ABCs, intubate if patient unable to protect their airway. Consider pretreatment with lidocaine for increased ICP
- Obtain STAT neurosurgical consult (or transfer to capable facility once patient is stabilized) to evaluate for emergent coiling, clipping or need for placement of external ventricular drain (EVD)
- Control ICP: Head of the bed elevated to 30 degrees. Ensure adequate sedation if intubated. Control pain (this increased SBP)
- Blood pressure control: Place arterial line to closely monitor blood pressure. Must balance maintaining adequate blood pressure to maintain cerebral perfusion and the need to lower blood pressure and reduce bleeding.
  - — Goal SBP <140
  - — Use nicardipine, labetolol, or hydralazine
- Discuss with consultants regarding preference for seizure prophylaxis unless patient has already had a seizure
  - — Keppra is the typical seizure prophylaxis medication→ loading dose is typically 750-1000mg IV x1
  - — Alternate agent is Fosphenytoin→dose is 10-20mg phenytoin equivalent per kg x1
- Prevent Vasospasm: A portion of SAH patients will have delayed vasospasm that will cause a secondary ischemia. This generally happens after patients are admitted early administration of oral Nimodipine (a calcium channel blocker) can improve outcomes. Discuss with the consulting team.
- Treat and reverse any coagulopathy. For elevated INR consider vitamin K, fresh frozen plasma, prothombin complex concentrate (PCC).
- Consider repeat imaging at 6 hrs to assess for progression of hemorrhage. Obtain repeat imaging earlier for any acute change in mental status.

IV continuous drip BP medications		
Medication	**Dosage**	**Comments**
Nicardipine	Initial rate of 5mg/hr IV. Increase by 2.5mg Q15min until desired BP. (Max 15mg/hr). Once goal BP achieved titrate down to 3mg/hr	Most commonly used medication to control BP in ICH. Use cautiously in patients with heart failure who are already taking beta blockers
Labetolol	20mg IV bolus followed by drip of 0.5-2mg/min	Caution in patients who are bradycardic
Nitroglycerin	Initial rate 5-20mcg/min. Can increase by 5mcg/min q5min until desired BP. Max dose 400mcg/min	NOT commonly used to control BP in ICH. Contraindicated in patients taking PDE-5 inhibitors

DISPOSITION

- All patients with a confirmed spontaneous SAH should be admitted to the ICU for frequent neurologic checks and close BP monitoring.

- The disposition of patients with traumatic SAH depends on their other injuries. Patients who are otherwise healthy and have an isolated traumatic SAH often can be discharged home.

- Consider admission for monitoring in patients who have a concerning headache story but negative non-contrast head CT and an equivocal LP, as they may warrant formal angiography.

- Discharge patients with negative CT and LP if pain is controlled and not concerned for other concerning etiology.

- RETURN IF: Sudden onset severe headache, persistent vomiting, fevers, neck pain or stiffness, changes in vision, any focal neurologic deficit, or any other new or concerning symptoms.

BEWARE...

ⓘ Do not be falsely reassured by the self-resolution of an otherwise concerning headache. This could represent a sentinel bleed.

Sources

Aisiku I, Abraham JA, Goldstein J, Thomas LE. Evidence based approach to diagnosis and management of aneurysmal subarachnoid hemorrhage in the emergency department. *EB Medicine Emerg Med Practice*. 2014;16(10):1-24.

Nentwich LM, Veloz W. Neuroimaging in acute stroke. *Emerg Med Clin North Am*. 2012;30(3):659-680.

Marx J, Hockberger R, Walls R. Rosen's Emergency Medicine: Concepts & Clinical Practice. 5th ed. Maryland Heights, MO: Mosby; 2002.

Notes

5 ▶ Temporal Arteritis

- Temporal arteritis, also known as giant cell arteritis, is a chronic vasculitis that affects medium to large vessels and has a strong association with polymyalgia rheumatic.

EVALUATION

- **High Yield History:** Patients may complain of vague constitutional symptoms such as low-grade fever, weakness, weight loss, and arthralgia.

Ddx
Acute angle glaucoma
CVA
Retinal artery occlusion
Retinal Vein occlusion
Lyme disease
Retinal detachment
Optic neuritis
Migraine

  — Consider in a patient over the age of 50 who complains of or is found to have:

    ▪ New headaches

    ▪ Abrupt onset of visual disturbances (acute painless vision loss, diplopia, visual field cuts) usually in one eye and subacute in onset

    ▪ Symptoms of polymyalgia rheumatica (aching and morning stiffness in the shoulder and hip girdles, neck, and torso)

    ▪ Jaw claudication (positive LR of 4.2)

    ▪ Unexplained fever or anemia

- **Exam:** Can have scalp tenderness and pulsations over temporal artery on affected side. Perform complete ocular exam, including visual acuity, visual fields, and intraocular pressures. Also perform thorough neurologic and cardiovascular exam for other etiologies.

- **Diagnostics**

  — Labs: ESR>50 (ESR value of < 50 mm/hr has a negative LR of 0.35), elevated CRP, and CBC, which may show normochromic anemia

  — Temporal artery biopsy (not done in ED; can be arranged as an outpatient test). Biopsy may reveal a necrotizing arteritis with a predominance of mononuclear cells or a granulomatous process with multinucleated giant cells.

MANAGEMENT

- 60mg of prednisone PO daily (start as soon as diagnosis is suspected, as it will not affect biopsy results in the first 48 hrs) for at least 2 weeks

- Patients require a long taper over many months (taper can be done as an outpatient)

- 1000 mg of methylprednisolone IV daily for 3 days for patients with vision loss, and then maintenance dose

- Aspirin 81mg/daily in order to reduce the risk of visual loss, transient ischemic attacks, or stroke

- Add PPI while on steroid therapy due to peptic ulcer risk

DISPOSITION

- May be admitted or may be discharged home, depending on strength of dispo plan.
- If patient is non-compliant, does not have a PCP, looks sick, **has acute visual loss, or focal neurologic deficits** → Consult rheumatology and then admit patient (consult neurology if patient has visual disturbances).
- Consult vascular surgery to help arrange temporal artery biopsy and call PCP. If biopsy arranged and PCP able to follow up with patient and test results and treatment management, you may discharge. Symptoms typically improve within 1-3 days.
- RETURN IF: You develop new or worsening visual symptoms, any severe headaches, focal weakness or numbness, or any severe or tearing chest or back pain.

BEWARE

(!) Treat vision loss aggressively, as patients seldom recover useful vision in an affected eye and some patients will continue to develop symptoms in the other eye.

(!) These patients are at increased risk for thoracic and abdominal aortic aneurysms.

Sources
Smetana GW, Shmerling RH. Does this patient have temporal arteritis?. JAMA. 2002;287(1):92-101.Nesher G, Berkun Y, Mates M, Baras M, Rubinow A, Sonnenblick M. Low-dose aspirin and prevention of cranial ischemic complications in giant cell arteritis. *Arthritis Rheum.* 2004;50(4):1332-7.

Notes

6 ▶ Venous Sinus Thrombosis

- Sinus venous thrombosis constitutes 0.5-1% of all strokes, and 5% of patients die in the acute phase.
- Dural venous sinus thrombosis forms, resulting in increased venous pressure. This leads to disruption of the blood-brain barrier, edema, and ultimately hemorrhage (if the vein ruptures).

EVALUATION

- **High Yield History:** Headache is the most frequent symptom and can be progressive over days. May also present with neurologic deficits (will not always correlate with a vascular territory), vomiting (from increased ICP), visual changes, and sometimes seizure.

Ddx
Migraine
Ischemic CVA
Hemorrhagic CVA
SAH
Optic neuritis
Seizure disorder
Meningitis
Idiopathic intracranial HTN

  — Risk factors: Prothrombotic states, birth control pills, pregnancy, systemic diseases, and malignancy. 80% of cases are in women of childbearing age.

  — Direct causes: Lumbar puncture, trauma, and infection (parameningeal infections)

  — In patients with lobar intracranial hemorrhage of otherwise unclear origin, with an infarction that crosses typical arterial boundaries, or with clinical features of idiopathic intracranial hypertension, a sinus venous thrombosis should be considered.

- **Exam:** Assess for signs of increased ICP (papilledema), focal neurologic deficits, cranial nerve exam, and any changes in mental status, including stupor or coma.

- **Diagnostics:**
  — Labs: Consider CBC, BMP. Coags and HCG
  — Imaging: CT-venography or MRI/MR venography(can provide early detection of ischemia)

MANAGEMENT

- ABCs, treat seizures with benzos
- Start anticoagulation with heparin or low molecular weight heparin (LMWH), even in the presence of hemorrhagic infarction.
  — Guidelines from the American College of Chest Physicians (ACCP) issued in 2012 recommend heparin or LMWH during the acute phase even in the presence of hemorrhagic infarction. However, for very large intraparenchymal hemorrhage, risk may outweigh benefit.
  — 2011 AHA/ASA guidelines conclude that initial anticoagulation with UFH or LMWH in full anticoagulant doses is reasonable, followed by vitamin K antagonists, regardless of the presence of ICH.
- If concerned for increased ICP or severe visual changes, consult neurosurgery for possible therapeutic LP or shunt.
- Consult neurology, and discuss consultant's preference for initiating prophylactic AEDs.

DISPOSITION

- Admit to neurology for long-term anticoagulation and pro-thrombotic screening.

BEWARE...

- ⓘ Be alert for signs or symptoms of increased intracranial pressure and neurological deterioration. If present consult neurosurgery.

- ⓘ These patients can have subtle seizure presentations. Start AED therapy early.

Sources

Kernan WN, Ovbiagele B, Black HR, et al. Guidelines for the prevention of stroke in patients with stroke and transient ischemic attack: a guideline for healthcare professionals from the American Heart Association/American Stroke Association. *Stroke*. 2014;45(7):2160-236.

Borhani haghighi A, Edgell RC, Cruz-flores S, et al. Mortality of cerebral venous-sinus thrombosis in a large national sample. *Stroke*. 2012;43(1):262-4.

Saposnik G, Barinagarrementeria F, Brown RD, et al. Diagnosis and management of cerebral venous thrombosis: a statement for healthcare professionals from the American Heart Association/American Stroke Association. *Stroke*. 2011;42(4):1158-92.

Lansberg MG, O'donnell MJ, Khatri P, et al. Antithrombotic and thrombolytic therapy for ischemic stroke: Antithrombotic Therapy and Prevention of Thrombosis, 9th ed: American College of Chest Physicians Evidence-Based Clinical Practice Guidelines. *Chest*. 2012;141(2 Suppl):e601S-36S.

Notes

7 ▶ Hypertensive Emergency

- **Hypertensive emergency** is hypertension that causes acute end-organ damage (ie, CHF or increased creatinine)
- Though generally defined at a BP >180/120 there is no absolute number that defines hypertensive emergency. The rate of BP increase is more important than absolute number.
- **Hypertensive urgency** is hypertension without the associated end-organ damage.
- Your goal is to determine if this is a 1) chronic elevation or acute change, and 2) if it's an acute change, is this a transient elevation from anxiety or pain (both very common in the ED).

Etiologies of HTN
• Essential HTN: Medication non-compliance
• Drugs: Sympathomimetics, serotonin syndrome, clonidine withdrawal, beta blocker withdrawal, cocaine, amphetamines
• Renal: Renal artery stenosis, glomerulonephritis
• Endocrine: Pheochromocytoma, thyrotoxicosis, Cushing's, primary hyperaldosteronism
• Vascular: Vasculitis, HUS, TTP
• Pregnancy: Pre-eclampsia, eclampsia
• CNS: Stroke, ICH, intracranial mass, head injury, spinal cord injury

EVALUATION

- **High Yield History:** In patients with markedly elevated blood pressure, first step is to re-check the BP with a correctly sized BP cuff.

  — Determine if the patient has a reason to have elevated BP from anxiety or pain; if so, treat and recheck.

  — Ask about signs or symptoms of end-organ damage (headache, chest pain, shortness of breath, edema, visual changes etc.).

  — Obtain history to assess for any precipitations (see table).

- **Exam:** Assess for physical manifestations of end-organ damage or clues to precipitants.

  — Fundoscopic: Papilledema or hemorrhages

  — Neurologic: Mental status, any neurologic deficits

  — Cardiovascular: Volume status, pulse exam

Acute End Organ Signs/Symptoms
• Neurologic: Encephalopathy, ICH or SAH, headache, stupor, seizures, delirium, agitation, visual disturbances
• Cardiac: Acute heart failure, ACS, aortic dissection, chest pain, back pain, shortness of breath
• Ocular: Hypertensive retinopathy, arteriolar narrowing, retinal hemorrhages, papilledema
• Renal: Acute renal insufficiency, proteinuria, elevated creatinine and microangiopathic hemolytic anemia

Diagnostics:

  — Labs: CBC, BMP, UA, EKG, troponin, BNP

  — EKG: Assess for LV hypertrophy or acute ST or T wave changes.

  — Imaging: CXR (for pulmonary edema), head CT if suspect intracranial process

MANAGEMENT

- For hypertensive emergencies, timeline of target blood pressures:
  - — 1-2hrs: Maximal reduction of in MAP of 20-25%
  - — 2-6hrs: Goal BP 160/100
- Potential antihypertensive agents
  - — Nitroglycerin 5-100 μg/min
  - — Labetalol 20-80mg IV bolus then 0.5-2 mg/min. Caution in bradycardia
  - — Nicardipine5 -15mg/hr
  - — Hydralazine 5-20 mg Q20-30min
- Abrupt drops in BP can lead to lost coronary, renal, or cerebral autoregulation; therefore, monitor BP closely.
- In a true hypertensive emergency use short-acting, titratable medications and place an A-line to monitor BP.
- For hypertensive urgency, rapid administration of antihypertensive therapy is unwarranted.
  - — Decrease BP over 24-48hrs with oral agents; if patient has missed home medications start there.
  - — Initiate a maintenance dose of an oral medication before discharge in patients with SBP ≥ 200mmHg, or DBP ≥ 120mmHg; this is optional for patients with lower blood pressure.

DISPOSITION

- Asymptomatic patients may be discharged home. It is not necessary to start treatment in the ED if that patient has close follow up.
- Patients with true hypertensive emergency generally are admitted to the ICU or a step down unit for continuous BP monitoring.
- RETURN IF: You have severe headaches, changes in vision, persistent vomiting, chest pain, shortness of breath, or any other new or concerning symptoms.

BEWARE...

- ⓘ There is no evidence to support a causal relationship between epistaxis and acute, severe HTN.
- ⓘ Always consider pre-eclampsia in pregnant or recently postpartum hypertensive patients.
- ⓘ Do not aggressively treat hypertension in acute stroke (want to continue to perfuse the penumbra) unless that patient is getting TPA or has other signs or symptoms of hypertensive urgency, such as acute heart failure or ischemia.

Sources

Kessler CS, Joudeh Y. Evaluation and treatment of severe asymptomatic hypertension. *Am Fam Physician.* 2010;81(4):470-6.

Decker WW, Godwin SA, Hess EP, Lenamood CC, Jagoda AS, American College of Emergency Physicians Clinical Policies Subcommittee (Writing Committee) on Asymptomatic Hypertension in the ED. *Ann Emerg Med.* 2006;47:237-49

8 ▶ Carotid/Vertebral Dissection

- Responsible for 20% of all strokes in people under 45 (most common cause in this age group)
- Occurs due to intimal tear of artery wall, normally penetrating media with hemorrhage into this space. This results in either intramural hematoma (thrombus compressing the lumen and causing occlusion), or aneurysmal dilation (compressing surrounding structures like sympathetic fibers and lower cranial nerves). Both of these can be sources of microemboli and mass effect.
- Vertebral dissection less common than carotid, and more than 50% of both are missed on presentation

Ddx
Migraine
Tension headache
Cluster headache
Cervical spine fracture
Retinal artery occlusion
Retinal vein occlusion
Stroke (hemorrhagic, ischemic)
SAH
TIA

EVALUATION

- **High Yield History:** Symptoms are headache (often sudden onset) with pain in face or neck (most often ipsilateral to dissection).
    - Patients can also have TIA symptoms from microemboli.
    - Risk factors: History of sudden neck movement or trauma (neck torsion, chiropractic manipulation, minor falls, MVCs, yoga, sports injury to neck), fibromuscular dysplasia, Marfan's, Ehlers-Danlos syndrome.
- **Exam**
    - **Carotid dissection:** Classic triad of unilateral headache, ipsilateral Horner's syndrome, contralateral hemispheric or lower cranial nerve finding (aphasia, neglect, visual change, hemiparesis). Can also present with amaurosis fugax.
    - **Vertebral dissection:** Young person with severe, unilateral posterior headache followed by rapidly progressive neurologic deficit (brainstem/cerebellar deficits – vertigo, vomiting, ataxia, diplopia, hemiparesis, facial weakness, tinnitus).
- **Diagnostics:** No specific lab data is truly helpful; this is a diagnosis made by imaging. However, can evaluate for other risk factors or other etiologies.
    - MRA: Lumen at affected level appears as a dark circle (no flow) smaller than original vessel caliber (which can be seen brightly in a crescent around it) – the crescent sign. MRI can also assess for any resultant ischemia.
    - CTA: Can demonstrate focal stenosis, intimal flap, or a dissecting aneurysm.

MANAGEMENT

- Aimed at stroke prevention!
- Location of dissection is extremely important to guide therapy: Discuss with neurology/stroke consult team prior to starting treatment
    - Extracranial dissection WITH ischemic neurologic symptoms→ Anticoagulation with unfractionated heparin (goal PTT 45-60 sec) or LMWH (enoxaparin 1mg/kg BID or dalteparin 100 U/kg BID)
        - This will usually be followed by either warfarin or antiplatelet therapy (consult or inpatient team will decide this) to bridge to outpatient therapy.

- Thrombolysis with alteplase should be considered if patient meets all ischemic stroke thrombolysis criteria.
— Extracranial dissection WITHOUT ischemic neurologic symptoms→ antiplatelet therapy with aspirin or Plavix
— Intracranial dissection → Antiplatelet therapy, NO anticoagulation
- Provide analgesia for local symptoms of head or neck pain.

DISPOSITION

- All patients with focal neurologic symptoms should be admitted to floor v. ICU.
- Consider discharge home in patients with small, asymptomatic extracranial dissections as long as they have close follow up and the ability to return if they develop ischemic symptoms.
- RETURN IF: You develop severe neck or head pain, have any new weakness, numbness or visual changes, vertigo, persistent vomiting, or any other new or concerning symptoms.

BEWARE...

(!) Always consider in differential, as many patients are missed on first presentation.

(!) Even trivial trauma (example: coughing), in the setting of predisposing factors (see conditions) can lead to dissection.

Sources

Schievink WI. Spontaneous dissection of the carotid and vertebral arteries. *N Engl J Med.* 2001;344(12):898-906.

Redekop GJ. Extracranial carotid and vertebral artery dissection: a review. *Can J Neurol Sci.* 2008;35(2):146-52.

Zane RD, Kosowsky JM, et al. Pocket Emergency Medicine. 2nd ed. Philadelphia, PA: Lippincott Williams & Wilkins; 2011.

Ma OJ, Cline D, Tintinalli J, et al. Emergency Medicine Manual. 6th ed. New York, NY: McGraw-Hill Professional; 2003.

Marx J, Hockberger R, Walls R. Rosen's Emergency Medicine: Concepts & Clinical Practice. 5th ed. Maryland Heights, MO: Mosby; 2002.

Hans L, Mawji Y. The ABCs of Emergency Medicine. 12th edition. Toronto, Canada: University of Toronto; 2012.

Medscape News & Perspective. New York, NY: http://emedicine.medscape.com.

Notes

9 ▶ Carbon Monoxide Poisoning

- Carbon monoxide (CO) binds hemoglobin with greater affinity (>200x) than oxygen →carboxyhemoglobin (COHb).

- CO impairs oxygen delivery to tissue and is a direct cellular toxin.

- It is an odorless, colorless, tasteless, and non-irritating gas, making detection difficult.

- Most common etiology of CO poisoning is smoke inhalation, but have a high suspicion in patients who present with headache and other vague complaints during colder months.

Ddx
Meningitis
Encephalitis
ICH
CVA
Migraine
Tox/Metabolic
EtOH ingestion
Tension headache
Viral Illness

EVALUATION

- **High Yield History:** Symptoms are highly variable and nonspecific. Diagnosis is suggested by history of exposure.

  — **Mild:** Headache, nausea, vomiting, dizziness, malaise, mild confusion, chest pain, or dyspnea

  — **Severe:** Coma, seizures, lactic acidosis, myocardial ischemia, arrhythmia, hypotension, or cardiac arrest

  — **Sources of exposure:** Structural fires, car exhaust, heating units, grills, indoor gas-powered generators, furnaces, and wood burning stoves

- **Exam:** Tachycardia and hypoxia may be present. Patient may be confused or encephalopathic.

  — Pathogenesis occurs through tissue oxygen deprivation, and physical exam findings are consistent with effects of hypoxemia.

  — While a well-known exam finding, "cherry red" lips is not sensitive and is most often a postmortem finding.

  — Pulse oximetry does NOT differentiate carboxyhemoglobin from oxyhemoglobin and will likely be normal. Special portable CO monitors do exist.

- **Diagnostics**

  — Obtain a carboxyhemoglobin level

    ▪ Level only weakly correlates with degree of toxicity.

    ▪ Baseline COHb in nonsmokers 3%, smokers 10-15%

  — Labs: ABG to evaluate acid-base status (expect normal PO2 but low measured O2 saturation), cardiac biomarkers if cardiac risk factors, chest pain, or age >65, and CN (cyanide) level in patients with smoke inhalation injury

  — EKG in all patients, looking for ischemia or arrhythmia

  — Imaging: Consider CT for AMS and CXR to rule out other causes of symptoms.

MANAGEMENT

- Airway assessment: If severely altered and not protecting airway, may require intubation.
- High flow oxygen: 100% oxygen if possible on NRB.
  — Elimination is dependent on oxygenation. Half-life on room air is 300min, high flow O_2 90min, 100% hyperbaric O_2 30 min.
- Hyperbaric oxygen therapy (HBOT) is controversial but recommended by many.
  — Criteria for HBOT (initiate within 6hrs): COHb >25% or >15-20% in pregnancy, severe metabolic acidosis (pH <7.1), end organ ischemia (EKG changes, chest pain, AMS), or if there is loss of consciousness.
- For smoke inhalation with coma, hypotension, or acidosis consider empiric treatment for concurrent CN toxicity with sodium thiosulfate 12.5g IV.
  — Sodium thiosulfate (25%) 1.65 mL/kg IV (maximum dose 12.5 g)
  — Hydroxocobalamin 70 mg/kg IV (5 g is the standard adult dose)

DISPOSITION

- Admit if persistent symptoms, EKG changes, seizures, or still symptomatic after several hours of oxygen therapy.
- Discharge home if asymptomatic and COHb <5% (non-smoker) or <10% (smoker).
- Consider discharge home if symptoms resolve with high flow O_2, no EKG abnormalities, and COHb <10.
- Ensure close follow up for potential delayed neuropsychiatric syndrome (2-40d after exposure).
- Perform home safety assessment and psych evaluation prior to discharge to ensure safe environment.
- RETURN IF: Your symptoms return, you have severe headache, chest pain, shortness of breath, you notice these symptoms in anyone you live with, or if you have any other new or concerning symptoms.

BEWARE...

(!) Have high suspicion for this diagnosis in patients presenting with vague symptoms in the winter months, especially if they are using a space heater.

(!) Ensure that patient's family members are also safe, as this is an environmental exposure.

Notes

Section XII.
Musculoskeletal
Complaints

1 ▶ Musculoskeletal Quick Guide

- **ALWAYS: Complete VS** and a thorough exam. IV, O2, and monitor if more severe injury or systemic symptoms
- **Can't-miss diagnoses:** Septic arthritis, fracture/dislocation with neurovascular deficit, compartment syndrome, vascular compromise, necrotizing fasciitis
- First branch point: Joint pain vs. bone pain vs. soft tissue pain. However, there is significant overlap.

JOINT PAIN

- **High Yield History:** Determine acute vs. chronic; inflammatory vs. non-inflammatory; mono- vs. polyarticular
  - Determine distribution of affected joints and assess for extra-articular symptoms or manifestations
  - Ask about history of previous trauma to that joint or a job/hobby that leads to repetitive stress and makes osteoarthritis, tendinitis, or bursitis more likely
  - Sexual history important to assess for infectious risk
- **Exam:** VS. Full MSK exam. Examine affected joint as well as joint above and below.
  - Assess for effusion, swelling of bursa, deformities, ROM in every axis, and stability. Compare to same joint on contralateral side.
  - Full skin exam for trauma, infection or breaks in the skin
  - Neuro exam including strength and sensation. Pulses below injury, murmur, neurovascular exam BEFORE manipulating extremity
- **Initial workup:** Start with EVERY joint pain patient gets UA, ESR/CRP, CBC, BMP, then peel off tests that are not indicated for your patient
  - X-ray if concern for fracture, dislocation, etc.
  - Bedside US: Localizes effusion and assists with arthrocentesis
  - Arthrocentesis: Think carefully about overlying cellulitis or prosthetic joints. Otherwise, tap every acute monoarthritis of unclear etiology (See procedures section).
- Pts therapeutic on warfarin are safe to tap

- Send synovial fluid for: Cell count with differential, Gram stain, culture, and examination for crystals

- Elevated synovial fluid lactate is reasonably specific for infection. Glucose and protein are non-specific—don't send.

- **Consults:** Consult orthopedics for fracture or infection involving prosthetic hardware. Also, any fracture that needs to be surgically repaired urgently (tri-mal, lisfranc, etc., or any that is unstable after splinting) or if there is difficulty reducing a dislocation. A native hip dislocation needs to be emergently reduced due to risk of avascular necrosis. Get consultants involved early.

Condition	Clarity	Viscosity	WBC	Crystals
OA	Translucent	High	<2,000	0
Trauma	Transparent, pink	High	<2,000	0
Pseudogout	Translucent/opaque	Low	15-30K	+ birefringent needle shaped
Gout	Translucent/opaque	Low	10-100K	- birefringent rod shaped
Septic arthritis	Opaque, purulent	Low	50-300K	0

BONE PAIN

- **High Yield History:** Assess for history of trauma to suggest fracture and ask about malignancy history or risk factors for primary or metastatic bone tumors.

  — Fevers, chills, or other infectious symptoms may suggest osteomyelitis. Patients with sickle-cell disease are at high risk for osteomyelitis.

- **Exam:** VS. Full MSK exam. Examine affected joint as well as joint above and below. Assess for obvious deformities, breaks in skin (open fracture), ecchymosis, or other signs of trauma. ROM and stability of joints above and below.

  — Remember certain bones (hip, forearm, and lower leg) act as a ring and usually more than one fracture site. Compare contralateral side. Full skin exam for trauma, infection, or track marks.

  — Neuro exam including strength and sensation, and check pulses below injury. Perform neurovascular exam before manipulating extremity.

  — Assess compartments.

- Imaging: Image any area of bony tenderness after trauma. Must have multiple planes.

  — Consider special views (scaphoid series for snuff box tenderness).

  — If there is high concern for fracture and x-ray inadequate, consider CT or MRI to assess for certain fractures such as an occult hip fracture or tibial plateau fracture.

  — Consider MRI to assess for osteomyelitis not visualized on x-ray.

- **Complications of fractures:** Osteomyelitis, avascular necrosis (femoral head, talus, scaphoid, lunate, capitate), hemorrhage (can hide 2L of blood in thigh), compartment syndrome, and fat embolism
- **Consults:** Consult orthopedics for open fractures (except Tuft fracture) and long bone fracture. Also for injuries with neurovascular compromise, injury, or infection involving prosthetic hardware. Also, any fracture that needs to be surgically repaired emergently (tri-mal, or any that is unstable after splinting)
- **Treatment:** Reduce and splint any displaced fractures to aide healing and provide pain relief. Provide pain control, tetanus, and antibiotics (cephalexin +/- gentamycin if contaminated) if open fracture. IV antibiotics if concern for osteomyelitis

Describing Fractures
— Open vs. closed (Does an injury to the skin communicate with the fracture?)
— Laterality (L vs. R), if applicable
— Bone name and location along the bone (humeral head, distal tibia, etc.)
— Direction of fracture line (transverse, oblique, spiral, comminuted)
— Displacement (in mm or % of bone) as well as direction (lateral, dorsal, etc.)
— Angulation (degrees off of midline of proximal fragment)
— Impaction (compression or telescoping of fragments into one another)
— Involvement of articular surface (estimate %)

SOFT TISSUE

- **High Yield History:** Ask about infectious symptoms such as fevers, chills, rash or immunocompromised status that may predispose to necrotizing soft tissue infection
    - Any history of IVDU, previous abscess or cellulitis. Any trauma, crush injuries, puncture wounds or animal bites
    - Any history of peripheral vascular disease, rest pain, or thromboembolic disease
- **Exam:** VS. Full MSK exam
    - Full skin exam to assess for infection and perfusion. Note that severe pain may preced the rash in herpes zoster.
    - Neurologic exam especially strength and sensation. Also check compartments.
    - Assess for DVT or arterial occlusion risk factors. Full pulse exam, and use Doppler if unable to palpate pulse.
- **Imaging**
    - X-ray to assess for foreign body associated with septic arthritis.
    - CT is useful for fluid collections or to assess for presence of necrotizing infection. CTA for arterial occlusion.
    - Ultrasound to assess for abscess, cellulitis.
- **Consults:** Consult surgery if abscess in high-risk location or concern for necrotizing soft tissue infection. Vascular surgery should be called immediately if concern for acute limb ischemia. Finally, if concern for compartment consult orthopedics vs. surgery for decompressive fasciotomy.

BEWARE...

⊙ A first presentation of a chronic arthritis may look "acute."

⊙ Patients with prosthetic joints, crystalline disorders, osteoarthritis, and rheumatoid arthritis have increased risk for septic arthritis, and septic arthritis is often polyarticular.

⊙ Always consider nerve and vascular injuries with fractures.

⊙ Patients on anticoagulation can develop severe complications from hematomas (infections, compartment syndrome, etc.).

Source

Ahmed I, Gertner E. Safety of arthrocentesis and joint injection in patients receiving anticoagulation at therapeutic levels. *Am J Med.* 2012;125(3):265-9.

Notes

2 ▶ Compartment Syndrome

- Limb-threatening, time-sensitive diagnosis that occurs when pressure within a facial compartment exceeds perfusion pressure, leading to ischemia and eventually infarction.
- Open fractures are not protective, as they produce only a small tear in fascia.

EVALUATION

- **High Yield History:** Consider in any patient with crush injury, fracture, prolonged down time
  - Most commonly associated with fractures; specifically tibial shaft, forearm, supracondylar fractures
  - Other etiologies include crush injury, reperfusion, arterial injury, burn, restrictive casts or bandages, IV infiltration, exercise, seizures, snakebites, and even small contusions in anticoagulated patients
- **Exam:** Classically the 6 Ps (pain, pallor, pulslessness, parasthesias, paresis, and poikilothermia); however most of these are late findings
  - Pain out of proportion to injury, poorly localized, with increasing analgesia requirement
  - Swollen and tense compartments; pain with passive stretch of muscles that pass through that compartment
- **Locations**
  - Most commonly occurs in lower leg, which has 4 compartments.
    - Anterior compartment is most common. Contains deep peroneal nerve
    - Lateral
    - Superficial posterior
    - Deep posterior
  - Can also occur in thigh, buttocks, hands, feet, forearms, and paraspinal muscles.
- **Diagnostics:** No specific labs or imaging will make diagnosis (can obtain pre-op labs or anything needed for evaluation of inciting injury)
  - Consider x-ray to assess for fracture and US to assess for blood blots or hematomas.
  - Compartment pressures are needed to confirm history and exam.

Pressure measurement

- Only objective measure of diagnosis is to obtain compartmental pressures. In the lower leg, check each compartment.
- Pressures should be obtained by experienced provider and with local anesthesia, as flexion of the muscles in the compartment will falsely elevate the compartment pressure.
  - Normal compartment pressure<12mmHg; elevated. >20mmHg. Still debated, but >30mmHg indicates need for fasciotomy.
  - Can also use pulse pressure (ΔP =Diastolic Pressure-Compartment Pressure) where <30mmHg indicates inadequate perfusion.

MANAGEMENT

- Early consultation: Orthopedics vs. vascular surgery vs. trauma surgery for fasciotomy. Consulting service depends on suspected etiology and hospital policies.
- Treat exacerbating factors:
  - Hypotension should be treated to raise diastolic BP and keep ΔP elevated.
  - Treat hypoxia and anemia to prevent further tissue ischemia.
- Patients who are at risk but not yet demonstrating symptoms should have frequent reassessments.
- DO NOT elevate a threatened limb, as this can decreased arterial flow and decrease the ΔP.

DISPOSITION

- Emergently to OR for fasciotomy.
- Admit for repeat exams if concerned but does not have elevated compartment pressures.
- If discharging someone home who could still be at risk (new cast, fracture, etc.) give clear and specific return instructions.
- RETURN IF: You have severe pain that is worsening, any new numbness or weakness, any severe pain with movement of your toes/fingers, or any other concerning symptoms.

BEWARE...

- ! Must have a high suspicion in certain traumatic mechanisms and diagnose early before permanent damage.
- ! High index of suspicion in intoxicated or obtunded patient or patient when you cannot rely on exam.
- ! The presence of an open fracture does NOT decrease the likelihood of developing compartment syndrome.
- ! Long-acting nerve blocks are generally safe and provide great pain relief. However, in patients at risk for compartment syndrome this can interfere with exam.

Source
Raza H, Mahapatra A. Acute compartment syndrome in orthopedics: causes, diagnosis, and management. *Adv Orthop.* 2015;2015:543412.

Notes

3 ▶ Septic Arthritis

- Bacterial infection of the joint space that represents approximately 8-27% of all acutely painful joint presentations

- Outcomes are poor even with treatment: 30% with poor joint function, up to 15% mortality.

- Source: gonococcal (young, sexually active adults) or staph, MRSA, strep, and Gram negatives. Usually is monomicrobial.

- Most common cause is hematogenous spread, but can happen from direct inoculation in trauma.

Ddx
Gout
Pseudogout
Lyme disease
Rheumatoid Arthritis
Cellulitis
Septic bursitis
Osteoarthritis

EVALUATION

- **High Yield Exam:** Generally monoarthritis. Will have a single hot, swollen joint. May complain of fever or other constitutional symptoms.
  - — 80% monoarticular, knee most common (>50%)
  - — Risk factors include DM, rheumatoid arthritis, prosthetic joints, age >80y, ETOH dependence, IVDU, recent procedure, history of steroid injection, overlying skin infection.

- **Exam:** VS may be notable for fever or tachycardia.
  - — Skin exam to assess for cellulitis, breaks in skin that serve as nidus for infection, or evidence of IVDU.
  - — Affected joint will be warm, erythematous, and have decreased and painful range of motion.

- **Diagnostics**
  - — Arthrocentesis: Never tap a prosthetic joint or through overlying skin infection. (see procedure section)
    - ▪ Send for Gram stain and culture, fluid cell count, crystals, and synovial lactate. Glucose and protein are rarely helpful but can be sent.
    - ▪ Large overlap in WBC counts for infectious (50-150K) versus inflammatory (8-75K) so the key deciding factors are Gram stain and your clinical suspicion.
    - ▪ No bacteria are found in 10-20% of cases.
  - — X-rays of the joint may show other causes of joint swelling/pain (calcium pyrophosphate deposition, DJD).
  - — No serum lab will make the diagnosis but consider lyme titer if suspicious. ESR and CRP (nonspecific) will often be requested by consult service. Consider also CBC, BMP, and pre-op labs if high suspicion.

MANAGEMENT

- Immediate treatment: If you suspect septic joint, treat with:
  - Gonococcus/Gram negative bacteria on Gram stain: Ceftriaxone 1gm IV daily
  - Gram positive on Gram stain, not immunocompromised: Vancomycin by total body weight
  - Immunocompromised or IVDU patient: Vancomycin + cefepime 2gm QD
  - Human or animal bite inoculation of wound: Ampicillin and sulbactam
- Orthopedics consultation for operative washout
- Splint joint in position of function (slight flexion)
- Pain control

DISPOSITION

- Positive tap needs OR for washout. Equivocal results will need admission with empiric abx coverage until fluid cultures grow out.
- RETURN IF: You have high fevers, severe joint pain, increasing redness or swelling, you are unable to move the joint, or any other new or concerning symptoms.

BEWARE...

- (!) Have a low threshold for arthrocentesis since crystal arthropathy and toxic synovitis can look the same as a septic joint.
- (!) Crystal arthropathies can have same synovial WBC count; key is in the Gram stain and crystals.

Sources

Shmerling RH, Delbanco TL, Tosteson AN, Trentham DE. Synovial fluid tests. What should be ordered?. *JAMA*. 1990;264(8):1009-14.

Kaandorp CJ, Krijnen P, Moens HJ, Habbema JD, Van schaardenburg D. The outcome of bacterial arthritis: a prospective community-based study. *Arthritis Rheum*. 1997;40(5):884-92.

Mikhail IS, Alarcón GS. Nongonococcal bacterial arthritis. *Rheum Dis Clin North Am*. 1993;19(2):311-31.

Goldenberg DL. Septic arthritis and other infections of rheumatologic significance. *Rheum Dis Clin North Am*. 1991;17(1):149-56.

Margaretten ME, Kohlwes J, Moore D, Bent S. Does this adult patient have septic arthritis?. *JAMA*. 2007;297(13):1478-88.

Notes

4 ▶ Acute Limb Ischemia

Sudden decrease in limb perfusion resulting in threatened limb viability. High morbidity and mortality; limb loss rates as high as 30%; hospital mortality as high as 20%

- **True vascular emergency** – Potentially irreversible neuromuscular damage within 6 hrs

- Caused by acute thrombosis of any artery or bypass graft, emboli, dissection, or direct trauma

- **Arterial emboli:** Majority from the heart (increased risk post MI or with AFib), however can also embolize from thrombus (from aneurysms or atherosclerotic lesions). Common locations of embolization are femoral, axillary, aortoiliac, and popliteal.

Ddx
Compartment syndrome
Peripheral vascular disease
Vasospasm
Trauma
DVT with phlegmsia cerulean dolens
Vasculitis

- **Arterial thrombosis:** Progressive narrowing of atherosclerotic vessel or intraplaque hemorrhage with resultant clot

- **Trauma:** Arterial trauma following cardiac or interventional procedures

EVALUATION

- **High Yield History:** Acute onset of lower extremity pain out of proportion to exam. Pain can be unheralded pain if cardioembolic source. History of claudication in that leg suggests thrombotic source.

    — Risk factors: History of Afib, recent MI, peripheral vascular disease, and recent surgery.

- **Exam:** Full neurovascular and musculoskeletal exam of the leg. The **5 Ps (pain, parasthesias, pulseless, pallor, paralysis)** are late findings. Initial exam may be notable only for decreased pulses.

    — Cardiac exam with attention to murmurs, irregular rhythms can give indication of etiology.

    — Perform a detailed neurologic exam (including sensory, motor, pinprick).

    — Assess for blue toe syndrome (sudden appearance of cool, painful, cyanotic toe with strong pedal pulses).

    — If unable to palpate distal pulses, use Doppler and mark skin where you hear location of pulses.

- **Diagnostics:**

    — **Doppler pulses** (including ABI: incompressible if > 1.4; normal if 1-1.4; borderline if 0.91-0.99; abnormal if < 0.9)

    — EKG assess for rhythm, specifically Afib due to risk for cardioembolism

    — Labs:

      ▪ Pre-op labs as likely to go to OR

      ▪ VBG, K^+, and CPK→ can get rhabdomyolysis and resulting kidney injury

    — Arteriography, CT angiography, or MR angiography per hospital protocol or consultant preference

- Cases where the limb is deemed "immediately threatened" (sensory loss extends beyond toes with pain at rest, no arterial Dopplers audible, and moderate muscle weakness) can be treated operatively without prior imaging.

MANAGEMENT

- Immediate IV heparin and aspirin followed by continuous heparin infusion (this can be done without diagnostic confirmation, based only on history and exam). This is vital to minimizing clot propagation.
- Vascular surgery consult for revascularization (+/- embolectomy, bypass graft) – ideal for patients with an immediately threatened extremity, as lytic therapy can take too long.
- Catheter based thrombolysis can be used for patients with "variable" ischemia (no sensory/muscle loss with audible arterial Doppler).

DISPOSITION

- To the OR.
- Patients who refuse surgery or are not surgical candidates should be admitted to a closely monitored setting, as they can become septic as the tissue dies and becomes infected. They can also develop significant metabolic derangements.

BEWARE...

- (!) This is a **TRUE SURGICAL EMERGENCY**. Have a low threshold for consulting surgery STAT.
- (!) Do not delay surgical consult if limb is threatened (sensory and motor changes).

Sources

Creager MA, Kaufman JA, Conte MS. Clinical practice. Acute limb ischemia. N Engl J Med. 2012;366(23):2198-206

Callum K, Bradbury A. ABC of Arterial and Venous Disease: Acute Limb Ischaemia. BMJ. 2000; 320: 764-767.

Notes

5 ▶ Gout

- Disorder of purine metabolism leading to increased uric acid in blood and precipitation of monosodium urate crystals resulting in joint inflammation

- Can be due to decreased renal elimination or overproduction of uric acid. Can be monoarticular or polyarticular.

- Exam can be difficult to distinguish from septic arthritis.

- **Pseudogout:** Deposition of calcium pyrophosphate crystals (polymorphic, rhomboid, and positively birefringent).

Ddx
Infectious: gonococcal, lyme, post-infectious, etc.
Hemorrhage: hemophilia, anticoagulation
Other crystal-induced: pseudogout
Cancer: bone cancer, metastatic disease
Trauma: fracture, overuse, ligament
Systemic: endocarditis, rheumatic fever, RA, SLE
Ischemia: avascular necrosis, vaso-occlusive

EVALUATION

- **High Yield History:** Classic presentation is middle-aged man with severe joint pain, redness, swelling, and warmth that progresses over hours to days. Onset generally over a few hours and more often overnight (due to lower body temperatures).
  - Precipitants: Chemo (high cell turnover and purine metabolism), EtOH, increased purine intake, joint trauma, diuretic use. Risk factors include obesity, HTN, HLD, kidney disease, and osteoarthritis.
  - Initial attack is usually monoarticular and occurs in the first metatarsophalangeal (MTP) joint (podagra); other sites include ankle, midfoot, knee, finger joints, wrist, and elbow.

- **Exam:** Perform head-to-toe exam because differential is broad.
  - Look for symptoms that may indicate alternative diagnosis.
  - Patient with gout may have tophi on other joints.

- **Labs:** WBC, uric acid level, and ESR/CRP rarely change Management
  - Arthrocentesis and synovial fluid analysis (WBC/cell count, diff, Gram stain/culture, crystals)
  - Crystals: *Needle-like shape, negative birefringence* under polarized light

- A clinical diagnosis can be made when typical features of inflammation affect the first MTP joint.

MANAGEMENT

- Relieve discomfort, prevent progression: NSAIDs (naproxen 500mg BID, indomethacin 50mg TID, ibuprofen 800mg QID)→ high initial dosing and then taper

- If contraindication to NSAIDs (bleed, renal failure) then consider steroids (PO, IV, IM, or intra-articular)

- Colchicine (contraindicated in end-stage renal disease, renal dialysis, or hepatic insufficiency): Low-dose course of 1.2mg (2 0.6mg tablets) followed 1hr later by 0.6mg (1 tablet), to give a total dose of 1.8mg. Warn patients of GI upset side effects (i.e. diarrhea).

- Don't use allopurinol or probenecid during acute exacerbations.

DISPOSITION

- Outpatient treatment unless the diagnosis is uncertain. Admit with orthopedics consult if concern for septic joint present.
- Counsel about EtOH, diuretics, and what foods to avoid (anchovies, sardines in oil, fish roes, herring, organ meat, legumes, mushrooms, spinach, asparagus, cauliflower)
- RETURN IF: You have high fevers, joint pain that is different than your gout pain, or any other new or concerning symptoms.

BEWARE...

(!) There is a large overlap in presentation with septic arthritis. Do not hesitate to initiate Abx and obtain orthopedics consultation early when concerned for septic arthritis.

(!) Consider joint infection in patients with pre-existing arthritis or immunosuppression.

Source

Roddy E, Mallen CD, Doherty M. Gout. *BMJ.* 2013;347:f5648.

Notes

6 ▶ Orthopedic Splints

- Majority of fractures we will see in the ED will require splinting. Whether the patient is going home and planning to follow up with orthopedics, or even going to the OR in the morning, stabilization is key.

EVALUATION

- Check neurovascular status before AND after splinting, and reduce the fracture as indicated.
- Look for any open areas of skin and or any potential pressure points. These should be dressed or provided with extra padding prior to splinting.

MANAGEMENT

- First apply stockingette with additional length at each end to tuck back under elastic bandage at end.
- When preparing a splint, you'll be putting your wet plaster/orthoglass between 2 strips of padding (7-10 layers of webroll to patient and 2-3 layers of webroll outside of splint). Provide extra padding on bony prominences, and try to avoid any creases.
- The splint will become warm as it dries. Using extra plaster gives off extra heat, and thermal burns can occur. If the patient complains of a burning sensation, take the splint off promptly. Avoid techniques that will cause extra heat to be generated, including wrapping the splint in towels or blankets to speed drying or using hot water to wet the plaster.
- Wrap with elastic bandage, tucking edges of stockingette under elastic, and document neurovascular exam after splint application.

DISPOSITION

- For patients going home, be sure to arrange appropriate orthopedic follow-up. Instruct the patient to keep the splint clean and dry, and give good return instructions for any neurovascular compromise. Provide additional adjuncts (i.e. crutches or sling) as needed.

Thumb Spica		Common injuries: Bennets/Rolando fractures Scaphoid/lunate fractures First metacarpal fractures De Quervain's tenosynovitis Application tips: Use 3- or 4-inch plaster Maintain wrist in "beer can" position with 20-30 degrees of extension

Ulnar Gutter		Common injuries: Ulnar styloid fracture 4th and 5th metacarpal fractures 4th and 5th phalanges fractures Application tips: Place cotton between 4th and 5th fingers Maintain wrist in 20-30 degrees of extension
Sugar Tong		Common injuries: Distal radius fractures Distal ulna fractures Application tips: Maintain wrist in neutral position Keep elbow at 90 degrees A double sugar tong splint adds a strap of plaster from proximal humerus medially around elbow to proximal humerus laterally. This limits flexion/extension and supination/pronation of the elbow joint.
Volar splint		Common injuries: Wrist sprains (extend splint to MCP) Metacarpal fractures (extend splint to DIP) Soft tissue injuries of the wrist and hand Application tips: Maintain wrist in 20 degrees of extension * Can extend to distal fingers to make a volar resting splint used in soft tissue injuries or infections
Posterior Long Arm		Common injuries: Distal humerus fractures Proximal humerus fractures Radial head and neck fractures Olecranon fractures Severe ligamentous injuries of the elbow Application tips: Maintain wrist in neutral position Keep elbow at 90 degrees Apply in a distal to proximal fashion

Posterior Leg/ Posterior Sugar Tong		Common injuries: Unstable ankle fractures Distal tib/fib fractures Midfoot fractures (metatarsal/tarsal) Application tips: Use larger plaster (4-5 inch) Extend from great toe to fibular head Have patient lie on stomach and flex knee 90 degrees for easier application.
Long Leg Posterior		Common injuries: Proximal tib/fib fractures Unstable knee fractures/injuries Femur fractures Application tips: Use 6 inch plaster Keep the ankle at 90 degrees and knee in 15 degrees of flexion Get some help for this one

Section XIII.
Shortness of Breath

1 ▶ Shortness of Breath Quick Guide

- ALWAYS: IV, O2, Monitor, **COMPLETE** VS (including temperature and pulse oximetry on room air or baseline home O2 unless in respiratory distress), EKG (arrhythmias or ischemia), fingerstick glucose, airway equipment nearby if needed.
- Can't miss diagnoses in first 2 minutes:
  — Flash pulmonary edema →BiPAP and nitroglycerin
  — Tension pneumothorax→ Needle decompression
  — Anaphylaxis →Epi-pen
  — Cardiac tamponade→ IVF for preload and emergent pericardiocentesis
  — Status asthmatics→ Albuterol and ipratropium nebs and steroids. If in extremis, consider magnesium and IV epinephrine.

Etiologies *Remember these broad categories as you approach patient*				
Pulmonary/ Airway	Cardiac	Neuromuscular	Metabolic/ Endocrine	Blood
PNA/aspiration	MI/ACS	Multiple sclerosis	DKA	Sepsis
Pulmonary edema	CHF	CVA	Toxic ingestion	Anemia
COPD/Asthma	Arrhythmia	ALS	Opioid overdose	Acute Chest
PE	Cardiomyopathy	Guillain-Barre	Electrolyte	Syndrome
Anaphylaxis	Tamponade	Organophosphate	abnormalities-K+,	Carbon monoxide
Foreign body/Mass	Valve rupture	poison	Mg, Phos	Blast crisis
Pneumothorax		Hyperventilation		
Pulmonary HTN		syndrome		
Flail chest		*diagnosis of		
Epiglottitis		exclusion*		

EVALUATION

- **High Yield History:** Any known pulmonary diseases and any clear precipitants (medication changes, missed medications, infection), onset of symptoms, any inhalers or diuretics used at home, any PE risk factors, recent viral infections or fevers, any thoracic trauma, or any chest pain or palpitations

- **Exam:** Airway assessment, any signs of respiratory distress (retractions, tripoding, etc.). Lung exam for wheezes, crackles, rhonchi, or absence of breath sounds
- **Initial workup**
  - Labs: CBC, BMP, ABG, D-dimer, Trop, BNP, fingerstick glucose
  - EKG: Ischemia, arrhythmia, R heart strain- S1Q3T3 (often mentioned but NOT sensitive or specific)
  - **Imaging:**
    - **CXR:** PTX, effusions (blood vs. infection), interstitial edema, air bronchograms (air space disease=consolidation in alveoli=blood, pus, mucus, cells, protein), Hampton's hump (PE), Westermark's sign (PE), mass, foreign body, diaphragm elevation, cardiac silhouette, subcutaneous air, blebs
    - **Bedside US (heart and lungs):** Global function (good vs. poor squeeze), pulmonary HTN (RV ≥ LV), valvular dysfunction, tamponade, PTX (absent sliding), pleural effusions. Diffuse B-lines in the lungs are suggestive of pulmonary edema.
    - **CT:** Trauma, PE (beware of renal function! Consider V/Q scan in renal failure), mass
  - Direct Visualization: Copious use of topical anesthetic in pharynx can allow for passage of nasopharyngeal fiberoptic scope= look for foreign body. Adding mild sedative to topical anesthetic can allow for direct laryngoscopy = look for foreign body or epiglottitis.

6 Causes of Hypoxia	A-a Gradient
V/Q mismatch	Increased
Hypoventilation	Normal
Altitude	Normal
Right to left shunt	Increased
Diffusion defects	Increased
Dysfunctional Hgb	Normal

Alveolar Gas Equation: $PAO_2 = (Patm - PH_2O)FiO_2 - (PACO_2/R)$

$= (713)FiO_2 - (PACO_2/0.8)$

*$R = 0.8$, $Patm = 760$, $PH_2O = 47$, FiO_2 room air 0.21

*$PACO_2$ and $PaO_2 \rightarrow$ obtained off ABG

*Each L O_2 on NC above room air increases FiO_2 by approximately .03 (i.e.1L NC = 0.24 FiO_2)

*Normal A-a gradient (PAO_2 minus PaO_2) is about 10

Easy Estimate A-a gradient: $FiO_2 \times 6 \approx PaO_2$ (If not then large A-a gradient present)

Source

Marx J, Hockberger R, Walls R. Rosen's Emergency Medicine: Concepts & Clinical Practice. 5th ed. Maryland Heights, MO: Mosby; 2002.

2 ▶ Airway Management

Airway management is the cornerstone of emergency medicine. Preparation is the key to success. You need to recognize when to advance airway management from positioning to bagging to oral/nasal airways to intubation when necessary. The fundamentals are listed here. For further information on equipment and intubation itself, please see the procedure section.

REASONS TO INTUBATE

- Failure to oxygenate
- Failure to ventilate
- Unable to protect airway
- Expected clinical course (i.e. worsening clinical condition, transport, worsening airway compromise)

EVALUATION FOR A DIFFICULT AIRWAY

- Difficult BVM (MOANS; Mask seal, Obesity/Obstruction, Age >55, No teeth, Stiff lungs)
  - Use proper positioning. Ideally have patient in sniffing position with a two person BVM. If concern for c-spine injury use jaw thrust.
  - Use adjuncts such as oral or nasal airways. Keep dentures in place while bagging if no contraindications
- Difficult Intubations (LEMON: Look externally, Evaluate 3-3-2 rule, Mallampati score, Obesity/Obstruction, Neck stiffness)
  - Assess patient for any external sign of difficult intubation including obesity, facial trauma and micrognathia
  - Assess mouth opening, mallampati score and look for any concerning or evolving oropharyngeal swelling or inhalation injury
- Difficult Cricothyrotomy (SMART: Surgery, Mass, Abscess/Anatomy, Radiation, Tumor)
  - Anything that significantly alters the normal anatomy or tissue plans can complicate a surgical airway
  - In the case of a anticipated, prepare for a possible surgical airway→ "double set-up." This can range from having the supplies at bedside to having the neck prepped.

Equipment and Preparation	Backup Devices
Bag valve mask (Ambu bag)	Bougie
Oral and nasal airways	LMA
Pre-oxygenate patient	Alternate video scope (ie, CMAC, Glidescope)
Laryngoscope (check light and/or monitor)	Regular laryngoscope (check the light source!)
Suction device	Bronchoscope
Call respiratory	Cricothyrotomy kit
Adequate IV access	
Calculate medication doses	

PREPARATION

RSI Checklist — SOAP-ME	
Suction	Have Yankauer suction ready, more if anticipate emesis
Oxygen	Start preoxygenation, have passive oxygenation ready, BVM and oral airway if needed
Airways	Have two ETTs of different sizes loaded with stylet and both balloons checked
Positioning	Ensure bed at correct height for you and patient is properly positisoned
Medication/Monitors	Ensure that patient is on telemetry, BP cuff, and has pulse oximetry. Also have end-tidal CO2 monitoring. Choose intubation and post-sedation meds
Equipment	Have your intubation equipment ready and working (check light sources or that video screen is on). Also have back-ups in the room.

- Preoxygenation
  - This is a critical portion of the intubation process. Critically ill patients (ie, the majority of patients you will intubate in the ED) will have rapid desaturations due to increased oxygen consumption. Also, the pulse oximetry reading will lag behind the patient's actual physiology by up to 1min.
  - For patients with SaO2 >90s, place on NRB at the maximal flow. For patients with SaO2 <90% NIPPV or BVM with PEEP valve attached. If able to tolerate, consider use of an oral airway.
  - Preoxygenate for at least 3min and then push your sedative and paralytic in quick succession. Consider preoxygenation in an upright position, especially in patients for whom you are intubating for failure to oxygenate or those who are unable to protect their airway.
  - Switch your O2 source to the nasal cannula previously placed in the patient's nares.
  - Remove the NRB, BVM, or NIPPV and maintain airway patency with jaw thrust if needed.
  - Intubate with nasal cannula in place.
- Positioning
  - Position patient in a recumbent position with the patient's head in the ear-to-sternal-notch position. In specific patient populations (ie, morbidly obese) consider pre-oxygenating in an upright position.
  - Utilize padding/ramping if necessary, especially in obese patients, and place a nasal cannula in the patient's nares.
- Equiment
  - A 7.5 endotrachial tube will work for most adults. Consider an 8.0 tube in larger male patients and a 7.0 tube in smaller female patients. Also use smaller tube choice if concerned for airway narrowing from airway edema, etc. A large tube can facilitate bronchosopy for patients who may need this as part of their hospital course.

INTUBATION MEDICATIONS

For the average expected uncomplicated intubation: (20mg etomidate, 120mg succinylcholine*)

Pre-Treatment Agents	Dose (typical)	For use in
Lidocaine	1.5 mg/kg (100 mg)	Increased ICP, reactive airways
Fentanyl	3 mcg/kg (200 mcg)	Increased ICP or risk from acute HTN response

Induction Agents	Dose (typical)	Comments
Etomidate	0.3 mg/kg (20 mg)	Minimal decrease in BP
Versed (midazolam) + Fentanyl	0.3 mg/kg (20 mg) 3 mcg/k (200 mcg)	Decreased BP
Propofol	1.5 mg/kg (100 mg)	Decreased BP
Ketamine	1.5 mg/kg (120 mg adult)	Hallucinations, good for peds and asthma

Paralytics	Dose (typical)	Comments
Succinylcholine* (depolarizing = fasiculations)	1.5 mg/kg (120 mg)	Onset <1 min, Short duration (4-6 min)
Rocuronium (non-depolarizing)	1 mg/kg (80 mg)	Onset < 2min, Medium duration (30-60min)
Vecuronium (non-depolarizing)	0.08-0.1 mg/kg (10 mg)	Onset 2-3 min, Medium duration (25-40min)
Pancuronium (non-depolarizing)	0.1 mg/kg	Onset 2-3 min, Long duration (60-100 min)

*Absolute contraindications to use of succinylcholine: History of malignant hyperthermia, burns >5 days old until they are healed, spinal cord injury, or stroke that occurred between 5 days and 6 months or neuromuscular disease

\# Note that the majority of these medications, including succinylcholine, are dose based on total body weight. However, rocuronium is based on ideal body weight.

BEWARE...

(!) Always anticipate a difficult airway and have a backup plan.

(!) Familiarize yourself with devices and locations of equipment. Assure that all are working properly.

Sources

Weingart SD, Levitan RM. Preoxygenation and prevention of desaturation during emergency airway management. *Ann Emerg Med.* 2012;59(3):165-75.e1.

Walls RM, Murphy MF. Manual of Emergency Airway Management. Lippincott Williams & Wilkins; 2012.

3 ▶ Asthma

Reversible airway obstruction. Bronchospasm and increased mucus production leads to increased work of breathing. Patient can fatigue and lead to hypoxemic respiratory arrest.

EVALUATION

- **High Yield History:** Symptoms (dyspnea, wheezing, cough, chest tightness)

  — Onset and timing of symptoms, triggers, current treatment regimen, med use prior to arrival and high-risk asthma history (prior intubations, ICU admissions, inhaler use/frequency, frequent ED visits, recent steroid use)

  — Triggers: Smoking, allergens, cold, stress, post-viral, exercise, medications (ie, NSAIDs, beta blockers, etc.), GERD

Ddx
CHF exacerbation
COPD
Upper respiratory infection
Pneumonia
Allergic reaction
Pulmonary Embolism

- **Exam:** VS (tachypnea, tachycardia, +/-hypoxia, pulses paradoxus >10mmHg) diaphoresis, AMS, accessory muscle use, determine baseline BS early, prior to treatment. **Wheezing may be absent in severe exacerbations. Also, evaluate airway for possible future intubation.

- **Diagnostics:** This is a clinical diagnosis. Your history and exam matter most.

  — Expiratory spirometry/FEV1 (i.e. Peak Flow): Best of 3 attempts (best / predicted). Some patients know their baseline FEV1 (predicted)

  — Peak flow should be done on all patients and is an objective marker of severity and to help assess for response to treatment.

    - *FEV1 > 70% = mild exacerbation
    - *FEV1 ≥ 40% = mild-mod severity
    - *FEV1 < 40% or unable to obtain due to clinical status = severe

  — Labs: CBC, BMP, or BNP if concern for comorbidities. ABG is not predictive of clinical outcome. Do not use as indication of need to intubate.

  — CXR: If concerned for infection, comorbidity, or complication (eg, PTX).

  — EKG: If patient also complaining of chest pain or other symptoms concerning for cardiac pathology.

MANAGEMENT

- First: ABCs. If sick appearing → O2, IV access, telemetry, pulse oximetry, EKG
- Is the patient maintaining an airway? What is their mental status? Continually reassess clinical status during ED stay. Start oxygen, early beta-agonists, and obtain baseline peak flow (see chart).
- Oxygen: Maintain SaO_2>90% (>95% in infants, pregnant women, CV disease). Can consider heliox if unresponsive to initial treatments below, but likely to have marginal benefit.
- Adrenergic Agents: B2 agonists ↑ cAMP → bronchial smooth muscle relaxation

  — Albuterol (MDI or Neb) 4-8puffs or 2.5-5mg Q15-30min x1hr then Q30min x additional 1-2hrs

- — MDI and nebulizer equally effective if used properly, but humidified air from nebulizer may ease patient's symptoms.
- — Long-acting beta agonists (ie, Salmeterol) not indicated in acute management.
- — If patient cannot tolerate inhaled therapy: Terbutaline 0.25-0.5mg SQ Q30min to max dose of 5mg over 4hrs or Epi (1:1000) 0.2-0.5 ml SC Q20-30min x3 doses
- Anticholinergic: ↓vagal-mediated bronchoconstriction in med-large airways and inhibit mucus secretions
  - — Albuterol/ipatropium x3 doses as substitute for first 3 doses of albuterol (preferred 1st line)
  - — Ipatropium Bromide MDI 2puffs or Neb: 0.5ml of 0.02% Onset 30+min, lasts up to 6hrs
- Glucocorticoids: Prednisone 40-60mg PO. If cannot tolerated PO, methylprednisolone 125mg IV
  - — Modulate inflammatory response. Indicated in mod-severe attack or poor response to initial beta agonists.
  - — Also consider early admin in patients on long-term steroids, recent relapse or prolonged symptoms prior to arrival
  - — PO has same efficacy and outcomes as IV
- Magnesium: Dose: 2-4g IV over 10-15minutes. For moderate to severe (i.e. considering admission intubation) asthma exacerbations

AIRWAY MANAGEMENT

- Decision to intubate based on clinical assessment, NOT labs or blood gases.
- Consider Bi-level Positive Airway Pressure (BiPAP) for pts with impending respiratory failure not responsive to therapy.
  - — Initial settings 8-10/3-5. Reassess for need for intubation.
- If intubation required, RSI with ketamine or etomidate, allow for permissive hypercapnea.
  - — Set initial vent settings to decrease barotrauma and dynamic hyperinflation (auto-PEEP); this usually requires decreased RR (~10/min).
  - — Tidal volume 7-8mL/kg ideal body weight, shorter inspiratory time and longer expiratory time (I:E ratio).
  - — Minimize PEEP. Also, better to use inhalers through ventilator than continuous nebs, as these can alter vent volume readings.

DISPOSITION

- Repeat Peak Flow after 3rd beta-agonist or 1hr.
  - — **Discharge:** FEV1>70%, tolerating room air, symptoms resolved, able to ambulate without dyspnea and hypoxia, improved pulmonary exam to near baseline
  - — **Admission:** Failure to respond to therapy → FEV1<40% predicted OR 40%<FEV1<70% with any: new onset asthma, multiple prior asthma admits or ED visits, history of CAD, social situation impeding adherence to meds.
  - — **ICU:** If severe exacerbation and not improving, even if not intubated.

- If poor effort on Peak Flow, use their clinical picture to guide your disposition decision.
- If patient received steroids in ED. Discharge on burst PO regimen. Prednisone 40-60mg PO daily x 3-7 days. If concern for poor compliance, alternative: Solumedrol 160mg IM x1 dose.
- Ensure patient has spacer for MDI and properly instructed on use.
- If not on inhaled corticosteroids, may benefit from addition if regularly symptomatic at home.
- Follow up with PCP within 1 week (ideally sooner).
- RETURN IF: You are using your inhaler more often than every 4hrs, feeling increasingly short of breath, you do not feel better after using your albuterol, if your peak flow numbers drop to a danger level (some patients will have an asthma action plan), or if you have any chest pain or fevers.

BEWARE...

(!) Search for alternative diagnosis in patient with no known history, especially older patients. "All that wheezes is not asthma."

(!) In children <2yrs old, cannot diagnose asthma given prevalence of bronchiolitis: 1st time wheezing and rhinorrhea.

Notes

4 ▶ COPD Exacerbation

- Chronic obstructive pulmonary disease (COPD) is a combination of irreversible alveolar destruction, airway inflammation, reversible bronchospasm and increased mucus production leading to the expiratory airflow limitation.

- An exacerbation is characterized by an increase in cough, sputum production, and/or bronchospasm. This occurs in the setting of chronically inflamed lung parenchyma, leading to increased work of breathing and hypercarbic respiratory failure, similar to asthma exacerbations.

Ddx
Asthma
CHF exacerbation
Upper respiratory infection
Pneumonia
Allergic Reaction
Pulmonary Embolism
ACS
Pericardial Effusion

EVALUATION

- **High Yield History:** Acute on chronic dyspnea, chest tightness, or wheezing, often in the setting of an identifiable trigger (URI -70%, pneumonia, medication noncompliance, seasonal allergies, and smoking).

  — High risk history: Prior noninvasive ventilation or intubation, ICU admissions, >2 annual COPD-related ED visits, recent admission, or steroid use.

  — If the patient does not carry the diagnosis of COPD, still consider it in any patient with significant smoking history.

  — Ask about home O_2 use, baseline pulse oximetry reading and any recent steroid tapers.

- **Exam:** Assess vitals for tachypnea and hypoxia – keep in mind patient's baseline O_2 sat may be 88-92; accessory muscle use, tripoding, unable to speak in full sentences; diffuse wheeze on lung exam.

  — Assess for signs of volume overload as many of these patients may also have CHF.

  — Determine mental status – may be altered due to hypercarbia.

- **Diagnostics:** Clinical exam most relevant in the ED

  — Labs to assess for alternative diagnoses including troponin or BNP. Consider ABG for CO_2 (VBG reliable for pH and CO_2, not PaO_2).

  — CXR to evaluate for concurrent pneumonia or signs of pulmonary edema.

  — EKG to assess for alternative diagnosis.

MANAGEMENT

- **ABCs:** IV access, telemetry, oxygen saturation, baseline peak flow.

- **Oxygen:** Attempt to correct to the patient's baseline SaO2. However, if unknown, aim for 90-94% to avoid suppressing respiratory drive.

  — If requiring more than 6LNC or ventimask, consider PE.

  — Monitor respiratory rate closely. Elevated (respiratory distress) and depressed (CO_2 narcosis) rates are concerning.

- **Noninvasive ventilation:** BiPAP should be used preferentially in patients with concern for impending hypercarbic respiratory failure to help resolve hypercarbia and prevent intubation.

- Initial settings of inspiratory pressure of 8-10mmHg and expiratory pressure of around 3-5mmHg
- Can increase end-expiratory pressure to assist with ventilation
- If severely obtunded due to hypercarbia, or if hypoxia is not improving with noninvasive ventilation, intubate.
  - Should be based on clinical status, not any one lab or vital sign.
  - Consider noninvasive if not responsive to nebs but mentating well.
  - RSI with ketamine (powerful bronchodilator) or etomidate.
    - Allow permissive hypercapnea – serial ABGs
- **Medication:** Treatment centers on treating the many components of an exacerbation, including the bronchoconstriction, airway inflammation, and mucus production.
  - B2 Agonists: bronchodilators
    - Albuterol nebulizer 2.5-5mg Q15 min x 1 hour (3 doses = stacked nebs), spacing as tolerated
    - Can be delivered in-line with BiPAP
  - Anticholinergic: inhibits mucus, inhibits bronchoconstriction
    - Ipratropium 0.5 mg of 0.02% solution q6h, often given with first dose of albuterol (also sometimes given with first three albuterol nebs)
    - Albuterol + ipratropium
  - Glucocorticoids: suppresses inflammatory response
    - Prednisone 60mg PO x1, or methylprednisolone 125mg IV x1 if unable to tolerate PO (bioavailability and effect are the same!)
    - If patient is on steroids at baseline, consider increasing dose.
  - Magnesium: 2-4mg IV x1, for moderate to severe exacerbations
  - Antibiotics: For moderate or severe exacerbations. Macrolides are thought to have an anti-inflammatory effect independent of their antimicrobial effect.
    - Uncomplicated COPD (Age<65, no comorbidities, FEV1>50, <3 exacerbations/year): azithromycin (Z-pack) or cefpodoxime or doxy or Bactrim for 5 days
    - Complicated (opposite of above): Consider a course of levofloxacin.
    - If Hospital Acquired PNA is trigger, follow that algorithm instead.
    - If severe exacerbation and clinically indicated: Consider oseltamivir for influenza.

DISPOSITION

- If patient has uncomplicated COPD exacerbation, can easily space to q4h nebs, and does not have an oxygen requirement after treatment, can consider dispo home.
  - Give prescription for prednisone burst: 40-60mg PO x3-5 days. If recent exacerbation, consider longer duration and taper doses, 7-14days.
  - Also prescribed remainder of antibiotic regimen, as well as any refills for nebs.
  - Follow up with PCP ideally before taper is completed.

- Indications for admission (observation if mild, inpatient if moderate or severe):
  — New or increased oxygen requirement (or needed noninvasive ventilation at any time in the ED).
  — Need for nebs more frequently than q4hrs or failure to improve on peak flow after treatment.
  — Altered mental status due to hypercarbia.
  — High risk comorbidities.
  — Inability to continue self-treatment at home (no nebulizer, poor support system) or poor follow up.
- RETURN IF: You are using a nebulizer more than q4h, fever, worsening shortness of breath, dizziness or lightheadedness, confusion, or any other new or concerning symptoms.

BEWARE...

(!) Keep your differential broad. Patients with COPD generally have multiple comorbidities and are at risk for many other processes that can mimic a COPD exacerbation.

(!) Initiate BiPAP early in patients that you are concerned are failing medical treatment. It has been shown to rapidly improve ventilation and prevent intubation.

(!) If the patient is severely altered, intubate early.

Sources

Sethi S, Murphy TF. Infection in the pathogenesis and course of chronic obstructive pulmonary disease. *N Engl J Med.* 2008; 359(22):2355

Bartlett JG, Sethi S. Management of infection in exacerbations of chronic obstructive pulmonary disease. In UptoDate. Sexton DJ (Ed), *UpToDate*, Waltham, MA.

Global strategy for the diagnosis, management, and prevention of COPD: Revised 2014. Global initiative for chronic obstructive lung disease (GOLD). http://www.goldcopd.org.

Notes

5 ▶ Anaphylaxis

- Anaphylaxis is defined as serious allergic reaction that is rapid in onset and may cause death.
- One of few life-threatening disorders seen in the ED where immediate diagnosis and treatment WILL save lives.
- It is under-recognized and undertreated. This is thought to be due to many mimics.
- Does NOT require skin manifestations as part of diagnosis.
- Epinephrine is the ONLY definitive treatment.

EVALUATION

- **High Yield History:** Inquire about trigger allergen (food, abx, insect sting, latex, exercise, temperature changes, injections of any type, contrast, blood transfusion). GI complaints present in up to 20% of cases.
- **Exam:** Presents as both vasodilatory and hypovolemic shock. Signs/symptoms by system below.
- **Diagnostics:** Diagnostics: Hives plus another system involvement, or 2 systems involved after exposure to allergen (min to hrs), or hypotension after-exposure to allergen.

  — Purely a clinical diagnosis; there's no time for any tests!

  — Even if no clear trigger, suspect anaphylaxis if there is: skin or mucocutaneous involvement, respiratory compromise, low BP, or signs of end-organ effect (ie, confusion).

Ddx
Vasovagal reaction
Vocal cord dysfunction
Angioedema
Allergic reaction
ETOH/drug intox
Serotonin syndrome
Mastocytosis
Asthma exacerbation
Scromboid poisoning
Sepsis

Clinical Signs and Symptoms					
Oral	**Cutaneous**	**GI**	**Respiratory**	**Cardiovascular**	**Other**
Pruritus of lips, tongue, or palate. Edema of tongue or lips Metallic taste in mouth	Flushing Pruritus Uritcaria Angioedema Morbilliform rash Pilor erecti	Nausea Abdominal pain (colic) Vomiting (large amounts of "stringy" mucus) Diarrhea	**Laryngeal** Pruritus and "tightness" in throat Dysphagia Dysphonia/ hoarseness Dry cough Itching in external auditory canals **Lungs** Dyspnea Chest tightness Wheezing	Feeling of faintness Syncope Chest pain Dysrhythmia Hypotension	Nose pruritus, congestion, rhinorrhea, and sneezing Periorbital pruritus Erythema and edema Conjunctival erythema and tearing Lower back pain and uterine contractions in women Aura of "doom"

MANAGEMENT

- Epinephrine is the ONLY definitive treatment. Use of other agents (diphenhydramine, albuterol, H2-blockers) is secondary and supportive only.

- There is NO absolute contraindication to use of epi. Use caution if history of cardiac ischemia or arrhythmias, but do not delay epi.

Treatment	Adults	Children
Epinephrine *Administer IV epi if refractory to IM epi	**IM epi (1:1,000):** 0.3-0.5 mL Q5min prn, titrate to effect (EpiPen= 0.3mL). Inject into anterolateral thigh ***In crisis situation:** take 1mL of 1:1,000 epi and mix into 1L NS (this gives you concentration of 1mcg/mL) and run at 1 to 4mcg/min with piggy-backed NS running wide open.	**IM epi (1:1,000):** 0.01 mL/kg Q5min prn, titrate to effect (EpiPen Jr= 0.15 mL). Inject into anterolateral thigh. ***In crisis situation:** take 1mL of 1:1,000 epi and mix into 1L NS (this gives you concentration of 1mcg/mL)
Diphenhydramine (H1 Blocker)	**IV or Oral:** 50 mg, up to 400mg/24hr, titrate to effect	**IV or oral:** 1mg/kg, up to 300mg/24hr, titrate to effect
Ranitidine (H2 Blocker)	**IV:** 50mg **Oral:** 150mg	**IV or oral:** 1mg/kg
Albuterol/Ipratropium Nebs	-Albuterol 2.5mg, diluted to 3 mL of NS, can give continuously OR -Levalbuterol 0.625-1.25mg, diluted to 3mL of NS AND -Ipratropium 0.5mg in 3mL of NS, repeat prn	-Albuterol 2.5mg, diluted to 3 mL of NS, can give continuously OR -Levalbuterol 0.31-0.625mg, diluted to 3mL of NS AND -Ipratropium 0.25mg in 3mL of NS, repeat prn
Methylprednisolone	**IV:** 125-250mg (onset of action is 4-6hrs)	**IV:** 1-2mg/kg

DISPOSITION

- All patients who receive epi should be observed for at least 4hrs due to the risk of rebound reaction.

- Consider admission if any of the following are present, as they increase the risk of biphasic (rebound) reaction and therefore the risk of death: asthma, persistent, chronic lung disease, anatomic airway obstruction, or cardiovascular disease.

- Discharge Criteria:

  — Has been monitored for appropriate time frame and did not require second dose of epi.

  — Is asymptomatic at time of discharge.

  — No wheezing or hypotension at any time during presentation.

  — Is safe for dispo (ie, can demonstrate understanding of discharge instructions, can fill prescriptions for any medications, and has ability to return if they develop a rebound reaction).

- Discharge Therapy:

  — First Line Therapy: Epinephrine auto-injector prescription (2 doses) and instructions on its use. (Adult injector for patients > 25 kg. Junior injector for patients < 25 kg.) Education on avoidance of allergen. Follow-up with PCP. Consider referral to allergist.

- Adjunctive Therapy, standard: H_1 antihistamine: diphenhydramine Q6-8 hrs for 2-3 days. Alternative dosing with a non-sedating 2nd generation antihistamine in the morning, plus diphenhydramine in the evening. Corticosteroids: prednisone daily for 2-3 days (consider 60mg, 40mg, 40mg).
- Adjunctive Therapy, supplemental:-H_2 antihistamine: ranitidine BID for 2-3 days, especially for sig. reaction with GI symptoms or marked hives.
- RETURN IF: You have any recurrent symptoms, shortness of breath, throat tightening, lightheadedness, chest pain, you need to use your epi-pen again, or develop any other new or concerning symptoms.

BEWARE...

(!) Consider anaphylaxis in any presentation of shock. Cutaneous manifestations are most common but not always present. Remember GI symptoms may occur too.

(!) Do not delay epinephrine administration. This is the ONLY life-saving treatment to this potentially fatal disease. Give epinephrine if suspect anaphylaxis.

Sources

Sampson HA. Anaphylaxis and emergency treatment. *Pediatrics*. 2003;111(6 Pt 3):1601-8.

Simons FE. Anaphylaxis: Recent advances in assessment and treatment. *J Allergy Clin Immunol.* 2009;124:625-36

Marx J, Hockberger R, Walls R. Rosen's Emergency Medicine: Concepts & Clinical Practice. 5th ed. Maryland Heights, MO: Mosby; 2002.

Notes

6 ▶ Angioedema

- Self-limited, localized subcutaneous swelling, typically affecting face, lips, larynx, or bowels that can progress to airway obstruction and may be a presenting sign of anaphylaxis.
- Several etiologies. Mediated by bradykinin pathway or mast cell activation with histamine release.
- Difficult to diagnose etiology in ED; **primary goal should be identification, stabilization, and securing airway.**

Ddx
Allergic reaction
Contact dermatitis
Inhalational Burn
Cellulitis
Facial lymphedema
SLE
Dermatomyositis
Sjogrens
Hypothyroid
SVC Syndrome
IBD
Tonsilitis

EVALUATION

- **High Yield History:** Time of onset (to get a sense of how rapidly it's progressing). Associated symptoms: shortness of breath, itching, rash, abdominal pain, nausea or vomiting
  - Trigger allergen, exposures, medications (especially ACE-inhibitors, calcium channel blockers, NSAIDs, aspirin), family history (hereditary angioedema).
- **Exam:** ABCs! Assess the airway. Look for respiratory distress, stridor, changes in voice, degree of lip and tongue swelling, uvular edema. Consider visualizing airway with nasopharyngeal scope if safe to do so. If anaphylaxis, patient may be tachycardic and hypotensive. Assess for wheezing, abdominal tenderness, and urticaria.
- **Diagnostics:** Labs are of little benefit for ED management. This is a clinical diagnosis! However, tryptase levels sent during acute phase can help inpatient team distinguish anaphylaxis (elevated tryptase) from other causes.

Hereditary/Acquired	Allergen Mediated	Drug Induced (ACEi)
C1 esterase deficiency/dysfunction →increased complement→ increased bradykinin	Mast Cell/IgE→ Histamine response	Exact mechanism unclear but thought to be bradykinin induced.
Family history of angioedema, precipitated by stress or trauma, recurrent, can have N/V/D, abdominal pain, usually no urticaria or pruritus	Classic allergic reaction with quick onset associated urticarial, pruritus and often a clear trigger	— ACEi most common but can occur with ARBs — More common in African-Americans — Can happen hours to years into treatment) — Generally limited to mucosal swelling, no skin involvement

MANAGEMENT

- IV/O2/monitor; airway equipment to bedside (know where your surgical airway equipment is located, and have difficult airway supplies handy).
- **ABCs!!** Special care if angioedema near or involving tongue, soft palate, or larynx. If intubation is needed, should be done by most experienced operator via specialized techniques (fiber optic,

nasal, etc.). Consider awake technique first, or anesthesia consult. Nasal intubation may be indicated to bypass edematous tongue.

- Treatment for bradykinin induced angioedema limited and generally supportive; therefore, if any question about etiology, treat as allergic.
- **Most patients get:**
  — Steroid (methylprednisolone 125mg IV or dexamethasone 10mg IV)
  — H1 Blocker (Diphenhydramine 50mg IV)
  — H2 Blocker (Famotidine 40mg IV or ranitidine 50 mg IV)
- Screen for anaphylaxis. If any doubt, give 0.3mg einephrine IM 1:1,000 (limited efficacy in ACE-inhibitor and hereditary etiology), caution in patients at risk for CAD as may precipitate ACS. Can progress to epinephrine drip if indicated and safe.
- **Targeted Therapies:**
  — *ACE-inhibitor induced angioedema*: Discontinue medication, protect airway, wait for symptom resolution (usually in 24-48hrs).
  — *Hereditary angioedema* (C1-inhibitor deficiency): May need FFP, as it will have active C1-inhibitor.

DISPOSITION

- Depends on severity of presentation. At the least, ED observation to be monitored for several hours. All admissions for "airway watch" go to ICU.
- If deemed appropriate to dispo home, needs close follow up with allergist/immunologist, prescription for an epinephrine injector pen, prednisone, and diphenhydramine.
- If stopping ACE-inhibitor, contact primary prescriber because patient will need alternative BP agent.
- RETURN IF: Your swelling returns, you have tightness in your chest, any difficulty breathing, or lip/tongue swelling.

BEWARE...

(!) Protect the airway: Watch for any involvement of tongue or soft palate or voice changes/hoarseness/dyspnea/stridor.

(!) Recognize anaphylaxis: Angioedema may be major presenting symptom of anaphylaxis. Consider early use of epinephrine.

Notes

7 ▶ CHF Exacerbation

- Left-sided heart failure (pulmonary congestion) vs. right-sided heart failure (JVD, edema, ascites, hepatomegaly).

- **Systolic dysfunction** (impairment of contractility (ie, myocyte destruction from MI) **vs. diastolic dysfunction** (normal EF- occurs due to impaired ventricle relaxation/filling, increased ventricular wall thickness, or accumulation of collagen in myocardium). Treatment tends to be the same for both systolic and diastolic dysfunction.

- Patients can present with subacute volume overload (increased oxygen requirement, increased weight gain but relatively stable), in extremis with acute pulmonary edema AKA "flash pulmonary edema" (hypertensive and severe pulmonary edema) or in cardiogenic shock (hypotensive, volume overloaded and with and cool extremities).

Ddx
COPD
Asthma
PE
PNA
ACS
Aortic stenosis
Cardiac tamponade
PTX
Anaphylaxis
Sepsis
Valvular disease
Hypovolemia/Shock

EVALUATION

- **High Yield History:** History of heart failure or similar past episodes, medication and diet adherence, orthopnea (# of pillows), PND, weight gain/leg edema, any medication changes, syncope, exercise tolerance changes, recent chest pain, dyspnea, or any palpitations.

  — Common precipitants: Systemic HTN (leading to "flash"), MI, dysrhythmia, dietary/pharmacologic non-adherence, infection, high output state (anemia, hyperthyroid, infection), acute valvular dysfunction, post-partum cardiomyopathy, PE (right sided HF), myocarditis/endocarditis, toxins (EtOH, cocaine), or medications (NSAIDs, chemo, steroids).

- **Exam:** Vital signs will vary based on precipitant and if the patient is compensated or decompensated.

  — Assess volumes status including crackles, elevated JVD, LE edema.

  — Extremity exam to assess peripheral perfusion (warm or cool?).

- **Labs:**

  — CBC: May show elevated WBC (consider infection) or anemia (consider high output CHF).

  — BMP: May show hyponatremia (indicative of severe failure) and elevated creatinine (mortality is increased in patients with heart failure who have a reduced GFR).

  — NT-proBNP or BNP

    ▪ NT-proBNP <300 pg/mL (NPV 98%) or BNP <100 pg/mL then UNLIKELY to be ADHF.

    ▪ NT-proBNP >1000 or BNP >400 suggestive of ADHF. BEWARE that optimal cutoff values of NT-proBNP vary with age (higher cutoff levels in older pts- age >75 then cutoff >800 pg/mL). Compare to previous values.

New York Heart Association Classification System
Class I: Asymptomatic on ordinary physical activity
Class II: Symptomatic on ordinary physical activity
Class III: Symptomatic on less than ordinary physical activity
Class IV: Symptomatic at rest
Patients with NYHA Class III or IV; 10% mortality risk at 60 days.

- ▪ There is an inverse relationship between BMI and BNP.
- ▪ Renal insufficiency leads to decreased clearance and, as a result, elevated BNP.
- — Troponin: Elevated troponin (severe failure and worse short term prognosis).
- — LFTs: Elevation can indicate hepatic congestion.
- — Also consider TSH, UA, and coags if indicated.
- EKG: To assess for current or past ischemia/infarction.
- **Bedside US:** May show pleural effusion, B-lines, and decreased EF. Eight zone ultrasound evaluating for B-lines that is completely positive (all zones show B-lines) or negative (all zones show absence of B-lines) had positive LR of infinite and a negative LR of 0.22. Beware of false positives in patients with chronic interstitial lung disease.
- **CXR:** May show interstitial edema, effusions, Kerley B-lines, hilar fullness, cephalization of pulmonary vessels (with clinical exam, 81% sensitivity, 92% specificity).

MANAGEMENT

- ABCs. Determine quickly: stable or unstable, and hypertensive or hypotensive.
- Elevate the head of the bed to help reduce venous return.
- Provide supplemental O_2 or start NIPPV.
- If **flash pulmonary edema** → goal to decrease afterload, provide respiratory support, and break the sympathetic drive.
  - — BiPAP with initial PEEP of 5-8 and titrate up.
  - — Nitroglycerin drip. Start BIG (ie, >25mcg/min) and titrate up.
- If **cardiogenic shock** (low output failure) → goal is to treat the etiology, get patient back on the Starling curve, and improve peripheral perfusion.
  - — If bradycardic, consider atropine or external pacing (see chapter).
  - — If hypotensive, first line treatment is norepinephrine; consider dopamine if norepinephrine not available.
  - — Consider milrinone or dobutamine for increased inotropy.
  - — If refractory to medical therapy, consider cardiology consult for intraaortic balloon pump (IABP).
- Volume overload → Give furosemide for diuresis. Give total daily home PO dose as IV dose (ie, if on 40mg PO BID, then give 840mg IV).
- For all patients, look for and treat the underlying etiology.

First-Line Therapies			
Medication	**Mechanism**	**Dosing**	**Caution/Comment**
Oxygen	Increases systemic O2 supply	Titrate to pulse oximetry	Can cause respiratory depression in COPD
Nitroglycerin	Decreases preload and (with higher doses) afterload.	Give 0.4mg of sublingual spray or tab for immediate relief Start 0.3-0.5 mcg/kg/min (typical starting dose is 25 mcg/min) Titrate up q3min **If no IV access:** • Can place 0.5-1.0 inch of nitro paste	Will cause decrease in BP and therefore is very efficacious in HTN, however, do not use if systolic BP < 95-100 **AVOID** in pt's: • Taking phosphodiesterase inhibitors • With severe aortic stenosis • With right sided MI
NIPPV (BiPAP)	Decreased LV preload and afterload due to raising intrathoracic pressure	Start with IPAP of 10 and EPAP/ PEEP of 5	Do not use in altered level of consciousness or unresponsive patients
Furosemide (Lasix = "lasts 6" hrs)	Loop diuretic/ venodilator	40-80mg IV bolus **or** an IV dose of pt's home PO dose (ie, if taking 840mg PO Qday then give 40mg IV bolus) Lasix IV to PO conversion→ 1:2 ratio (i.e. 20mg IV is equivalent to 40mg PO)	• Can cause electrolyte abnormalities (hypokalemia, hypocalcemia, hypochloremia). • Peak diuresis 30 min Lasix 40mg = Torsemide 20mg = Bumex 1mg
Second-Line Therapies			
Milrinone	Phosphodiesterase inhibitor that inhibits breakdown of cAMP leading to increased inotropy, afterload reduction, decreased pulmonary vascular resistance	Bolus 50mcg/kg IV over 10 min then start 0.375 mcg/kg/ min IV and titrate up	For use in low-output HF and **refractory** pulmonary edema. Can cause hypotension and arrhythmias. Obtain cardiology consult
Dobutamine	Pure Beta-1 agonist leading to increased myocardial inotropy and chronotropy	Start 2.5 mcg/kg/min IV and titrate upward slowly (max 15mcg/kg/min)	For use in low-output HF and **refractory** pulmonary edema. Can cause tachycardia, arrhythmias, and hypotension. Obtain cardiology consult
Dialysis	Corrects volume overload not responsive to medical management.	Call a renal consult	Indications for dialysis in general: Acidosis, Electrolytes, Ingestion, **Overload**, Uremia. Add on coags to blood work

DISPOSITION

- Almost all patients require admission given the morbidity and mortality associated with acute diastolic heart failure.

- Admit to medicine/cardiology if improving after initial treatment.

- Depending on the institution, may admit to ED observation unit/clinical decision unit.

- Admit to ICU if patient requires NIPPV or intubation, pressors, emergent dialysis.

BEWARE...

⚠ Acute Coronary Syndrome: Provide aspirin and go through ACS algorithm with early PCI. TPA generally ineffective given low output state.

⚠ Caution giving nitrates or over-diuresing in patients with aortic stenosis, as it may lead to irreversible hypotension.

⚠ If in decompensated heart failure, give medications through the IV. Many patients will have bowel edema and will not absorb PO meds as well.

Sources

McAlister FA, Ezekowitz J, Tonelli M, Armstrong PW. Renal insufficiency and heart failure: prognostic and therapeutic implications from a prospective cohort study. *Circulation* 2004;109(8):1004-9.

Kociol RD, Pang PS, Gheorghiade M, Fonarow GC, O'Connor CM, Felker GM. Troponin elevation in heart failure prevalence, mechanisms, and clinical implications. *J Am Coll Cardiol*. 2010;56(14):1071-8.

Liteplo AS, Marill K a, Villen T, et al. Emergency thoracic ultrasound in the differentiation of the etiology of shortness of breath (ETUDES): sonographic B-lines and N-terminal pro-brain-type natriuretic peptide in diagnosing congestive heart failure. *Acad Emerg Med*. 2009;16(3):201-10

Gillespie ND, McNeill G, Pringle T, Ogston S, Struthers AD, Pringle SD. Cross sectional study of contribution of clinical assessment and simple cardiac investigations to diagnosis of left ventricular systolic dysfunction in patients admitted with acute dyspnoea. *BMJ*. 1997;314(7085):936.

Pang PS. Acute heart failure syndromes: initial management. *Emerg Med Clin North Am*. 2011;29(4):675-688.

Kosowsky, Chan. Acutely decompensated heart failure: diagnostic and therapeutic strategies. *EB Medicine Emerg Med Practice*. Dec 2006.

Marx J, Hockberger R, Walls R. Rosen's Emergency Medicine: Concepts & Clinical Practice. 5th ed. Maryland Heights, MO: Mosby; 2002.

Notes

8 ▶ Pericardial Effusion and Tamponade

- Pericardial effusion is the accumulation of fluid (transudate/ exudate/blood/clot) in pericardial space.

- Tamponade occurs when the effusion causes maximum pericardial stretch→ reduction in heart chamber size and myocardial diastolic compliance reduced→ impaired cardiac filling→decreased cardiac output→equalization of mean diastolic pericardial and chamber pressures.

- Consider tamponade in patients with undifferentiated shock and history of renal failure, cancer, recent cardiac surgery, or autoimmune disease.

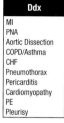

Ddx
MI
PNA
Aortic Dissection
COPD/Asthma
CHF
Pneumothorax
Pericarditis
Cardiomyopathy
PE
Pleurisy

EVALUATION

- **High Yield History:** Unexplained shortness of breath, chest discomfort, malaise, lightheadedness, anorexia, dysphagia, cough, fatigue.

  — Past medical history to assess for likely etiology. Ask about history of malignancy, renal disease (uremia), autoimmune or collagen vascular disease, recent viral illnesses, recent MI (Dressler's Syndrome or catheterization complication), or prior effusions.

  — Trauma assessment (see trauma chapters).

  — Medications. Anticoagulants and other specific medications (eg, doxyrubicin) are risk factors for effusion.

- **Exam**: Tachycardia (>90 beats/min) is almost always present (except for bradycardia due to uremia or patients with hypothyroidism), many have low-grade fever, tachypnea, or hypotension. A pericardial friction rub may also be present, and some patients may have epigastric tenderness from diaphragmatic irritation.

  — **Beck's triad:** Hypotension, distended neck veins, muffled heart sounds.

  — **Pulsus paradoxus:** Inspiratory systolic fall in arterial pressure of 10 mmHg or more during normal breathing. Ddx of pulsus paradoxus: severe COPD/asthma, massive PE, severe hypovolemic shock, obesity, tense ascites. Not often done at bedside.

- **Diagnostics**

  — Labs: No lab data can make this diagnosis. However, they can direct you toward etiology and evaluate for any end-organ hypo-perfusion. Consider CBC (infection) BMP (uremia), coags (especially if planning on placing a drain), and troponin (myocarditis).

  — EKG: May show low voltage (limb QRS ≤ 5mm, precordial QRS ≤ 10mm) or electrical alternans (most often in V6). May show signs of pericarditis (1) Diffuse ST elevation and PR depression, (2) Diffuse TWI, (3) Normal EKG.

  — CXR: Cardiomegaly only present if at least 200mL of fluid has collected.

  — Bedside Ultrasound: The presence of an effusion (right atrial diastolic collapse / RV diastolic collapse / IVC plethora), heart swinging, and volume of most non-hemorrhagic effusions that cause tamponade is moderate to large (300mL-600mL).

MANAGEMENT

- Cardiac monitor, IV, supplemental O2
- AVOID positive airway pressure (BiPAP or intubation) as these further decrease cardiac output from decreased preload to RV.
- Give IV crystalloid resuscitation with the goal to maintain cardiac preload. Consider vasopressor if hypotension persists, but fluid is the 1st line treatment.
    — If stable, initiate diagnosis-specific treatment:
    — Subcritical uremic tamponade can be initially treated with intensified renal dialysis.
- Start aspirin for Dressler's syndrome.
- Emergent surgical consult for traumatic effusions or those associated with a Type A aortic dissection.
- If tamponade or large effusion is present, consult cardiology to have pericardial drain placed. Patients with recurrent effusions may require a pericardial drain.
- Pericardiocentesis by needle paracentesis is the primary treatment→Performed by cardiology if patient is stable and best under echo guidance.
    — Circulatory collapse is an indication for emergent ED needle pericardiocentesis without imaging.
    — Use a paraxiphoid approach, as this is usually the closest to the largest fluid pocket.
    — Insert the needle at a 15° angle to the skin (to bypass the costal margin) between the xyphoid process and the left costal margin.
    — Once the costal margin is bypassed then depress the hub of the needle towards the skin so that the tip of the needle is advanced towards the left shoulder. Slowly advance needle tip while aspirating until the pericardium is pierced and the fluid is aspirated. Save fluid for testing.

DISPOSITION

- Traumatic effusions and those secondary to type A dissection go immediately to the OR.
- ICU admission for patients who are symptomatic or concerns for tamponade. Medical floor admission for effusions that are mildly symptomatic but no concern for tamponade.
- Patients who are otherwise well and had incidentally discovered or small effusion can be discharged home with close follow up with PCP and repeat echo to assess for resolution.
- RETURN IF: You develop any worsening shortness of breath, chest pain, you pass out, have any high fevers, or any other new or concerning symptoms.

BEWARE...

(!) It is important to consider this diagnosis in any patient in with hypotension. It is a form of obstructive shock.

(!) Effusions can have a subtle presentation but have rapid decompensation.

(!) The volume of effusion is not as important as the rate of accumulation. The rapid accumulation of a small amount of fluid does not give the pericardium time to stretch and therefore tamponade can occur with small effusions.

(!) Arrange for pericardiocentesis in a timely manner (if patient is stable a cardiology or cardiothoracic surgery consult should be obtained to perform pericardiocentesis).

Sources

Bandinelli G, Lagi A, Modesti PA. Pulsus paradoxus: an underused tool. *Intern Emerg Med*. 2007;2(1):33-5.

Kapoor T, Locurto M, Farina GA, Silverman R. Hypotension is uncommon in patients presenting to the emergency department with non-traumatic cardiac tamponade. *J Emerg Med*. 2012;42(2):220-6.

Nagdev A, Stone MB. Point-of-care ultrasound evaluation of pericardial effusions: does this patient have cardiac tamponade? *Resuscitation*. 2011;82(6):671-3.

Spodick DH. Acute cardiac tamponade. *N Engl J Med*. 2003;349(7):684-90

Marx J, Hockberger R, Walls R. Rosen's Emergency Medicine: Concepts & Clinical Practice. 5th ed. Maryland Heights, MO: Mosby; 2002.

Notes

9 ▶ Pulmonary Embolism

- Unexplained dyspnea, tachypnea, or chest pain or the presence of risk factors for pulmonary. Due to the embolization of DVT, air, fat, amniotic fluid, or vegetations (in tricuspid valve endocarditis or in patients with indwelling catheters).

- The embolus can cause an increase in pulmonary vascular resistance, which increases the right ventricular afterload. If the afterload is increased severely, right ventricular failure may ensue.

- Smaller clots typically travel more distally, occluding smaller vessels in the lung periphery. These are more likely to produce pleuritic chest pain by initiating an inflammatory response adjacent to the parietal pleura but are rarely hemodynamically significant or cause hypoxia.

- Large embolic lodge in the central vasculature and are more likely to cause hemodynamic changes and hypoxic but are less likely to have associated pleurisy unless they fragment into smaller pieces.

Ddx
ACS
Pneumonia
Pneumothorax
Anxiety
Asthma/COPD
Aortic Dissection
Arrhythmia
Pericarditis

Low Risk PE	Submassive PE	Massive PE
An acute PE without RV dysfunction, myocardial infarction, EKG changes, echo changes or hypotension	PE with signs/symptoms of RV strain or myocardial infarction (as evidenced by changes in Echo, EKG or elevated troponin or BNP) but no associated hypotension.	An acute PE associated with sustained hypotension, other signs/symptoms or shock or cardiac arrest

EVALUATION

- **High Yield History:** Shortness of breath, pleuritic chest pain, dyspnea on exertion, palpitations, cough, hemoptysis, lower extremity pain or asymmetrical swelling, syncope (15% of PEs present with syncope), malaise/weakness or nonspecific symptoms

  — Risk Factors: previous PE/DVT, hypercoaguable disorders or states, hormone use, cancer history, recent surgery/immobilization, indwelling catheters, or exogenous estrogen use.

- **Exam:** Hypoxia, tachypnea, tachycardia. Patients can have low-grade temp. Assess for lower extremity unilateral tenderness/swelling, elevated JVD, murmur suggestive of endocarditis. Wheezing is NOT common in PE (does not exclude PE but makes less likely).

- **Diagnostics**

  — Use PERC rule or Wells' criteria to determine probability and need for testing.

  — Labs: Consider CBC, BMP and an ABG.

PERC rule (Pulmonary Embolism Rule Out Criteria) should ONLY be applied to pts with LOW pretest probability of PE	
Age < 50	No unilateral leg swelling
Pulse rate less than 100 beats/min	No recent major surgery or trauma
Oxygen saturation >94%	No prior pulmonary embolism or DVT
No hemoptysis	No hormone use
Sensitivity of 97.4% and specificity of 21.9%. In pts who fulfill all 8 criteria, the likelihood of PE is low and no further testing is required.	

- **D-dimer** (cutoff depends on assay, typically >500 ng/mL is abnormal) - Highly sensitive (95%) but not specific (around 50%). Useful if low clinical suspicion and normal coags. Several conditions elevate the D-dimer (therefore lowering specificity): advanced age (beginning at age 40), active malignancy, pregnancy, recent operation, rheumatologic disease, sickle-cell disease.

- **Troponin and BNP**: Useful to evaluate for other etiology of symptoms or right heart strain.

— Ultrasound

- Bedside echo: Evidence of RV dilation and hypokinesis. Can also visualize a pleuthoric IVC.

- Lower extremity ultrasound: If pregnant or CT not feasible (a negative LE US does not exclude diagnosis, but can rule in DVT).

- Echocardiogram - **McConnell's sign**: Akinesia of the right ventricle mid-free wall but normal motion of the apex. If the right ventricle is equal or larger in size than the left ventricle suggesting right heart strain.

Assess clinical pretest probability of PE using Wells criteria	
Clinical Characteristic	**Score**
Clinical signs of deep vein thrombosis	+3
Alternative diagnosis less likely than pulmonary embolism	+3
Previous pulmonary embolism or deep vein thrombosis	+1.5
Heart rate >100 beats per minute	+1.5
Recent surgery or immobilization (within the last 30 d)	+1.5
Hemoptysis	+1
Cancer (treated within the last 6 months)	+1
Clinical Probability of Pulmonary Embolism	**Score**
Low	0-1
Intermediate	2-6
High	≥6

— Imaging

- Gold standard: PE CT or chest CT angiogram.

- V/Q scan: If allergic to IV contrast or renal insufficiency. Interpretation depends on your pretest probability and are of low utility in patients with underlying lung disease.

— **EKG:** Usually normal. Most common finding is sinus tachycardia or non-specific ST segment or T waves changes. Can also see a right-axis deviation or a new bundle-branch block. S1Q1T3, while famous, is uncommon and not specific.

MANAGEMENT

- ABCs. Always provide O2 and analgesia.

- Airway management. In patients with respiratory failure requiring intubation, RSI with either etomidate or ketamine for induction is preferred given that other induction agents may depress cardiac function or reduce preload which can precipitate severe hypotension.

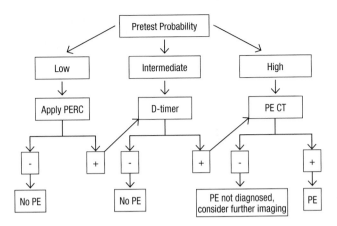

- Anticoagulation is used to prevent clot propagation; resolution of small emboli usually occurs rapidly during the first 2 weeks of therapy (see chart).
- Short-term anticoagulation should be started for:
  — Confirmed PE.
  — Empiric anticoagulation if diagnosis likely to be delayed.
  — Ultrasound evidence of DVT in patient with signs or symptoms of PE (ie, pleuritic chest pain, shortness of breath, palpitation, tachycardia, or any evidence of right heart strain on EKG or cardiac echo).
- In the case of contraindication to anticoagulation:
  — Consider vascular surgery consult for urgent IVC filter placement and/or embolectomy.
  — If above cannot be performed within 12hrs, consider performing baseline head CT and then starting unfractionated heparin infusion at 18 units/kg/hr (without a bolus) and admitting patient to the ICU for close monitoring and frequent PTT checks.

Anticoagulation Options	Dose/Comments
Unfractionated Heparin	80 units/kg IV bolus followed by 18 units/kg/hr IV infusion (goal PTT 60-85 sec). If no weight available, 5000u bolus, 1000u/hr drip in average sized pt. *Reversible with Protamine (dosage depends on time of heparin administration)
Fractionated Heparin (LMWH)	Enoxaparin: 1 mg/kg SC Q12 hrs Dalteparin: 100 units/kg SC Q12hrs OR 150 units/kg SC q24hr **Contraindications:** Renal insufficiency (CrCl <30), HIT, weight <50kg or >100kg, recent or planned procedure.
Fondaparinux Factor Xa inhibitor	5-10 mg SQ injection (dose depends on body mass), safe in pts with HIT **Contraindications;** renal insufficiency (CrCl <30), if <50 kg given 5 mg sc
Rivaroxaban Factor Xa inhibitor	15mg PO BID **Contraindications;** Renal insufficiency (CrCl <30), moderate to severe hepatic impairment
Argatroban: Direct thrombin inhibitor	2 mcg/kg/min IV → if hepatic dysfunction 0.5 mcg/kg/min **Call hematology consult prior to administering** given dosing variability. Effects are NONREVERSIBLE.
Warfarin Vitamin K antagonist	Do not start warfarin prior to starting short-term anticoagulation given ↑ risk of recurrent DVT/PE Should be overlapped with short-term anticoagulation for a minimum of 5 days **AND** until INR is therapeutic (INR 2.0-3.0) for 24hrs. Typical initial dose is 5mg PO for the first two days and then adjusted according to INR. Lower initial doses should be used in elderly patients. **MANY** medications interact with warfarin; be sure to review patient's med list.

- **Thrombolysis**: Use of thrombolytic therapy in PE is controversial given increased risk of bleeding and should only be considered in following situations:

  — Massive PE confirmed by CT with hypotension (systolic BP <90 mmHg for > 15 min.) not attributable to another cause.

  — Empirical use (no CT confirmation) may be considered in a patient under the following circumstances:

    ▪ Clinician can state their clinical probability of PE exceeds 50%.

    ▪ Persistent profound shock.

    ▪ Patient is hemodynamically too unstable or is unable to undergo confirmatory testing.

Contraindications to Anticoagulant Therapy

Absolute Contraindications

Active bleeding
Severe bleeding diathesis or platelet count ≤20,000/mm³
Neurosurgery, ocular surgery, or intracranial bleeding within the past 10days
Recent large cerebral infarction

Relative Contraindications

Mild-to-moderate bleeding diathesis or thrombocytopenia
Brain metastases
Recent major trauma
Major abdominal surgery within the past 2 days
GI or GU bleeding within the past 14 days
Endocarditis
Severe hypertension (systolic BP ≥ 200mm Hg, diastolic BP ≥ 120mm Hg) at presentation

- Bedside cardiac ultrasound showing a dilated, hypokinetic right ventricle supports the decision for empirical thrombolysis.

- Thrombolytic dosing:
  - Alteplase (tPA) 15 mg IV bolus followed by 2 hour infusion of 100 mg. Discontinue heparin during infusion. (IF pulseless 50mg IV bolus over 2-3 min, additional 50mg IV bolus can be given 30 minutes later.)
  - Streptokinase 250,000 units infused over 30 min followed by 100,000 units/hr IV over 24 hrs.

- Consider consultation for surgical or catheter embolectomy in high-risk patients or those with contraindications for thrombolysis.

DISPOSITION

- Depending on patient comorbidities and hemodynamic stability. Almost all patients will be admitted.

- Consider ICU or step-down unit for any patient with hemodynamically significant PE, evidence of RV dysfunction, or myocardial infarction.

- Consider outpatient treatment in patients who are younger, do not have significant comorbidities (ie, cancer, CHF, or chronic lung disease), stable and reassuring vital signs, and have good follow up. Must be able to arrange home anticoagulation.

- RETURN IF: You develop severe shortness of breath, chest pain, you pass out, have black, tarry stool, severe headache, any focal weakness, or any other new or concerning symptoms.

BEWARE...

ⓘ More than a quarter of patients with DVT, but no symptoms of PE, are found to have PE on CT.

ⓘ Most pulmonary emboli are multiple, and the lower lobes are involved more commonly.

ⓘ Embolus can persist on CT for months to years. Chronic pulmonary hypertension may occur with failure of the initial embolus to undergo lyses or in the setting of recurrent thromboemboli.

Sources

Church A, Tichauer M. The Emergency Medicine Approach to the Evaluation and Treatment of Pulmonary Embolism. *Emerg Med Pract.* Dec 2012; 14(12).

Fesmire FM, Brown MD, Espinosa JA, et al. Critical issues in the evaluation and management of adult patients presenting to the emergency department with suspected pulmonary embolism. *Ann Emerg Med.* 2011;57:628-52

Jaff MR, et al. Management of massive and submassive PE, iliofemoral DVT, and chronic thromboembolic pulmonary hypertension: a scientific statement from the AHA. Circulation. 2011;123(16):1788-1830.

Ouellette DW, Patocka C. Pulmonary embolism. Emerg Med Clin North Am. 2012;30(2):329-375.

Davis, Melnick. Management of massive and submassive pulmonary embolism in the emergency department. EB Medicine Emerg Med Practice. Nov 2011.

Marx J, Hockberger R, Walls R. Rosen's Emergency Medicine: Concepts & Clinical Practice. 5th ed. Maryland Heights, MO: Mosby; 2002.

Section XIV.
Skin Emergencies

1 ▶ Rash Quick Guide

- ALWAYS: **Complete VS**, complete skin exam and full ROS
- Can't-miss diagnosis in the first 2 minutes: Meningococemia, Stevens-Johnson syndrome(SJS), Toxic Epidermal Necrosis (TEN), measles, pemphigus vulgarus, and smallpox

Ddx by Rash Type				
Maculopapular	**Petechia/ Purpura**	**Diffuse Errythema**	**Vesicular/ Bullous**	**Pustular**
Toxic shock	Meningococcemia	Toxic shock	Pemphigus vulgaris	Bacterial
Erythema multiforme	Rocky Mountain	syndrome	Bullous pemphigus	folliculitis
Drug reaction	spotted fever	Staphylococcal	varicella	Gonorrhea
Viral exanthem	Henoch-Schonlein	scalded skin	Herpes zoster	Acne vulgaris
(rubeola,	purpura	Kawasaki disease	Contact dermatitis	Impetigo
adenovirus,	Vasculitis	Hypersensitivity drug	Necrotizing soft	Pustular
Epstein-Barr,	ITP	reaction	tissue infection	psoriasis
enterovirus)	TTP	Cellulitis	(late)	
Lyme disease	DIC	Necrotizing soft	Stevens-Johnson	
Pityriasis		tissue infection	syndrome (late)	
Rocky Mountain		Eczema	Toxic epidermal	
spotted fever		Psoriasis	necrolysis (late)	
Scabies		Candidiasis		
Eczema/psoriasis				

EVALUATION

- **High Yield History:** When did the rash first appear? How did the rash first appear? Has it changed in appearance or location? Associated symptoms such as pain or itching? Systemic symptoms such as fevers, sore throat, or vomiting? Has the patient tried any treatments? Does anyone else have similar rashes? Has the patient ever had this same rash before? Any recent new medications, personal care products, occupational exposures, or recreational exposures? What does the patient think the rash is from?
- High risk findings: Hypotension, fever, immunocompromised state, adenopathy, systemic illness, mucosal involvement, petechial/purpura, or arthralgias.
- Rashes can take a variety of appearances depending on where they are in their clinical course and the presence of secondary lesions.

- **Exam**
  - HEENT: Conjunctiva or oral mucosa involvement (SJS/TEN)? Roth spots on fundoscopic exam (endocarditis)? Conjunctivitis with perilimbic sparing (Kawasaki's)?
  - Cardiovascular: Tachycardia (systemic involvement)? Murmur (endocarditis)?
  - *Nikolsky's sign*: The dislodgement of the intact superficial dermis by slight pressure on the skin. Occurs in TEN and pemphus vulgaris.
  - *Koebner phenomenon*: Skin lesions that occur in linear pattern along the site of trauma (ie, scratching). Some examples include vitiligo psoriasis and lichen planus.
- **Initial Workup:** Laboratory testing only indicated if patient appears toxic or febrile.
  - CBC, BMP, LFTs, PT/INR, PTT, consider BCx (if admitted), consider ESR/CRP, ASO titer. Serologies indicated if certain infectious causes suspected (eg, Lyme IgM, IgG).

Primary Lesions: terms to describe the first visual lesion/skin changes	Secondary Lesions: evolved changes of the skin disorder
Macule: Nonpalpable lesions that vary in pigmentation from the surrounding skin and are less than 2cm in diameter. There are **no** elevations or depressions.	**Excoriation:** Superficial skin erosion caused by scratching
Patch: Same quality as a macule except diameter is >2cm. Macules can coalesce to create patches	**Lichenification:** Increased skin markings and thickening with induration secondary to chronic inflammation caused by scratching or other irritation
Papule: Palpable, discrete lesions measuring ≤5mm in diameter	**Scale:** Superficial epidermal cells that are dead and cast off from the skin
Nodule: Palpable, discrete lesions measuring ≥6mm in diameter	**Crust:** Dried exudate. Also known as a scab
Tumor: Large nodule	**Fissure:** Deep skin split extending into the dermis
Plaque: Large (>5mm) superficial **flat** lesions. Can be formed by a confluence of papules	**Erosion:** Superficial, focal loss of part of the epidermis
Pustules: Small, circumscribed skin papules that contain **purulent** material	**Ulceration:** Focal loss of epidermis that extends down into the dermis
Vesicles: Small (<5mm diameter) circumscribed skin papules that contain **serous** material	**Atrophy:** Decreased skin thickness due to skin thinning
Bullae: Large (≥6mm diameter) vesicles	**Scar:** Abnormal fibrous tissue that replaces normal tissue after injury
Wheal: Irregularly elevated edematous skin areas that are often erythematous and migratory in nature	**Hypopigmentation:** Decreased skin pigment
	Hyperpigmentation: Increased skin pigment
Telangiectasia: Dilated superficial blood vessel	**Depigmentation:** Total loss of skin pigment

Specific Rashes and Treatments		
Diagnosis	**Clinical Syndrome**	**Treatment**
Staphylococcal scalded skin	Children, due to endotoxins of *s. aureus*. Widespread, fluid-filled blisters, erythroderma, and desquamation	Treat the underlying staph infection (naficillin or vancomycin), antipyretics, IVF, and wound care

Toxic shock syndrome	Caused by toxin of s.*aureus*. Fever, hypotension and sunburn like diffuse erythematous rash involving palms, soles, mucus membranes with desquamation in 1-2 weeks. Associated with tampon use	Infection control (drain abscess, remove source i.e. tampon or nasal packing), antibiotics against staph (Vancomycin, cephalosporin or PCN) IVF and supportive care. Floor versus ICU admission
Stevens-Johnson syndrome (SJS)/ Toxic epidermal necrolysis	Severe mucocutaneous reactions with extensive necrosis. Usually at least 2 mucosal surfaces involves (oral, eye or genital). Most often a drug reaction (sulfa) or from infection. SJS and TEN have same pathology but is called **SJS when <10%TBSA involved** and **TEN when >30% TBSA**	Stop suspected culprit medication (most commonly antibiotics, AEDs, NSAIDs) **Dermatology consult** (and ophtho or gyn if those systems involved) Likely Burn ICU admission for aggressive fluid/electrolyte Management Early intubation may be needed if significant airway involvement. ED treatment mostly supportive; consider cyclosporine, plasmapheresis, IVIG
Measles (Rubeola)	A specific type of viral exanthema. Infection characterized by coryza, cough, conjunctivitis, fever, and rash that spreads from head to toe. Also with oral lesions called Koplik's spots	Increasing case numbers due to decreased vaccination. Self-liming and generally just supportive care. **Highly infectious**: Report all suspected cased to the CDC,
Erythema multiforme (major or minor)	**Minor**: Raised, edematous targetoid lesions with acral distribution **Major**: Similar to minor but with involvement of mucus membranes involving <10% TBSA Causes include infection, medications, vasculitis or malignancy	Treat underlying illness; stop offending medication, topical steroids. **Dermatology consult** and ophthalmology if there is ocular involvement
Meningococcemia	Vaccine preventable, from Neisseria meningitis. Petechial rash usually over trunk and lower extremities that can progress to purpura and ecchymosis	Ceftriaxone 2gm IV, isolate and treat sick contacts
Scabies	Small, pruritic, erythematous papule with excoriation and associated with liner lesions (burrows). Distributed over extensor surfaces, waist, and web spaces of fingers	Ivermectin 200mcg/kg PO x 1 and then again in 2 weeks. Or, permethrin 5% cream
Eczema	Pruritic, erythematous, scaly, and crusted lesions over flexor surfaces. Patients generally have a history of atopy or had an allergic contact exposure (soaps, etc.)	Moisturizures or ointments. Antihistamines for pruritus, and topical steroids.
Necrotizing fasciitis	Infection of the deeper tissues, rapidly progressive	See chapter. Surgery consult, broad-spectrum abx
Pemphigus vulgaris	Chronic autoimmune disease. Flat bullae with positive Nikolsky sign. Involves the mucus membranes, often painful	Admit, dermatology consult, systemic steroids, supportive care

Henoch-Schonlein purpura	Children, with associated arthalgia, hematuria, and GI symptoms. Palpable purpura in lower extremities and buttocks	Symptomatic treatment. If systemically ill, admit.
Herpes Zoster (shingles)	Reactivation of varicella zoster from a sensory ganglia → erythematous papules along a unilateral sensory dermatome that evolve into grouped vesicles. Pain-only dermatome may precede rash.	Acyclovir 500mg 5x/day x 7-14 days or valacyclovir 1000mg PO TID x 7-14 days Pain control

MANAGEMENT

- Treatment based on rash etiology.
  - — Viral exanthema → supportive care
  - — Candidiasis → 1% Clotrimazole cream or 1% terbinafine. If extensive, consider oral agent.
  - — Contact dermatitis or eczema → 1% hydrocortisone cream
  - — Treat pruritus with diphenhydramine hydroxazine
- When documenting or speaking to a consultant, **use words to create the picture** by including: location of lesions, type of lesion, shape of lesion, arrangement of lesions (ie, scattered, grouped, linear, solitary, clusters), color, border, and secondary changes.

Rashes involving Palms and Soles
Meningococcemia
Rickettsia
Syphilis
Toxic shock syndrome
Ehrlichia
Coxsackievirus
Kawasaki disease

DISPOSITION

- Majority of rashes will be benign and will be safely discharged home with close primary care follow-up and referral to dermatology if indicated.
- If patient is toxic-appearing or febrile, more severe pathophysiology must be suspected, with low threshold for admission for observation to ensure a more dangerous process is not evolving.
- RETURN IF: High fevers, severe pain, rash is not improving or is progressing, spreads to mouth or genitals, or any other new or concerning symptoms.

BEWARE...

- ! Always examine mucosal membranes.
- ! Concerning symptoms/signs include severe pain, high fevers, hypotension, rapidly progressive, at BSA >10%, involvement of the mucosa, positive Nikolsky sign, or any petechial/purpura.
- ! Treat TEN as a burn and provide appropriate fluid resuscitation, electrolyte repletion, and pain control.
- ! Rash in setting of fever, hypotension, and recent foreign body (ie, tampon or nasal packing, etc.) → Think about toxic shock.

Further Reading

Nguyen T, Freedman J. Dermatologic Emergencies: Diagnosing and Managing Life-Threatening Rashes. *EMPractice.net*. September 2002;4:9.

Usatine RP, Sandy, N. Dermatologic Emergencies. *AAFP*. October 2010;82:7.

2 ▶ Abscess

Abscess: Localized collection of pus, with or without a component of surrounding cellulitis

EVALUATION

Ddx
Cellulitis
Necrotizing soft tissue infection
Cyst
Hematoma
Lymph node
Hidradenitis suppurativa

- **High Yield History:** Ask patients about (1) any trauma preceding the infection (cuts from glass or punctures from metal, suggesting the need to look for a foreign body in the abscess cavity); (2) animal bites or certain exposures such as saltwater/freshwater, which might require different antibiotics for associated cellulitis; and (3) comorbidities such as diabetes.

- **Exam:** Fever and tachycardic suggest an alternate diagnosis or more complicated infection.

  — Determine whether there is surrounding induration, or red streaking of the skin proximally (which would suggest lymphangitis/spreading of the infection via lymphatics/overlying cellulitis). Pain out of proportion to exam or crepitus suggests necrotizing fasciitis.

  — Fluctuance (ie, when you apply digital pressure over the area, you can push and feel a "give", indicating the presence of fluid underneath).

  — Pointing (the abscess center starts to stick up, as the overlying skin starts to thin from the pressure of fluid underneath).

- **Imaging:** X-rays are only needed if an underlying foreign body is suspected. Soft-tissue ultrasound can be helpful; this is best done with a high-frequency linear probe, since most abscesses are superficial. If you do ultrasound the area, take note of the width and depth of the abscess cavity to help guide the size of your incision.

MANAGEMENT

- Surgical I&D is the DEFINITIVE treatment of a soft-tissue abscess; antibiotics alone are ineffective. In uncomplicated cases, the drainage of a suppurative focus results in resolution of symptoms and antibiotics are not necessary.

- DON'T BE SHY! You want to open the abscess cavity enough to drain it completely and prevent reformation.

EQUIPMENT

**NOTE: Although sterility is impossible during I&D, avoid contamination of surrounding tissue.

- ~ Standard suture tray
- ~ No. 11 blade scalpel
- ~ Packing gauze
- ~ Hemostat
- ~ Dressing supplies (wound dressing or dry gauze with tape)

- ~ Local anesthetic (1% lidocaine)
- ~ Sterile gauze
- ~ Skin antiseptic agent
- ~ Syringe with 25-gauge needle for anesthetic

PROCEDURE

- **Anesthesia**
  - Local anesthetic often does not work well, in part because the amount of pressure in the abscess cavity makes it hard to infiltrate a large-enough amount, and in part because of the poor function of local anesthetic in the low pH of the infected tissue.
  - Therefore, in areas where it is feasible, a REGIONAL NERVE block or a RING/FIELD block can provide better anesthesia than local infiltration directly over the site of incision.
  - NOTE: Lack of adequate anesthesia is the most common limiting factor in ED I&D. If the abscess cannot be fully I&D'ed because of inadequate local anesthesia, providers should consider procedural sedation or move to the OR for management under general anesthesia.

- **I&D:**
  - Make a longitudinal incision through the most fluctuant part of the abscess. WHEN possible, make the incision along the plane of/parallel to Langer's lines, to improve cosmesis once the abscess opening heals.
  - Use the tips of a clamp to explore the abscess cavity, to open /disrupt individual pockets of pus, and to ensure thorough drainage.
  - Pack the wound with a strip of gauze packing **IF the abscess is >5cm in diameter**, if a pilonidal abscess was drained, or if the patient is immunocompromised or has diabetes. There is no clear benefit to packing abscesses <5cm in healthy patients and it may increase pain.

- **Post-Procedural Care:**
  - Where possible, patients should elevate the affected area.
  - Gauze packing should remain in place for at least 1 day, but ideally until the first follow-up visit in 1-3 days.
  - At the next visit, patients can be taught to remove the gauze and repack it themselves. (If you think a patient will be unable to do this, because of pain or anxiety, then a family member or friend may be taught how, or the patient may need further follow-up in a wound care clinic or the ED.)

The LOOP technique for abscess I&D is an alternative option. This consists of making two small incisions (~5mm each) at opposite ends of the most fluctuant area of an abscess, threading a vessel loop or thin Penrose drain through (usually with the help of a curved hemostat or a needle driver), and then tying the loop ends to secure it into a circle.

- Vessel loops are thin, rubbery strings made of silicone that surgeons often use to tie around and mark vessels in their surgical field. Since this method is still relatively new, you will probably not find large quantities of vessel loop material stocked in your ED. If you can't find it in your procedural area or supply room, ask a charge nurse or ED coordinator if they can request if for you from the OR.
- The advantages of the LOOP technique include:
  - Less scarring (2 small incisions instead of 1 long one)

- Easier care for patients. Many abscesses are in locations that are hard for patients to see themselves (ie, back of the legs, buttocks). The loop can be felt and moved periodically by the patient to enhance drainage
- The loop will stay in as long as the knot is secure and the loop is not cut, allowing for continued drainage and preventing abscess reformation
- For more instructions on how to do this procedure, see the video by Dr. Rob Ormon of ER Cast: http://vimeo.com/19580472.

CLINICAL PEARLS

- MRSA has now become the most common identifiable cause of community-acquired skin and soft-tissue infections in many metropolitan areas in the United States.
- In some cases a patient may seek treatment for a draining abscess that appears to have already undergone spontaneous rupture, or that a patient has tried to puncture themselves to attempt drainage. In most cases, a formal I&D and packing procedure in the ER will be helpful in eliminating the infection, even though there may not be copious drainage of pus.

ANTIBIOTICS

- Consider antibiotics for immunocompromised patients (ie, patients with AIDS or diabetes, patients receiving chemotherapy or steroids, transplant recipients, and alcoholic patients) and for the immunocompetent patient with "significant" cellulitis, lymphangitis, or systemic symptoms, such as chills or fever.
- Because the bacteriology of abscesses is complicated and multifactorial, no SINGLE antibiotic can be recommended.
  - When cutaneous CA-MRSA infection presents as an abscess, incision and drainage remains the mainstay of therapy. Antibiotics are not indicated for many patients. However, they may be helpful to limit the spread of infection. Therefore, after I&D of suspected or confirmed CA-MRSA skin abscesses, initiation of empirical or culture-guided therapy with a systemic antimicrobial agent can be considered. A minimum of 10-14 days of therapy is usually necessary.
  - In geographic areas with high rates of outpatient MRSA infections, use oral antibiotics to which most strains of MRSA are susceptible (ie, sulfamethoxazole/trimethoprim, clindamycin, or tetracycline) for empirical treatment.
- For abscesses with a cellulitis component related to cat or dog bites, treatment should include an antibiotic that will cover for Pasteurella species (amoxicillin/clavulanate or cefuroxime). Consider adding coverage for pseudomonas species.
- For human bite-related infections, augmentin can be used if the injury is treated early before infection develops; otherwise, IV ampicillin/sulbactam or ticarcillin/clavulanate should be used.
- For seawater/shellfish-related infections, cover for Vibrio species with tetracycline or an aminglycoside. For freshwater exposures, cover for Aeromonas hydrophila by using a fluoroquinolone or sulfamethoxazole/trimethoprim.

Sources

Available at http://www.proceduresconsult.com/medical-procedures/incision-and-drainage-of-cutaneous-abscesses-EM-029-procedure.aspx#.

Fitch MT, Manthey DE, Mcginnis HD, Nicks BA, Pariyadath M. Videos in clinical medicine. Abscess incision and drainage. *N Engl J Med*. 2007;357(19):e20.

Ladde JG, Baker S, Rodgers CN, Papa L. The loop technique: a novel incision and drainage technique in the treatment of skin abscesses in a pediatric ED. *Am J Emerg Med*. 2014.

Notes

3 ▶ Animal Bites

- In mammalian bites (including humans!), must assess for damage to the underlying structures as well as the infection risk.

- Dog bites are often crush and avulsion injuries due to duller teeth and stronger jaw.

- Cats have sharper teeth and weaker jaw; therefore, these injuries tend be puncture wounds than can inoculate joints or bones.

- Should keep high suspicion for fight bites in anyone who presents with a laceration to the hand or a boxer's fracture.

Considerations/Ddx
Infection
Retained foreign body
Crush injury→compartment syndrome
Joint inoculation
Tenosynovitis
Rabies exposure
HIV, Hep B, Hep C exposure
Fracture
Nerve or arterial damage
Child abuse

EVALUATION

- **High Yield History:** Time and location of event, type of animal and its health status (rabies vaccination history, behavior, whereabouts), number and location of wounds, any signs or symptoms of infection, any parasthesias, numbness, or weakness distal to injury.

  Past medical history: Immunocompromised, peripheral vascular disease, DM, immunization history (rabies, tetanus).

- **High Yield Exam:** Check distal neurovascular exam. Assess for tendon involvement, bone injury, joint space violation, visceral injury. Assess for retained foreign bodies or teeth. Assess for signs of infection.

- **Inspection:** Identify depth of wound (visualizing bottom), exclude injury to deeper structures.

- **Diagnostics:**

  — Laboratory testing usually not indicated UNLESS significant trauma or signs of systemic illness. Wound cultures are generally unhelpful unless obvious infection.

  — X-ray or US for deep wounds or those near joints to assess for retained foreign body, joint involvement, or to assess for SQ air or other signs of infection. Also obtain x-ray if concerned for traumatic injury.

  — In young children with dog bites to the head, consider a head CT to assess for skull fracture.

MANAGEMENT

- If significant trauma→ ABCs, apply direct pressure to active bleeding, and treat as blunt or penetrating trauma (see sections).

- **Wound Care:** Remove any foreign bodies and perform copious irrigation.

  — Debridement: Remove devitalized tissue, particulate matter, and clots, because they serve as nidus for infection!

- **Closure:** Consider delayed primary closure or healing by secondary intention.

  — Factors to consider: Cosmetics, function, risk factors for infection (animal and patients medical history)

- — Consider closure for:
    - ▪ The face has an excellent blood supply, and cosmesis is important.
    - ▪ Simple bite wounds (particularly dog) that are early (<12hrs), without signs of infection, and not on the hand or foot.
- — Do not close:
    - ▪ Extremities, especially wounds to the hands and feet.
    - ▪ Deep puncture wounds or crush injuries, especially those by a cat.
    - ▪ Older wounds (>12hrs) or those in patients at higher risk for infection.
- Consider surgical consultation for large or high-risk wounds.
- Tetanus shot if last one >10yrs ago.
- **Rabies PPx**
    - — If the animal can be isolated and monitored for 10 days or can be tested for rabies → No need for PPx; alert animal control and monitor animal.
    - — If animal unavailable, acting abnormally or tests positive:
        - ▪ If not previously vaccinated:
        - ▪ Rabies immunoglobulin 20units/kg injected directly into wound. If cannot fit entire volume, remainder is IM injection.
        - ▪ Rabies vaccine on days 0, 3, 7, and 14 (if immunosuppressed, add day 28).
        - ▪ If previously vaccinated, just rabies vaccine on days 0 and 3.
- **Antibiotics:** PPx only in high-risk wounds (ie, immunocompromised patients, deep puncture wounds, crush injures [devascularize] or wounds to hands, feet, or face). Infected wounds generally require IV abx.
    - — Want to cover usual skin flora as well as P. multocida and anaerobes.
    - — **Oral agents:**
        - ▪ Amoxicillin-clavulanate 875mg/125mg BID
        - ▪ Doxycycline 100mg BID or sulfamethoxazole/trimethoprim 1DS tab BID *PLUS* metronidazole 500mg TID or clindamycin 450mg TID
    - — **IV agents:**
        - ▪ Ampicillin-sulbactam 3gm Q6hrs
        - ▪ Piperacillin-tazobactam 4.5mg Q8hrs

DISPOSITION

- Typically patients can be discharged home with close follow-up within 1-2 days, especially for open wounds.
- Admit if: High-risk wound, infection present, or other traumatic injuries.
- RETURN IF: Any fever, redness or purulent drainage from wound, numbness or weakness distal to wound, severe pain or swelling, any other new or concerning symptoms.

BEWARE...

(!) **Do not** use skin glue to close these wounds. If they do become infected, closure with skin glue can interfere with treatment.

(!) Treat deep animal scratches as similar to bites, because of similar infection risk and organisms (animals lick their paws).

Sources

Rupprecht CE, Gibbons RV. Clinical practice. Prophylaxis against rabies. *N Engl J Med.* 2004;351(25):2626-35.

Endom EE. Initial Management of Animal Bites. In: UpToDate. Danzl DF (Ed), *UpToDate*, Waltham, MA.

Notes

4 ▶ Cellulitis

Cellulitis: Skin infection involving that extends into the deeper layers of the skin including the deer dermis and the subcutaneous fat.

Erysipelas: Infection involving the more superficial layers of the skin specifically the upper dermis.

Ddx
Burns
Toxic shock syndrome
Septic arthritis
Contact Dermatitis
Acute gout
Vasculitis
Osteomyelitis
Herpes Zoster
DVT
Erythema-Migrans
Bursitis
Venous stasis
Necrotizing soft tissue infection

EVALUATION

- Generally occurs due a break in the skin (ie, penetrating wound, insect bite, IVDU, or in cases of a pre-existing skin condition such as eczema). However, pts often will not call recall any trauma or breaks in skin.

- Patients with venous stasis are at increased risk due to poor venous return. This makes it even more difficult to differentiate between worsening stasis and infection.

- **High Yield History:** Cellulitis tends to have a slower onset and is rarely associated with systemic symptoms.

  — Attempt to identify the cause: trauma, puncture wounds, breaks in the skin, lymphatic or venous stasis, immunodeficiency, and foreign bodies.

  — Risk factors for complications: IVDU, DM, immunosuppressed or immunocompromised, recent surgery, venous stasis.

- **Exam:** This is a clinical diagnosis - erythema, swelling, and tenderness. May have associated purulence or drainage.

  — Look for streaking (lymphangetic spread) or lymphadenopathy nearby.

  — If on the extremities, always compare to the other side.

  — Red flags: fever/tachycardia (sepsis, toxic shock), pain out of proportion (necrotizing infection), pain with ranging of joint (septic arthritis).

- **Diagnostics:** Again, this is a clinical diagnosis; any diagnostic testing is to evaluate for alternative diagnoses.

  — X-ray: If concerned about foreign body or subcutaneous air.

  — US: To look for fluid consistent with abscess vs. cobble stone appearance of cellulitis.

  — No blood cultures for uncomplicated appearing cellulitis.

MANAGEMENT

- Elevate the affected area and outline erythema with a skin marker to monitor progression. Label with time and date for future providers.

- IV abx if systemically ill, rapid progression, or have risk factors for complications. Otherwise can treat with oral regimen for 7-10days.

- IDSA Guidelines: If no purulence, treat for beta-hemolytic strep and MSSA; if concern for purulence, treat for MRSA.

- Consider treatment for both in high-risk patients, or if a high rate of community acquired MRSA with linezolid, clindamycin, or combination.

	Non-Purulent	Purulent
Bacteria	**Beta-hemolytic strep and MSSA**	**MRSA**
Oral Antibiotic	Cephalexin 500mg Q6hrs Clindamycin 300mg QID Augmentin 875mg PO BID	Clindamycin 450mg QID Sulfamethoxazole/trimethoprim 2 DS tab BID Doxycline 100mg BID Linezolid 600mg BID
IV Antibiotic	Cefazolin 1-2mg Q8hrs Naficillin 2gm Q4hrs Clindamycin 900mg IV Q8hrs	Vancomycin 15-20mg/kg Q8-12hrs Linezolid 600mg q12HRS Ceftaroline 600mg Q12hrs

DISPOSITION

- Uncomplicated cellulitis can be discharged home on oral antibiotics with PCP or ED follow up in 2 days. Ensure that the area of erythema is outlined prior to discharge for ease of monitoring progression.

- In high risk patients (DM, IVDU, etc.), consider admission for IV antibiotics.

- RETURN IF: You develop any high fevers, develop nausea or vomiting, have spreading redness beyond the outlined margins, or severe pain at the infection site.

BEWARE...

(!) In patients with systemic symptoms, consider alternative diagnoses such as a necrotizing skin infection or osteomyelitis.

(!) A rapidly spreading erythema while in the ED (well outside the margins you outlined with your marker) is highly concerning for a necrotizing skin infection → Surgery consult.

Notes

5 ▶ Necrotizing Soft Tissue Infection

Necrotizing Soft Tissue Infection (NTSI): Rapidly progressive, life- and limb-threatening infections of the soft tissue characterized by significant local tissue destruction and, in some cases, systemic toxicity. NTSI is a term that encompasses all necrotizing infections. Can be classified by their depth in tissue involvement (ie, necrotizing fasciitis) or their location on the body (ie, Fournier's gangrene). ED management is similar amongst all, thus they will be discussed as a single entity.

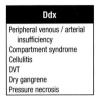

Ddx
Peripheral venous / arterial insufficiency
Compartment syndrome
Cellulitis
DVT
Dry gangrene
Pressure necrosis

BACKGROUND

- Higher rates seen in obesity, peripheral vascular disease, smokers, ETOH abuse, diabetics, and immunocompromised (neutropenic, etc.), but can occur in any patient population, including the young and healthy.

- Can occur via direct inoculation of breaks in skin or mucosal surface (surgical site, trauma, IVDU, insulin injection sites, ulcers, abscesses); less common via hematogenous spread or idiopathic.

- Three types:
  - *Type I:* Polymicrobial (gram negative rods, gram positive cocci, and anaerobes), patients often older, diabetic. More likely in trunk or perineum.
  - *Type II:* Monomicrobial (group A strep +/- staph), generally younger patients, located in extremities, associated with trauma, IVDU, and surgery, can have associated systemic symptoms such as toxic shock.
  - *Type III:* Not agreed upon. Per some sources, NSTIs from vibrio species found in warm coastal waters.

EVALUATION

- **High Yield History:** Rapidly progressive infection (over hours) and classically "pain out of proportion to exam." Past medical history including DM and how well-controlled.
- **Exam:** Initially appears similar to cellulitis or abscess→ High mortality due to initial deceptively benign physical exam.
  - Can sometimes visualize rapid spread over course of ED stay→ Use skin marker to delineate border early.
  - Exam variable due to pathogen and depth of infection, but commonly erythema, edema, and low-grade fever, tachycardia. Edema/induration beyond margins of erythema due to deep tissue spread.
  - Crepitus, bullae, ecchymosis, necrosis, or systemic toxicity are late and ominous findings.

- **Diagnostics**
  - Labs: CBC, BMP, coags, VBG, lactate, and gram stain/wound culture. Pre-op: CXR, EKG and type and cross-match.
  - ****LRINEC score** (laboratory risk indicator for necrotizing fasciitis) utilizes WBC, Na, glucose, creatinine, CRP, Hgb, and WBC to risk stratify patients. Use as additional data point and to communicate with the surgeons. *Don't* use as sole diagnostic tool.
  - Imaging: X-ray / CT / US to assess for SQ air can assist in diagnosis, but should NEVER delay immediate surgical evaluation for debridement.
  - Non-con CT findings of fluid tracking, facial/muscle edema, lymphadenopathy, and SQ edema can assist in diagnosis.

MANAGEMENT

- High suspicion and early recognition!
- Definitive care is early surgical debridement→ Consult surgery early if any clinical suspicion and urology if located in perineum →Fournier's gangrene.
- Early resuscitation with IVF and antibiotics: Cannot distinguish pathogen or depth of involvement based on exam, so must treat aggressively and with broad spectrum abx covering gram positive cocci, gram negative rods, and anaerobes based on local resistance patterns.
- One suggested abx regimen:
  - Vancomycin 20mg/kg IV AND clindamycin 900mg IV AND [meropenem 1g IV or Zosyn 4.5g IV].
  - Can also use penicillin G, vancomycin, clindamycin, and gentamycin (vs. fluoroquinolone if significant renal impairment).
  - Clindamycin is a protein synthesis inhibitor and shown to reduce mortality in group A strep NSTI by reducing toxin production.
  - Can add cephalosporin or fluoroquinolone if suspect vibrio.

DISPOSITION

- To OR vs. admission to surgery with serial exams.

BEWARE...

⚠ This diagnosis can easily be missed during early stages. Always initiate broad-spectrum antibiotics and obtain surgical consultation early.

Sources

Ustin JS, Malangoni MA. Necrotizing soft-tissue infections. *Crit Care Med.* 2011 Sep;39(9):2156-62

Sarani B, Strong M, Pascual J, Schwab CW. Necrotizing fasciitis: current concepts and review of the literature. *J Am Coll Surg.* 2009;208:279–288.

Wong CH, Chang HW, Pasupathy S, Khin LW, Tan JL, Low CO. Necrotizing fasciitis: clinical presentation, microbiology, and determinants of mortality. *J Bone Joint Surg Am.* 2003;85(8):1454e1460.

Zacharias N, Velmahos GC, Salama A, et al. Diagnosis of necrotizing soft tissue infections by computed tomography. *Arch Surg.* 2010; 145(5):452e455

6 ▶ Laceration Repair

EVALUATION

- **High Yield History:** Time of injury (most wounds should not be closed > 6hrs after incident), last tetanus, possible foreign body, mechanism of injury (Dirty wound? Did they have syncope causing them to cut themselves?), risk factors for adverse wound healing (diabetes, renal insufficiency, malnutrition, immunocompromised, connective tissue disorders).

- **Exam:** Location, muscle function, tendon involvement, vascular injury, nerve injury, foreign material.

  — Always examine distal neurovascular function and document prior to anesthesia or repair.

  — If overlying a joint, examine for joint involvement.

  — Note tension on wound or if any tension/gaping with movement of underlying muscle as part of consideration fur suture or glue repair.

- **Diagnostics:** X-ray and/or ultrasound if foreign body suspected.

MANAGEMENT

- Anesthesia

  — Topical analgesia for pediatrics (onset 20 min, duration 20-30min), avoid mucus membranes, fingers, toes, nose, or other end-organs.

  — Lidocaine without epi for most lacerations (onset 4-10 min, duration 30-120 min).

  — Lidocaine WITH epi for scalp or other vascular areas (onset 4-10 min, duration 60-240 min). Although the risk of ischemia is low, you should avoid fingers, toes, and nose.

  — Local anesthesia or regional nerve block for sensitive areas like the hands, feet, or face.

- Clean periphery (avoiding betadine in wound itself).

  — Irrigate (100cc/cm) by 60cc syringe with splash guard, goal is serial dilution with volume and high pressure

  — Debride devascularized or contaminated tissue

- Suture repair: Avoid in bite or puncture wounds, or wounds under high tension.

  — Nonabsorbable: Used in most skin closures. Material: Nylon, polypropylene.

  — Absorbable: Useful in mouth, tongue, nailbed, or deep closure as well as pediatric pts. Material: Surgical gut, chromic gut, monocryl, vicryl

- Staple repair: Higher rates of scarring; do not use for cosmetic wounds. Ideal for scalp, especially if need to obtain hemostasis quickly.

- Tissue adhesives: Useful for wounds that are well-approximated, smaller, and not under tension.

- Antibiotics are rarely indicated. Consider in the following cases:

  — Delayed presentation (hand/foot >8 hrs; face > 24hrs; others >18 hrs).

  — Crush mechanism with devitalized tissue.

  — Puncture wounds, bite wounds (see chapter), or large wounds > 5cm.

— Gross contamination that cannot be adequately cleaned, or foreign bodies.
— Open fractures, joints, tendon involvement.
— Poorly controlled DM, renal/hepatic dysfunction, chemo, chronic steroids.

SPECIAL CONSIDERATIONS

- If patient is a high risk for poor follow up, consider placing deep sutures and then using steri-strips to close wounds. Can tack down ends of the steri-strips to help them stay in place longer.
- Large avulsion wounds in patients with thin, atrophic skin (elderly and those on chronic steroids) can be difficult to repair → The skin tears easily and patient at higher risk for infection.
    — Consider lining wound edges with steri-stripes and suturing through them to add strength and stability to wound margins.
    — Obtain surgical consult for large avulsion wounds or those under high tension.
- For facial wounds, where cosmesis is important, use nerve block or topical analgesia if able, as local infiltration of anesthetic can distort anatomy.
- Scalp lacerations: If hemodynamically stable, consider hair ties → Using the patient's own hair and skin adhesive to repair.

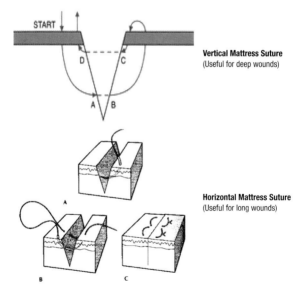

Vertical Mattress Suture
(Useful for deep wounds)

Horizontal Mattress Suture
(Useful for long wounds)

Location	Suture Suggestions	Specific Consideration	Duration (days)
Ear (pinna)	6-0 nylon/polypropylene	Compression dressing to prevent hematoma	4-6
Extremities	4-0/5-0 nylon/polypropylene	Splint if wound is over a joint	7 (10-14 if over a joint)
Eyelid	6-0 fast absorbing gut	Rule out globe rupture, optho consult, horizontal mattress	3-5
Face	6-0 nylon/polypropylene	Layered if under tension (ie, chin)	3-5
Foot-sole	4-0 nylon/polypropylene	Horizontal mattress if tension	7-10
Hand – palm/ dorsum	4-0/5-0 nylon/polypropylene	Splint if wound over joint	7
Lip – vermillion border	6-0 fast absorbing gut on cutaneous portion; 5-0 chromic gut on vermillion	Layered closure	Dissolve
Nailbed	5-0/6-0 Absorbable suture or chromic gut	Replace nail under cuticle as splint	Dissolve
Oral Cavity (and tongue)	4-0/5-0 Absorbable suture or chromic gut	Only if gaping, bleeding or food sticking (otherwise, will often heal quickly on own)	Dissolve
Scalp	Staples		5-7
Trunk	4-0/5-0 nylon/polypropylene		7-10

Tetaus Prophylaxis		
Prior tetanus toxoid immunization	Clean minor wound	All other wounds
Uncertain	TD or Tdap	Tdap or Td and TIG (separate injection sites)
> 10 years	Td or Tdap	Td or Tdap
< 5 years ago	None	None
Between 5-10 years ago	None	Td or Tdap

DISPOSITION

- Majority are discharged home, with follow up needed only at time of suture removal, or sooner if signs of infection develop.
- Discharge care:
  - Consider topical abx and wound coverage for first 24hrs, then can leave open to air.
  - Keep wound clean and dry. Do not soak. Pat dry after shower.
  - Keep out of sun to help prevent scar formation.
  - Wound can take up to 1yr to fully heal and scar.

- If laceration crosses a joint, that joint should be immobilized and patients should be sent home in a splint.
- If wound to bottom of foot or deep wound to leg, provide crutches.
- RETURN IF: You develop signs of infection (fever, pus, warmth, or redness), numbness, severe pain, or persistent bleeding.

BEWARE...

(!) Always do a thorough neurovascular exam prior to providing local anesthesia or nerve block.

(!) Take care when applying a tissue adhesive to make sure your gloves or instruments do not become glued to the patient.

Sources

Zane RD, Kosowsky JM, et al. Pocket Emergency Medicine. 2nd ed. Philadelphia, PA: Lippincott Williams & Wilkins; 2011.

Ma OJ, Cline D, Tintinalli J, et al. Emergency Medicine Manual. 6th ed. New York, NY: McGraw-Hill Professional; 2003.

Marx J, Hockberger R, Walls R. Rosen's Emergency Medicine: Concepts & Clinical Practice. 5th ed. Maryland Heights, MO: Mosby; 2002.

Hans L, Mawji Y. The ABCs of Emergency Medicine. 12th edition. Toronto, Canada: University of Toronto; 2012.

Medscape News & Perspective. New York, NY: http://emedicine.medscape.com.

Boston Children's Hospital Resident Laceration Repair Guide.

Notes

7 ▶ Thermal Burns

CLASSIFICATION

Superficial (1st degree): Involves only the epidermis. Painful, dry, red, blanches with pressure, NO blisters. Example: sunburn.

Partial Thickness (2nd degree): Includes portions of the dermis, characterized as superficial or deep.

- **Superficial**: Forms blisters within 24 hrs. Painful, red, weeping, and blanches with pressure.
- **Deep**: Blisters, painful to pressure only, wet or waxy dry, mottled colorization from patchy, cheesy white to red, DOES NOT blanch with pressure.

Full Thickness (3rd degree): Burn eschar present. The skin is dry, inelastic, anesthetic or hypoesthetic, does not blanch with pressure, and no blisters develop.

4th Degree: Extend to deep tissue such as fascia, bone, muscle, and tendon.

Ddx	Consider Associated Diagnoses
— Bullous pemphigoid — Toxic Epidermal Necrosis Syndrome (TENS) — Stevens-Johnson syndrome (SJS)	— Traumatic injury — Airway edema/compromise — Corneal burns — CO/cyanide poisoning — Intentional injury (by self or other) — Substance abuse — Superimposed infection — Chemical burns

EVALUATION

- **High Yield History:** Circumstances of burn, including presence of flash/explosion, structure fire, enclosed space, or steam injury because these have risk of airway injury. Time of fire, chemicals involved, exposure time, enclosed space, throat symptoms, voice changes, visual impairments at the scene and in the department. Less common sources of burn injury include electrical, chemical, and radiation.
    - Be suspicious for other injuries from the trauma, and direct your questions appropriately. Investigation of burn should include witnesses and correlation with physical findings (particularly in pediatrics, elderly, and when abuse is suspected).
    - EMS/police provide very useful history regarding the scene.
- **Exam**
    - Vital signs (particularly O2 saturation and temperature). If CO exposure, BEWARE that pulse oximetry may falsely reassure.
    - Comprehensive airway, oral pharynx, and lung exam, including presence of burn to mouth or nose, singed nose hairs, oropharyngeal edema, voice change, or black sputum. Expose all skin fully, identify additional injuries, and remove any agents that may be continuously contributing to burn (tar, exothermic dressings, chemicals, etc.).

- All burns to the face/chest/upper extremities should have a low threshold for corneal examination given risk for corneal burns; this includes welders who can present with diffuse punctuate abrasions from UV burns.
- **Labs:** CBC, BMP, LFTs (for albumin, ALT/AST), coags (to assess hepatic function), UA, CPK (rhabdomyolysis), type and screen if admission possible. Consider ABG and carboxyhemoglobin levels if respiratory symptoms or mechanism present.
- **Imaging**
  - CXR if symptomatic, hypoxic or high risk.
  - Consider nasopharyngeal scope if airway symptoms or high risk to look at the cords for degree of edema.
  - Burn has strong association with trauma and certainly may constitute a "distracting injury." Often patients will need additional extremity imaging, head or C-spine imaging, etc., depending on mechanism.
- **Assessment of severity**
  - **Mild:** <10% TBSA in adults; <5% in pediatric and elderly with <2% full thickness
  - **Moderate:** 10-20% TBSA in adults; 5-10% in pediatric and elderly with <5% full thickness; high voltage; inhalation; circumferential; co-morbid disease
  - **Severe:** Criteria beyond moderate

MANAGEMENT

- **Severe burns:** Establish access for resuscitation (think GI bleed – 2 large bore IVs or central access), O2 monitoring, and assessment/preparation for intubation for suspected airway compromise.
- **Escharotomy:** May be indicated in circumferential extremity injury to prevent compartment syndrome 12-24hrs following injury, and chest wall escharotomy may be indicated during initial assessment if burns interfere with mechanics of respiration. Use NG tube for gastric decompression to facilitate breathing.
- **Airway:** Burn airways should be managed with the regular airway management – with one exception: All burn patients with facial involvement requiring intubation should be assumed difficult due to the risk of airway edema. A smaller than expected ETT should be immediately available.
- **IVF:** Appropriate crystalloid resuscitation (use lactated ringers):
  - **Parkland formula**: **4mL x (%TBSA burn) x (weight in kg)** → Use in severe burns >20% TSA
  - Should be administered over first 24hrs with ½ in first 8hrs and ½ during the following 16 hrs. This often overestimates fluid needs and should be titrated to each patient in discussion with burn team.
  - Do not forget to include any pre-hospital or outside hospital fluids already administered.
  - Consider Vitamin C Protocol in pts >30% TBSA burn.
- **Minor burns:** Cool skin with saline-soaked towels. Open any blisters with high risk of rupture (larger than the size of a quarter) and clean already ruptured blisters. Leave small clean blisters alone (act as biologic bandage). Cover partial-thickness burns with silver sulfadiazine ointment

(or bacitracin) and dry or xeroform dressing. Facial burns may be covered with bacitracin and left uncovered.

- **All burns: Pain control is essential**. Combine NSAIDs with opioids to improve control. If the pt has an IV for fluid resuscitation or if debridement is likely, use IV opioids. Addition of anxiolytic (0.5-1mg lorazepam) will increase analgesia. Acetaminphen +/- oxycodone should suffice for minor burns. Consider regional anesthesia or procedural sedation if extensive debridement is required. Tetanus immunization if >5yrs.

Assessment of Burn Size

- Can use patient's palm surface as 1% total body surface area (TBSA) to estimate small burns.

- For large burns use rule of 9s where head or entire arm = 9%, chest or back or entire leg = 18%, genitalia = 1%.

- **Peds (under 1yr) rule** of 9s has head + neck = 18%, back or chest = 16%, each leg = 15%, each arm = 10%.

- Toddler/child BSAs are average of ped and adult values, with "adult" reached at approx. age 6-9.

- **Important to remember that only 2nd, 3rd, and 4th degree burns included in calculation. DO NOT include 1st degree burns.**

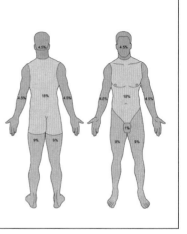

DISPOSITION

- 95% of all burn patients (mild burns) get discharged to home with pain control and follow-up appropriate to the injury (PCP vs. burn clinic). Be sure to provide adequate dressing supplies to cover until follow up appt. Consider a visiting nurse if the burn is extensive or to a hard-to-reach area.

- Patients with moderate burn or minor burn with intractable pain are appropriate for inpatient admission.

- **American Burn Association burn center referral/admission criteria are**:

  — 3rd degree burn >5% BSA

  — 2nd degree burn >10% BSA

  — Any burn >15% BSA in adults and 10% BSA in children

  — Any 2nd or 3rd degree burn to face, hands, feet, genitals, perineum, or skin over major joint

- Consider psych or social work consult as appropriate for pts where self-injury or abuse is considered.

BEWARE...

(!) Always consider injury to airway and respect hidden manifestations of burn injury; have a low threshold for intubation.

(!) Treat these patients like trauma patients; make sure to identify all associated injuries.

(!) Adequately treat pain and arrange appropriate follow-up, use your hospital's burn services for immediate and follow-up management.

(!) The Parkland formula is for burns >20% TBSA; use caution in fluid resuscitation in patients with less extensive burns because of complications of over-resuscitation.

(!) If having difficulty ventilating, consider abdominal compartment syndrome (bladder pressure >20 mmHg with dysfunction of at least one organ) or need for chest wall escharotomy.

Sources

Perel P, Roberts I, Ker K. Colloids versus crystalloids for fluid resuscitation in critically ill patients. *Cochrane Database Syst Rev.* 2013;2:CD000567.

Taira BR, Singer AJ, Thode HC, Lee C. Burns in the emergency department: a national perspective. *J Emerg Med.* 2010;39(1):1-5.

Singer AJ, Brebbia J, Soroff HH. Management of local burn wounds in the ED. *Am J Emerg Med.* 2007;25(6):666-71.

Notes

Section XV.
Trauma

1 ▶ Trauma Quick Guide

Initial Assessment	
Preparation (major trauma)	**If you get advance warning**: Consider: Airway (video/direct laryngoscope first, have a "plan B" like bougie, and "plan c" like surgical airway), chest tube setup and Pleurovac (know where a blade is), trauma cooler (prepare for massive transfusion), Broselow tape (peds), thoracotomy tray, trauma team ready and know everyone's role, gown/shield/gloves, **breathe**!
As they roll in	IV, O2, monitor, **complete** VS, EKG, fingerstick glucose (if altered), airway equipment close by
Key questions for EMS	(Leader takes report): Time and mechanism of injury, changes in VS/mental status (known baseline? onset before or after injury?), IV access, "any other EMS interventions?" and response to interventions
Initial approach (primary survey)	**A** (and c-spine stabilization): If pt can answer his name clearly, A pretty much clear **B** (and ventilation): Auscultate, look at rate/depth of breaths, make sure O2 on **C** (and hemorrhage): Pulses, and major sources of hemorrhage (chest/abdomen/pelvis/long bones/floor), WRAP pelvis if unstable, because pts can exsanguinate **D** (disability): GCS, pupils **E** (exposure): Undress, logroll, prevent hypothermia
Can't miss signs, symptoms, and diagnosis in first minutes	Need for intubation (not protecting airway, GCS<8 = intubate), airway obstruction, tension PTX (needle it!), pre-hospital ETT not in place, cardiac tamponade, obvious head injury, or catastrophic hemorrhage (pressure/tourniquet!) → shock (most often hemorrhagic)
Adjuncts to primary survey	IV access (and fluids/blood), monitor, reassess after interventions EKG, CXR/pelvis X-ray, FAST, ABG, Foley

Secondary survey	This is where you go over patient in detail, but with focused, efficient exam from top to bottom (look, listen, and feel). Also includes AMPLE History (**A**llergies, **M**eds, **P**MH, **L**ast meal, **E**vents [what happened] including specifics of injury mechanism). Adjuncts to secondary survey: Blood, glucose (if AMS), anticoagulation reversal, hang Abx (cefazolin 1-2gIV for anything >superficial wounds), TDaP, other imaging (CXR, pelvis if indicated)	
	Head/ maxillofacial	Lacs, cephalhematomas, stability of midface, crepitus of mandible, hemotympanum, nasal septal hematoma, CSF rhinorrhea, battle signs, raccoon eyes, thorough eye exam (globe rupture, retrobulbar hematoma, hyphema, etc.), foreign body in mouth, oral/dental trauma
	C-spine/neck	Anterior hematomas, carotid bruits, tracheal deviation, SQ emphysema, C-spine step offs, penetrating wounds obscured by c-collar
	Chest	Bilateral chest excursion, breath sounds, ecchymosis, crepitus, SQ emphysema
	Abdomen	Ecchymosis, distended, tenderness, peritonitis
	Pelvis	Stable (if unstable on primary exam and have wrapped, do NOT re-examine, because this can cause more bleeding)
	Perineum	Contusions, hematomas, urethral bleeding
	Extremities	Obvious deformities, firm compartments, pulses, cap refill, bony tenderness, ROM
	Neuro	GCS (again), strength, sensation, rectal tone
	Back	Likely examined during log roll, entire spine for tenderness, step offs, skin exam

EVALUATION

- **High Yield History:** (Motor vehicle collision) Restrained? Airbag deployment? Position in vehicle, rate of speed, area and level of damage to vehicle, extrication time, how are other passengers doing? (Penetrating injury) size of object? Associated blunt trauma? (Head trauma) Fall: How high, witnessed, LOC (and how long), seizure activity? Anticoagulation/anti-platelet therapy? Ambulatory after? Previous falls? Reason for fall?

- **Initial labs:** Most patients with a serious mechanism will need type and screen (cross if bleeding significantly). CBC, VBG (base deficit!) UA, BMP, HCG, Tox. Consider LFTs, lipase, troponin, CPK, PT/INR if on anticoagulation

- **Imaging:** Based on a combination of mechanism and patient presentation. Patients with a severe mechanism of injury often get a pan scan

GCS		
Eye Opening	Spontaneous	4
	To voice	3
	To pain	2
	None	1
Verbal	Oriented	5
	Confused	4
	Inappropriate words	3
	Incomprehensible	2
	None	1
Motor	Obeys commands	6
	Localizes pain	5
	Withdraws to pain	4
	Decorticate	3
	Decerebrate	2
	None	1
	Add "T" if intubated	

(brain, c-spine, chest, abdomen/pelvis CTs). Plain films for every area with focal tenderness or deformity. UIS can be used as an adjunct to the primary survey.

DISPOSITION

- Case-by-case, however patients with minor injuries that are successfully addressed in ED and normal mental status may be selectively discharged home. The rest will likely be admitted and have tertiary survey performed by inpatient team.

Notes

2 ▶ Blunt Trauma

- The presentation varies widely depending on the mechanism of injury. The most common presentations are falls, motor vehicle collisions, pedestrian versus automobile, and bicycle accidents.

- Patients may have a depressed mental status, which makes it more difficult to assess their injuries. In most cases, however, the patient is able to communicate where they have pain, which can offer some guidance on the location of injuries. The general rule in trauma is to be suspicious for injury and, when in doubt, image.

Ddx
- The initial trauma evaluation is the same for every trauma case: primary survey (ABCs) and secondary survey (head to toe survey to assess for injuries)
- Several patterns of injury are seen, depending on the mechanism of injury. For example, rapid deceleration (as in an MVC) is associated with aortic injuries and solid organ lacerations.
- 30% die within a few hours. **These are the critical diagnoses to make in the ED:**
— Massive hemorrhage: Liver, spleen, pelvic fracture, aortic rupture
— Major head injury (especially ones that are amenable to OR (subdural and epidural hematoma)
— Tension pneumothorax
— Massive hemothorax
— Cardiac tamponade

EVALUATION (ALSO SEE TRAUMA QUICK GUIDE)

- Beware of increased bleeding risks from anticoagulation, anti-platelet drugs, and aspirin.

- **PRIMARY SURVEY** comprises the initial priorities of assessing/securing the airway, maintaining ventilation, and controlling hemorrhage. Airway protection should be initiated early for patients with GCS<8. Consider intubation if neck or facial trauma may cause impending obstruction. Place all trauma patients on supplemental O2.

- Place chest tubes if pneumothorax or massive hemothorax is suspected by absent breath sounds WITH hypotension.

- Apply direct pressure to actively bleeding wounds.

- Obtain 2 large-bore IVs, or intraosseous access. Permissive hypotension is maintained in patients with suspected acute hemorrhage, so as to avoid blowing off the clot that may have formed. Aim for SBP of 90-100. Higher blood pressures and anti-coagulant effects of IV normal saline can dislodge clots and lead to worsening hemorrhage.

- Ultrasound can be used as an adjunct to the primary survey in assessing for intra-abdominal hemorrhage, hemo/ pneumothorax and cardiac tamponade. Perform an E-FAST on all patients with dangerous mechanism, chest pain, abdominal pain, or difficulty breathing.

- **SECONDARY SURVEY** comprises the history and thorough evaluation for other injuries not discovered on the primary survey. Obtain an AMPLE history (allergies, medications, past medical history, last meal, environment, and events). Perform a head to toe exam looking for contusions, lacerations, and other pertinent abnormalities.

- **Trauma series:** CXR and pelvis screen for acute injury, followed by CT scans as indicated by the survey and mechanism.

MANAGEMENT

- Many aspects of the management occur simultaneous to the primary and secondary surveys, such as securing the airway and controlling hemorrhage, IV access, monitor.
- Other definitive management of injuries depends on their nature and degree. Any life-threatening ongoing internal hemorrhage should be taken to the OR/IR suite as soon as possible. This is arranged in discussion with the surgery team.
- Diagnostic testing and management decisions should be in collaboration with your trauma team.
- A positive FAST in hypotensive blunt abdominal trauma patients is indication for emergent exploratory laparotomy prior to imaging.
- **For head injuries:** See traumatic head injury chapter
- **Spinal Fractures:** Unstable fracture or presence of neurologic deficits is indication for surgical management, otherwise stabilize and obtain MRI to further evaluate ligamentous and cord injuries.

Blunt Thoracic Injuries

- Injuries can occur from direct trauma to chest wall or from rapid deceleration (see chart).
- Must take into consideration the mechanism/energy of injury, and the comorbidities of the patient.
- Always think anatomically. A rib fracture should raise concern for underlying injuries (eg, splenic lacerations or pulmonary contusions)
- In the case of high energy injuries (sternal fractures) must search for associated injuries and have low threshold for further workup.

Blunt Thoracic Injuries		
Injury	**Presentation**	**Management**
Pulmonary Contusion	Injury to lung parenchyma leading to collection of blood and edema in the alveolar spaces. CXR findings (irregular nonlobular opacifications) and hypoxia develops over first 24hrs.	Pain control and pulmonary toilet. May progress over time and patients may require intubation. Complications include PNA and ARDS.
Rib Fractures	Pleuritic chest pain, chest wall crepitus. If 3 or more adjacent ribs fractured in two places →concern for flail chest.	Older patients, those with cormorbidities or 3 or more fractures have a high morbidity from fractures (splinting→ PNA) and require admission.
Diaphragmatic Rupture	High-energy mechanism. Left-sided more common than right. CXR may demonstrate abdominal viscera or NGT in the thorax.	Most will require surgical management. However, given the high-energy mechanism, priority in ED should be to identify associated injuries.

Injury	Presentation	Management
Blunt Aortic Injuries (BAIs)	Majority die prior to arrival in ED. No specific signs or symptoms. Must maintain high suspicion and obtain CT if there is a high-energy mechanism and any CXR abnormality or other thoracic injury (other injuries in this chart).	While in ED goal HR <100 and goal SBP <100mmHg. Majority need operative management; small intimal tear can be medically managed.
Cardiac Contusion	Persistent tachycardia, arrhythmias, or new conduction abnormalities on EKG. Unclear utility of biomarkers.	Telemetry, serial EKGs and echo if concerned for acute heart failure or valvular injury. Treat arrhythmias per ACLS.
Hemothorax	Similar to symptoms of pneumothorax. Ultrasounds during FAST can be useful to visualize pleural fluid.	Tube thoracostomy (see procedure section). Immediate return of >1500ml is an indication for surgical thoracotomy.
Pneumothorax	Diminished breath sounds, shortness of breath, poor chest excursions, often in the presence of rib fractures, should be suspected before CXR obtained.	If unstable (concern for tension PTX) perform needle decompression with 14g angiocath in 2nd/3rd intercostal space on midclavicular line. Must follow with immediate tube thoracostomy (see procedure section).

Blunt Abdominal Injuries

- The spleen and liver are the most commonly injured solid organs, but the pancreas, bowel, mesentery, bladder, diaphragm, kidney, and abdominal aorta should also be considered, though they are less common. Concern for bleeding from solid organs and rupture of hollow viscus.

- Injuries can occur from compression, shearing forces, or secondary to factures (rib or pelvis).

- Physical exam should focus on findings associated with blunt abdominal trauma:
  - Seat belt sign: Bruising along the sites of the lap belt.
  - Rebound tenderness, abdominal distension, and peritonitis, which can indicate visceral injury or bleeding.

- **Splenic Injuries:** Unstable patients with positive FAST will likely have emergency ex-lap.
  - In patients with low grade splenic injury and no extravasation of contrast on CTA, observation is appropriate.
  - IR embolization should be considered for patients with extravasation on CTA.
  - Grading system for injuries:
    - Grade I: Capsular tear <1cm or subcapsular hematoma <10% surface area
    - Grade II: Parenchymal laceration 1-3cm or intraparenchymal hematoma <5cm
    - Grade III: >3cm laceration or intraparenchymal hematoma >5cm
    - Grade IV: Laceration or segmental or hilar vessels
    - Grade V: Shattered spleen or devascularizing injury

- **Liver Injuries:**
  - — Grading similar to splenic injuries except Grade IV (parenchymal disruption of 25-75% of hepatic lobe), Grade V (parenchymal disruption of >75% of hepatic lobe), and grade VI (avulsion).
  - — Majority of patients who are HD stable and do not have other indications for ex-lap can be observed.
- Non-operative management had become the standard for blunt abdominal trauma; however, immediate ex-lap should be considered in patients with unexplained hypotension and concern for intra-abdominal trauma persistent peritonitis, CXR with signs of diaphragmatic rupture or free air.
  - — Unstable Patients:
    - If FAST positive→OR
    - Treat other hemodynamically significant injuries, serial FAST exams and consider abdominal imaging once stable
  - — Stable patients:
    - If FAST positive → Obtain CT imaging
    - If FAST negative: Serial exams and obtain imaging if any changes in exam or if concerned due to mechanism.

Pelvic Injuries

- **Pelvic Fractures:** If pelvis unstable during trauma survey, place pelvic binder and do not continue to test stability (can exacerbate injuries).
  - — Hemodynamically significant bleeding from a pelvic fracture can be retroperitoneal and will not show up on FAST
  - — Management depends on fracture pattern and patient stability. Conservative vs. pelvic packing vs. IR embolization
- **Urogenital injuries:** Findings of a high riding prostate on rectal exam, blood at the urethral meatus, or difficulty passing Foley should raise suspicion for urethral injury. Also should be concerned for possible urethral or bladder injury in patients with pelvic fractures.
  - — Pelvic fracture evaluation takes precedence, especially if patient is unstable.
  - — If patient does not require intervention for pelvic fracture, obtain retrograde urethrogram and cystogram.
  - — If concern for kidney injury or blood in urine and negative urethrogram/cystogram, consider CT scan.

Extremity Injuries

- Evaluate for crush injuries, monitor CPK and potassium due to potential for rhabdomyolysis.
- Evaluate for fractures, reduce, and stabilize with splint. Patients can have hemodynamically significant bleed from femur fractures.
- Check neurovascular exam before and after reduction.
- Monitor for compartment syndrome (see chapter).

DISPOSITION

- If immediate hemorrhage control is needed, the patient goes to the OR/IR suite, then to the SICU or surgical floor.

- Depending on the severity of injury, if the patient is not going immediately to the OR, they are admitted to the SICU or surgical service.

- If the injuries are minor and the patient is stable with minimal risk for decompensation, you can consider discharging them home with appropriate follow up. They should have clear instructions to return with any new or worsening pain in their chest or abdomen, as delayed bleeding has been described, especially with splenic lacerations. Cervical and back muscle spasms are to be expected 24-72 hrs after an MVC.

BEWARE...

(!) Remember to expose everything and look at every inch of the body to identify all injuries, including the scalp below the c-collar, the back, and perineum. Palpate every joint and compartment if any suspicion for injury exists or if patient is altered.

(!) Have a higher suspicion for injury (especially pelvic fractures) in the elderly.

(!) Serial FAST exams can increased sensitivity and should be performed in cases of changes clinical status.

Notes

3 ▶ Penetrating Trauma

- Presentation depends on the mechanism of injury and body parts affected. Most commonly, the injury is a gunshot wound (GSW) or stab wound.
- Patients may be critically ill secondary to massive blood loss, or stable and looking well. Young patients have a lot of reserve and may look relatively well until they decompensate quickly.
- Wounds may appear small on the outside, but be life-threatening on the inside, so be suspicious!

Ddx
• Injuries from stab wounds generally stay along the path taken by the blade. The length of the blade is helpful to know, but cannot rule out deeper injury.
• Gunshot wounds can ricochet inside the body, taking unpredictable courses and damaging organs far from the entry and exit wounds. They cause damage by direct laceration, crush injury, shock waves, and cavitation.
• Remember that projectiles in otherwise blunt trauma can cause significant penetrating trauma. This includes glass shards in MVC or shrapnel in an explosion.

EVALUATION

- Penetrating traumas are evaluated in a similar manner as blunt traumas, according to ATLS guidelines. (See blunt trauma for further description of the primary and secondary surveys.)
- The ultrasound E-FAST should be a part of your primary survey in identifying intra-abdominal hemorrhage, hemo/pneumothorax, or cardiac tamponade. If penetrating wound to the thoracoabdominal area, E-FAST should start with the cardiac view to evaluate for a cardiac injury.
- Never probe a wound – unless it is obviously superficial, assume that deeper structures are involved.
- Stabilize any impaling object to prevent displacement – never remove it!
- Exposure is key! Ensure that a thorough skin exam is performed, and examine axilla, perineum, scalp, and skin folds.
- Difficult to differentiate entrance and exit wound, but the total number of gunshot wounds (odd or even) should be noted.

MANAGEMENT

- As with blunt traumas, many aspects of the management occur simultaneous to the primary and secondary surveys, such as securing the airway and controlling hemorrhage.
- Control active bleeding quickly.
  - If there is a scalp wound, staple it to achieve hemostasis; you can re-do the repair later when the patient is more stable.
  - Apply pressure to any other external wound.
  - Apply tourniquet to extremities if direct pressure is not successful in controlling active hemorrhage.

- — Any life-threatening, ongoing internal hemorrhage should be taken to the OR/IR suite as soon as possible. This is arranged in discussion with the surgery team.
- If the FAST exam identifies significant intra-abdominal hemorrhage or pericardial tamponade, and the patient is hypotensive, they should proceed to the OR/IR suite without CT scanning.
- The blood bank should be called to release emergency blood: O+ (male) or O- (female of childbearing age).
  - — As with blunt trauma, permissive hypotension is maintained in patients with suspected acute hemorrhage, so as to avoid blowing off the clot that may have formed. Aim for SBP of 90-100. Higher blood pressures and anti-coagulant effects of IV normal saline can dislodge clots and lead to worsening hemorrhage.
  - — If available, consider giving transexamic acid (which inhibits fibrinolysis) to patients with severe hemorrhage who require at least 1 unit of PRBCs.
- Check a base deficit and lactate on trauma patients as indicators of hypovolemic shock and mortality.

PENETRATING NECK TRAUMA

- C-spine injuries from penetrating wounds are rare and c-collars can interfere with evaluation and management. C-spine immobilization is only necessary if there is a focal neurologic deficit or unable to obtain accurate exam.
- Zones of the neck:
  - — Zone 1: Sternal notch to below cricoid cartilage
  - — Zone 2: Between cricoid cartilage and angle of mandible
  - — Zone 3: Above angle of mandible to base of skull
- "Hard signs" of vascular injury in Zone II are indication to go directly to the OR:
  - — Bruit or thrill
  - — Expanding or pulsatile hematoma
  - — Pulsatile or severe hemorrhage
  - — Pulse deficit (usually in upper extremity)
- Have low threshold to intubate early, especially with signs of stridor, voice changes, expanding hematoma, or distortion of neck anatomy.
- If intubating, have a double setup: Prep the neck for cricothyrotomy while you set up for RSI.
- Any wound that violates the platysma should be evaluated by a trauma surgeon.
- Zone II most common injury but penetrating wounds can span more than one zone.

PENETRATING THORACOABDOMINAL TRAUMA

- The movement of the diaphragm with respirations makes it difficult to predict potential organs involved; can be thoracic or intra-abdominal.
- Injuries to the lungs, heart, and great vessels that are encountered should be managed during the primary survey.
- Management depends on weapon and type of wound.

— If stabbed with small blade and CXR reassuring, can consider local wound exploration. Obtain CT for gunshot wounds or large blades.

— Place chest tube for hemo or pneumothorax. If large, persistent air-leak and concerned for tracheobronchial injury or immediate return of >1500ml of blood → OR for thoracotomy.

— If clinical or US signs of cardiac tamponade (hypotension, JVD, and muffled heart sounds) give preload and → OR.

- For pts who present pulseless, but with signs of life, an ED thoracotomy is recommended. Other pulseless pts with penetrating injury may have a thoracotomy performed on a case-by-case basis. In any pt with unstable VS and evidence of a pericardial tamponade, an emergency pericardiocentesis should be performed.

PENETRATING ABDOMINAL TRAUMA

- HD instability, peritonitis, or eviscerated bowel are indications for emergent exploratory laparotomy.
- Cover eviscerated bowel with damp sterile gauze to prevent desiccation.
- **Stab wounds:** Non-operative management and serial exams have become more common, even in instances of peritoneal violation.
  - If patient is HD unstable, has peritonitis, or eviscerated bowel → OR.
  - If stable, assess for peritoneal penetration via CT scan or local wound exploration by an experienced surgeon (usually the attending).
    - If no peritoneal violation, patient may qualify for discharge home from ED.
    - If peritoneal violation and reliable patient (no head injury, etc.), can observe for 24hrs with serial exams by the same provider.
- **Gunshot wounds:** Local wound exploration has small role in GSW compared to stab wounds due to local tissue destruction and absence of clear wound tract. Same indications for emergent laparotomy as stab wound.
  - Majority of patients should have CT scan with IV contrast.
  - In the carefully selected patients with a reassuring CT scan and abdominal exam, nonoperative management can be considered.

PENETRATING EXTREMITY TRAUMA

- Major concern is for vascular injury that is life- or limb-threatening.
- Obtain good pulse exam and use Doppler if needed.
  - If concern for HD significant bleed, place direct pressure on bleeding source.
- Hard signs of vascular injury and indications for surgical management include: hemorrhage, expanding or pulsatile hematoma, bruits over wound, absent distal pulses, and extremity ischemia.
- In patients w/o hard signs, but abnormal exam, obtain Ankle-Brachial Index. An ABI<0.9 should prompt further evaluation to rule out vascular injury
- In stable patients with equivocal exam, obtain angiogram of the affected extremity.
- These patients are at risk for compartment syndrome.

DISPOSITION

- OR vs. trauma service vs. ICU vs. home depending on severity of injury

BEWARE...

(!) Especially with gunshot wounds, the injuries from shock waves and cavitation can be very distant from the course of the bullet.

(!) Have low threshold to intubate early in penetrating neck injuries and be prepared for a surgical airway if needed.

(!) **Never** remove an impaled object; secure in place.

(!) Do not be distracted by extremity injury. If bleeding, apply direct pressure or tourniquet and continue with primary and secondary survey.

Notes

4 ▶ Hemorrhagic Shock

- Inadequate tissue perfusion as the result of loss of circulating blood volume from hemorrhage, which leads to hemodynamic disturbances and end-organ damage. At the cellular level sufficient oxygenation of tissue is not achieved and aerobic metabolism shifts to anaerobic metabolism, which leads to lactate production (ie, increased base deficit→ decreased serum bicarbonate from baseline)

Ddx
Cardiac tamponade
Pneumothorax
Hemothorax
Pulmonary contusion
MI or myocardial contusion
Spinal cord injury/neurogenic shock
Drug effects
Sepsis
Vasovagal event

EVALUATION

- **High Yield History:** Majority of these patients will be trauma patients. Obtain full trauma history (see chapter)
    - Not all hemorrhage is the result of trauma. Patients can hemorrhage from other source, such as post-partum hemorrhage or retain products of conception (vaginal bleeding), melena or hematochezia (GI bleed), back pain (AAA), or abdominal pain (delayed splenic bleed, post-operative complications, ectopic pregnancy).
    - Past medical history including bleeding diathesis, history of previous bleeding such as GI bleeds, last menstrual period (ruptured ectopic), EtOH use (variceal bleeds), or any comorbidities such as CAD that may make patient less tolerant of anemia
    - Medications: Ask all patients about anticoagulation medications. Also ask about beta-blocker use that may mask vital sign changes.
- **Exam:** Frequent reassessment of vital signs. (see chart)
    - In all cases, goal is to identify locations of major potential hemorrhage and examine those locations.
        - In trauma: scene (floor), scalp, pelvis/retroperitoneal, long bones, abdomen, chest
        - In other etiologies: similar locations but do not forget GI and genitourinary tracts
- **Diagnostics**
    - Labs are generally of low utility as initial HCT can be falsely elevated and will unlikely have an effect on initial management. The most important labs to send are a type and cross match, coags in patients of anticoagulation, and obtain a base deficit.
    - Imaging: In trauma obtain portable chest and pelvis x-rays
        - **Ultrasound all patients.** US can be used to evaluate for causes of shock in these pts through evaluating for free fluid in the abdomen or the size of the abdominal aorta.
        - CT scan: If stable enough and safe to send to scanner. Usually only a CTA of the chest and abdomen indicated based on likely bleeding source.
    - Consider placing a Foley to measure urine output or an arterial line to monitor blood pressures.

- ATLS describes 4 classes of shock, though further studies have shown that many patients have falsely reassuring vital signs in the setting or large volume blood loss.

Classifications of Shock				
	Blood volume loss	Blood Pressure	Heart Rate	Other
Class I	≤15%	No change	Normal to min elevated	No change in RR or pulse pressure
Class II	15-30%	Min change	HR 100-120	RR 20-30, decreased pulse pressure, cool/clammy skin
Class III	30-40%	SBP ≤90 or drop of >20% from BP on presentation	HR 120 -140 and thready pulse	RR > 24, cool/clammy skin, cap refill delayed, decreased UOP, anxious patient
Class IV	≥40%	SBP <90	HR >140	AMS, cold/pale skin, minimal UOP, decreased pulse pressure

MANAGEMENT

- Initial goals (as in all cases of shock):
    — Identify and treat the cause: Obtain control of the bleeding and minimize ongoing volume loss.
    — Support the patient: Obtain large bore IV access and provide blood/IVF resuscitation.
- Control the bleeding: Majority of intra-abdominal and thoracic causes will ultimately require surgical repair.
    — For external bleeding, Apply direct pressure, staple any large scalp wounds.
    — Use a tourniquet for arterial bleeding from an extremity that is not controlled by direct pressure.
    — Pull traction on any long bone fracture (especially femur) that is causing significant blood loss.
    — Bleeding from a pelvic fracture can be temporized with a pelvic binder.
    — In exsanguinating upper GI bleed, consider placement of a Blakemore tube.
- Support the patient.
    — IV access: Obtain 2 large bore 16g IVs. Cordis (single lumen) central line or IO device can be placed if unable to obtain peripheral access.
    — Permissive hypotension: Aggressive resuscitation to a goal "normal" blood pressure is associated with worse outcomes. Allow for lower blood pressures: systolic BP >90 or MAP >65.
    — Be sure to **AVOID hypothermia** as it can potentiate coagulopathy.
- Vasopressors should be used with caution, as they may be harmful in hemorrhagic shock. Patients need intravascular volume, not peripheral squeeze. May be used in cases with hypotension with head injury or to prevent hypotension related to intubation.

- Resuscitate
  - **Step 1**: Determine if trauma is severe and unlikely to be controlled quickly (ie, projected requirement of 4u PRBCs within first hour)→**If YES** then initiate massive transfusion and bypass steps 2-4. **If NO** then go to Step 2.
  - **Step 2**: Be sure type and cross was sent. For hemorrhagic shock the key is locating and stopping the site of hemorrhage. Primarily use blood products for resuscitation. Use IV fluids while awaiting the availability of blood products.
  - **Step 3**: If BP not at goal then give 2u PRBCs. (If uncrossed PRBCs then Rh negative for girls and women of childbearing age.)
  - **Step 4**: Additional transfusion: Used for significant ongoing hemorrhage (ie, >4u PRBCs over a few hours) and inability to achieve BP goals. Continue transfusing at a 1:1:1 ratio of PRBCs, FFP, and platelets in the same manner as you would for the massive transfusion protocol.
  - **Massive Transfusion (1:1:1):** Initiate 1:1:1 resuscitation with equal quantities of PRBCs, FFP, and platelets.
  - Goal is to transfuse based on hemodynamics; you are not transfusing to a hematocrit level.
- Minimize ongoing bleeding.
  - Tranexamic acid (TXA- antifibrinolytic agent)
    - If <3 hrs since time of trauma: Give TXA 1000mg IV over 10min followed by 1000mg IV over 8hrs.
    - If >3 hrs since time of trauma: **Do not** give TXA; studies suggest a trend toward harm.
  - Cryoprecipitate: If patient is in ED for prolonged time with continued bleeding from trauma and fibrinogen <100mg/dL, then give 10units of cryoprecipitate.
  - Reverse any pre-existing coagulopathies. Given FFP to reverse elevated INR or platelets in patients with thrombocytopenia or dysfunctional platelets.
- Consult the appropriate service for hemorrhage control. GI for a GI bleed, Ob/Gyn for vaginal bleeding or ruptured ectopic, vascular surgery for AAA, or surgery for intrabdominal or traumatic bleed. If operative repair is needed for hemorrhage control, involve the consulting service ASAP and in parallel with your other resuscitation efforts.

DISPOSITION

- To OR or IR for definitive hemostasis, if not achieved or concern for likely re-bleed.
- Most of these patients should be admitted to the ICU for close hemodynamic monitoring and serial HCT.
- Patients for whom definitive hemostasis achieved in the ED, low concern for potential re-bleeding, and minimal comorbidities can be admitted to the floor.

BEWARE...

⚠ Failing to recognize that altered mental status or agitation in trauma patients is due to hemorrhagic shock and **not intoxication**.

⚠ Waiting for SBP to drop before considering resuscitation; at this point a patient may have lost up to 40% intravascular volume! Be cautious in interpreting vital signs, especially in older patients, well-trained athletes, and children.

⚠ Achieve early control of external bleeding. Patients can exsanguinate from scalp wounds!

Sources

Morrison JJ, Dubose JJ, Rasmussen TE, Midwinter MJ. Military application of tranexamic acid in trauma emergency resuscitation (MATTERs) study. *Arch Surg.* 2012;147(2):113-119

Neal MD, Marsh A, Marino R, Kautza B, Raval JS, Forsythe RM, et al. Massive transfusion: An evidence-based review of recent developments. *Arch Surg.* 2012;147:563–71

Cocchi MN, Kimlin E, Walsh M, Donnino MW. Identification and resuscitation of the trauma patient in shock. *Emerg Med Clin North Am.* 2007;25(3):623-642.

Cherkas. Traumatic hemorrhagic shock: advances in fluid management. *EB Medicine Emerg Med Practice.* Nov 2011.

Marx J, Hockberger R, Walls R. Rosen's Emergency Medicine: Concepts & Clinical Practice. 5th ed. Maryland Heights, MO: Mosby; 2002.

Notes

5 ▶ Cervical Spine and Head CT Rules

HEAD CT RULES

- Patients with a moderate to severe head injury obviously need to have a head CT. The more difficult decision is which patients with a seemingly mild head injury need further imaging.
- **Canadian Head CT rule**
  — Higher specificity than New Orleans criteria.
  — Head CT is only required for patients with minor head injury (witnessed LOC, amnesia, or witnessed disorientation in patients with a GCS 13-15) **with** any one of the following:

High risk (for neurosurgical intervention)	Medium risk (for brain injury on CT)

• GCS < 15 2h after injury
• Suspected open or depressed skull fracture
• Any sign of basal skull fracture hemotympanum, raccoon eyes, CSF rhinorrhea, Battle's sign)
• Vomiting ≥ 2 episodes
• Age ≥ 65 years
	• Amnesia before impact > 30min
	• Dangerous mechanism
	  — Ped struck by motor vehicle
	  — MVC with ejection
	  — Fall > 3 feet or 5 stairs

  — This rule does not apply in pediatric patients (<16yo), if there was no head trauma, the GCS< 13, there is an obvious open skull fracture, or if the patient is on blood thinners or has a known bleeding disorder (eg, hemophilia).

- **New Orleans Head CT rule**
  — Head CT is required for patients with minor head injury (LOC with normal CNII-XII and extremity strength and sensation) and ED arrival GCS of 15 and any one of the following:
    - Seizure
    - Visible trauma above the clavicles
    - Drug or EtOH ingestion
    - Headache
    - Vomiting
    - Age >60

C-SPINE RULES

- Used in blunt neck trauma for patients who are in stable condition with a GCS of 15
- The Canadian C-Spine Rule is more sensitive and specific than Nexus criteria (99.4% sensitivity vs. 90.7%) and (45.1% vs. 36.8%)
- **Nexus Criteria:** Caution in elderly (were only a small portion of the patient population)

A dangerous mechanism
Fall from >3 feet/5 stairs
Axial load to head
A bicycle collision
Motorized recreational vehicle
High speed MVC (>100km/hr rollover or ejection)

- — A C-spine CT is indicated unless the patient meets all of these criteria:
    - No posterior midline cervical tenderness
    - Is not intoxicated
    - Is awake and alert
    - Does not have any focal neurologic deficits
    - There are no painful distracting injuries (as defined by the provider)
- **Canadian C-Spine Rule**
    - — If ANY high risk factors (age>65yo, dangerous mechanism** or parasthesias) are present, obtain imaging.
    - — If ANY of the following low risk factors are present, can proceed to test range of motion; if none, get imaging.
        - Simple rear-end MVC (not pushed into traffic, hit by bus or large truck, hit by high speed vehicle, and no rollover)
        - Sitting in ED
        - Ambulatory at any time
        - Delayed onset of neck pain
        - Absence of midline C-spine tenderness
    - — If NO high risk factors and ANY low risk factors, check active ROM 45 degress in both directions. If unable, get imaging.
    - — If NO high risk factors, ANY low risk factors and is able to range neck → No imaging

Sources

Haydel MJ, Preston CA, Mills TJ, Luber S, Blaudeau E, Deblieux PM. Indications for computed tomography in patients with minor head injury. *N Engl J Med.* 2000;343(2):100-5.

Hoffman JR, Mower WR, Wolfson AB, Todd KH, Zucker MI. Validity of a set of clinical criteria to rule out injury to the cervical spine in patients with blunt trauma. National Emergency X-Radiography Utilization Study Group. *N Engl J Med.* 2000;343(2):94-

Stiell IG, Clement CM, Mcknight RD, et al. The Canadian C-spine rule versus the NEXUS low-risk criteria in patients with trauma. *N Engl J Med.* 2003;349(26):2510-8.

Stiell IG, Wells GA, Vandemheen K, et al. The Canadian CT Head Rule for patients with minor head injury. *Lancet.* 2001;357(9266):1391-6.

Notes

6 ▶ Traumatic Head Injury

- Suspect in any patient with traumatic injury, particularly those with dangerous mechanism or altered mental status, headache, etc.
- High-risk diagnosis associated with high mortality. Primary irreversible injury occurs at time of impact. Goal is to reduce secondary injury through appropriate brain perfusion and ICP. Must avoid hypotension, hypoxia, hypoglycemia!

EVALUATION

- Big picture: Look for and prevent things that increase ICP, ischemia or CNS metabolic demand: hypoxia, hypo/hypertension, hypo/hypercarbia, hyperthermia ("the H-bombs"), hematoma, cerebral edema, infection, anemia, seizure
- **High Yield History:** PAST MEDICAL HISTORY, anticoagulant/anti-platelet use, EtOH and illicits, mechanism of injury (speed, height, etc.), LOC, return to baseline after LOC

Ddx
Hemorrhage: SDH (most common), traumatic SAH, epidural (least common, most lethal)
Blunt trauma: Cerebral contusion, Diffuse axonal injury (DAI)
Penetrating cranial injury
Primary medical injury leading to trauma: CVA, ACS, Syncope, seizure, intoxication, etc.
*Also consider other traumatic injuries as this is still a trauma patient!a

- Exam:
  — A-B-C-D-E. Don't focus just on the head injury.
  — C-spine: Assume C-spine injury unless NEXUS/Canadian negative (see C-spine section)
  — GCS (with frequent re-evaluation)
  — Look at pupils to establish baseline
  — Herniation syndromes:
    ▪ Cushing's triad (poor sensitivity): HTN, bradycardia, and irregular respirations
    ▪ Anisocoria (>1mm difference) or dilated and unresponsive pupils
    ▪ Extensor posturing on motor exam
    ▪ Drop in GCS of >2 points
- Labs: Fingerstick glucose if AMS (STAT), CBC (anemia and thrombocytopenia), BMP (Na+ and Cr for potential imaging), Coags (consider Xa if on LMWH), ABG (paO2 and CO2), type and screen, consider UA / tox as appropriate
- Imaging: Non-contrast head CT and C-spine (if not cleared). CTA if penetrating injury.

MANAGEMENT

- Big picture: The goal in TBI is NORMAL: BP, HR, O2 sat, temperature, paCO2, paO2. Avoid extremes in all cases. Get Neurosurgery on board early if you suspect herniation/bleed.
- **Airway:** Intubate if patient not protecting airway, expected course, or if need to secure airway prior to definitive treatment or diagnostics.
  — Attempt complete sensory, motor, and mental status exam BEFORE sedation.

- Use video laryngoscopy or fiberoptic if available to minimize C-spine movement.
- Pretreatment:
  - Consider Lidocaine 1.5mg/kg (Same dose as Succinylcholine) 3min prior to intubation
  - Fentanyl (3mcg/kg – 200mcg in normal adult): Indicated, but can cause hypotension. Use with caution.
- RSI Meds:
  - Induction: Etomidate (0.3mg/kg, 20mg in normal adult) can cause hypotension. Ketamine (1.5mg/kg – 120mg in normal adult) is safe in head trauma.
  - Paralysis: Succinylcholine (1.5mg/kg, 120mg in normal adult) is preferred, although may increase ICP. Roc (1mg/kg – 80mg in normal adult) is alternative.
- Sedation:
  - Midazolam (0.04-0.2 mg/kg/h). Avoid propofol as hypotension.
  - Fentanyl (1-3mcg/kg/h) – titrate slowly to avoid hypotension.
- Vent settings:
  - ARDS-Net settings (start with 6-8 mg/kg Ideal Body Weight), plateau pressures < 30
  - Goal $PaCO_2$ 35-45mmHg (frequent gasses)
  - Down-titrate FiO_2 to < 0.6 to prevent O_2 toxicity but maintain O_2 sat >90

- **Blood pressure control:** In ED assume ICP of 20, so maintain MAP 70*-20 to keep CPP > 50 and avoid catastrophic hypertension (particularly in setting of bleed). *Some studies have shown benefit to minimum SBP >110 (Approx. CPP>70 and MAP >80).
  - Monitoring: A-line
  - Hypotension: Use crystalloid until euvolemic then vasopressors (Phenylephrine drip, starting at 10mcg/min)
  - Hypertension: Nicardipine drip (starting at 2.5mg/hour)
- **ICP Control:**
  - Head of bed to 30 degrees (okay if C-spine not yet cleared)
  - Ensure c-collar not too small (can decrease venous return and increase ICP)
    - Hyperosmolar agents:
      - Hypertonic saline – In patients with severe TBI give 23.4% over 20min if patient exhibits lateralizing signs or has an ICP>20.
      - Mannitol (1g/kg) – Place Foley, match ins and outs to prevent hypotension.
- **Seizure prophylaxis:** Levetiracetam (1gm) and Phenytoin (15mg/kg) are equivalent; base on hospital policy or consultant preference.
- **Control of bleeding:**
  - Platelets: If PLT <20 or recent aspirin/clopidogrel, give 1unit
  - Vitamin K (10mg IV) / FFP (15-20 cc/kg): If coagulopathy (INR >1.5 and head bleed)
  - Protamine 0.5mg-1mg per 100u Heparin or 1mg LMWH (max 50mg)
  - PCCs if available and patient is on coumadin
- **Antibiotics** if penetrating injury (cefazolin or vancomycin; discuss with your consultants)

- Tylenol 1gm PR, PRN fever
- Neurosurgical consult for emergent decompression/evacuation or need for invasive monitoring device

DISPOSITION

- These patients go to an ICU if intubated, obtunded, or have an arterial line, either trauma, neurosurgical, or neurologic ICU, depending on hospital availability and presence of other injuries.
- Patients with small amount of blood that is stable on repeat CT and are otherwise stable can be admitted to the floor.
- A small group of these patients be discharged home (mild TBI, otherwise healthy, GCS 15, have a safe home environment where they can be monitored, and have good follow up). These patients should be referred to an outpatient TBI clinic if available, to identify any additional neurocognitive testing and discuss return to sports.
- RETURN IF: You have severe headaches, persistent vomiting, changes in vision, or any other new or concerning symptoms.

BEWARE...

(!) Even a single episode of hypotension or hypoxia can lead to bad outcomes.

(!) Many of the agents and interventions we provide can lead to hypotension, so be careful.

Source

Zammit C, Knight WA. Severe traumatic brain injury in adults. *Emerg Med Pract*. 2013;15(3):1-28.

Section XVI. Urogenital Complaints

1 ▶ Male Quick Guide

- ALWAYS: Complete VS, complete exam including testicular, rectal, and perineal exam.
- Can't-miss diagnosis in first 2 minutes: Testicular torsion, priapism, paraphimosis, Fournier's gangrene, and scrotal trauma.

Ddx
Urethritis (STIs)
Balanitis
Balanoposthitis
Penile fracture
Phimosis
Entrapment injury

EVALUATION

- **High Yield History:** Acute vs. chronic, past medical history, medications, any recent trauma, fever, sexual activity
- **Exam:** VS, full genitourinary and abdominal exam. Examine unaffected areas first.
- Initial workup: Varies by differential diagnosis and is often clinical; however, UA and US are often first line.

Can't-Miss Urogenital Diagnoses		
Diagnosis	**Presentation**	**Initial approach**
Testicular torsion	High-riding testicle, transverse lie, absence of cremasteric reflex. Often <1yr and 10-15yrs old. Sudden onset of pain.	If suspected, call urology and THEN order testicular ultrasound. "Time is testicle."
Priapism	Unwanted erection for >4hrs. Often related to meds, malignancy, sickle-cell disease	O2 in sickle-cell disease. Otherwise phenylephrine or PO terbutaline (5mg Q15min)
Paraphimosis	Uncircumcised patient with foreskin caught in retracted position→decreased blood flow to glans	ED Reduction
Fournier's gangrene	A perineal necrotizing soft tissue infection → "pain out of proportion" to exam. Ill-appearing patient. DM, elderly or immunocompromised	Immediate surgical/urological consultation. Treat as sepsis. Cover with Zosyn IV + Vanco by nomogram
Penile / Scrotal trauma	History of trauma. Tender scrotum or penis, loss of erectile function	Remainder of trauma survey, immediate urology involvement. Caution with foley placement

Subacute diagnoses for scrotal pain and swelling			
Complaint	**Signs / Symptoms**	**Diagnosis**	**Treatment**
Appendage Torsion	Pain localized to head of testicle. Often age 3-13yo	Clinical, "blue dot" on scrotum. Difficult to clinically distinguish from testicular torsion	Conservative: NSAIDs, ice, scrotal support
Epididymitis	Teenagers and older, gradual onset of pain, dysuria, pyuria	Clinical, UA (helpful only if positive), increased blood flow on US.	<35y: ceftriaxone 250mg IM once + doxy 100mg PO BID x10d. >35y: Cipro 500mg PO BID x 14d
Epididymo-orchitis	As above + fever	As above	As above
Orchitis	Gradual onset of pain and swelling. May be bilateral. Fever, malaise.	Clinical. Consider mumps as possible Ddx.	Conservative: NSAIDs, ice, scrotal support
Hydrocele / Hematocele	Painless swelling	Scrotal ultrasound. Transillumination is NOT helpful.	Surgical consultation of >1yr old. Urgent if testicular compromise from mass effect
Scrotal Cellulitis	Tenderness, erythema	As general cellulitis	As general cellulitis
Tumor	Gradual onset of symptoms, often painless	Ultrasound	Oncology consultation
Varicocele	Painless proximal swelling	"bag of worms" on exam, US	Surgical consultation

BEWARE...

! Consider abdominal processes in the ddx such as incarcerated inguinal hernia, AAA, renal colic, appendicitis.

! Always consider non-accidental trauma in GU complaints in children.

! Assess for urethral injury in testicular trauma.

2 ▶ Priapism

Persistent, painful erection lasting more than 4hrs, independent of sexual arousal. If untreated →
erectile dysfunction, penile fibrosis, and urinary retention. Goal of management is to achieve
detumescence and preserve erectile function.

- **Ischemic (low flow).** Majority. Abnormal vasoconstriction or
  prolonged relaxation of smooth muscle→ occlusion of venous
  drainage. Firm corpus cavernosa, painful, fully erect penis.
  Urologic emergency.

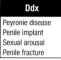

Ddx
Peyronie disease
Penile implant
Sexual arousal
Penile fracture

- **Nonischemic (high flow)** Trauma/Neurologic → unregulated
  cavernous arterial inflow (arteriovenous fistula). Typically the
  penis is neither fully rigid nor painful. Does not require emergent treatment.

EVALUATION

- **High Yield History:** Degree of pain, past history of priapism (causes and previous treatment),
  etiologies, evidence of trauma, duration
  — Causes: ~50% idiopathic. Remainder include: sickle cell, leukemia, thalassemia,
    cocaine, phenothalines, calcium channel blockers, alpha-antagonists, SSRIs, trazodone,
    intracavernous injections (papervine, prostaglandin E1)
- **Exam:** Degree of tumescence and any signs of trauma
- **Diagnostics:** Only indicated for first episode. Does not dictate care but can influence outpatient
  management. If 1st ischemic episode → CBC, consider urine tox and sickle cell labs (ie,
  reticulocyte count; see chapter). If etiology unclear consider a corpus cavernosa blood gas.

MANAGEMENT

- See flowchart.
- IV access, monitor oxygen, and provide adequate pain control!
- If secondary to sickle-cell disease, treat for vasocclusive crisis (see chapter) and per specific
  treatments.
- Involve urology consult early.
- Goal is to use alpha-agonists to constrict the smooth muscles of the corpus cavernosa and
  allow outflow of venous blood. Beta-agonists also facilitate venous outflow but through less
  clear mechanisms.
- Can start with an oral agent such as terbutaline, but most patients will require direct injection of
  an alpha-agonist.

DISPOSITION

- Patients with priapism from vasocclusive process or those with failure to achieve
  detumescence should be admitted.
- Most patients can be discharged home:
  — Apply compressive wrap to prevent hematoma and detumescence.

— May discharge with pseudoephedrine 60mg PO Q6hr x 3 days to prevent recurrence.

— Provide pain control as needed.

— Urology appointment within 1 week.

• RETURN IF: Tumescence recurs, you have severe pain, urinary retention, any chest pain or lightheadedness, or any other new or concerning symptoms.

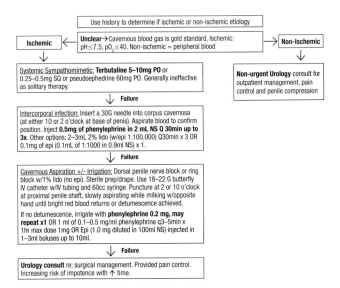

BEWARE...

(!) Ensure adequate pain control throughout ED course.

(!) Attach to monitors prior to any vasoactive meds.

(!) In a trauma patient the presence of priapism should raise the concern for a spinal cord injury.

Sources

Roberts JR, Price C, Mazzeo T. Intracavernous epinephrine: a minimally invasive treatment for priapism in the emergency department. *J Emerg Med.* 2009;36(3):285-9.

Vilke GM, Harrigan RA, Ufberg JW, Chan TC. Emergency evaluation and treatment of priapism. *J Emerg Med.* 2004;26(3):325-9.

3 ▶ Phimosis/Paraphimosis

Phimosis: The inability to retract the foreskin proximally over the glans penis

Paraphimosis: The inability to reduce the proximal edematous foreskin distally over the glans

To remember the distinction between these terms "paraphimosis" and "phimosis," you can think of the Greek translation for "para," which means "BESIDE" → In "paraphimosis," the foreskin has been retracted proximally and is on the "SIDES" of the penis, rather than down over the glans... OR "para" is the emergency and needs a PARAmedic!

PHIMOSIS

- Contracted white ring may be visible at orifice.
- Usually occurs due to distal scarring of foreskin (possibly secondary to poor hygiene, recurrent balanitis, forceful retraction of foreskin causing microtears, or in the elderly due to decreased skin elasticity and fewer erections).
- Emergent therapy is usually NOT indicated.
- Topical steroids can be helpful (0.1% betamethasone or 1% hydrocortisone BID for 4-6 weeks) in reducing the rate of required circumcision.
- Outpatient urologic referral/follow-up is recommended to monitor response to steroids, and to consider circumcision if not improving or if causing urinary outflow obstruction.

PARAPHIMOSIS

- Can occur: (a) when a patient, caretaker, or child forgets to replace the foreskin back over the glans after retraction, (b) in the elderly with chronic catheters, (c) after vigorous sexual activity or with penile piercings.
- Is a true **urologic EMERGENCY** because resulting glans edema and venous engorgement can eventually progress to arterial compromise and gangrene.
- Pathophysiology: Impairment of venous and lymphatic flow to the glans →venous engorgement, which worsens swelling → arterial supply compromise → penile infarction/ necrosis → gangrene; and lastly → auto-amputation.
- The goal of treatment is **reduction** (replacement) of the foreskin to its naturally occurring position over the glans.

Management Options for Paraphimosis

- MANUAL REDUCTION: To optimize success with this technique, you need to:
  — **Pre-treat** to help reduce the edema of the glans and/or foreskin. Various ways to pre-treat /reduce surrounding tissue edema:
    ▪ Wrap the glans with 2 x 2 in. elastic bandages for 5mins.
    ▪ Place the penis in a glove filled with ice for 5mins.
    ▪ Make several puncture wounds (up to 20!) in the foreskin, with a small 22-25 gauge needle, to help express the edema/fluid from the puncture sites during manual compression.

- Aspiration: Apply a tourniquet to the shaft of the penis. Use a 20-G needle to aspirate 3-12 mL of blood from the glans (going parallel to the urethra). This can reduce the volume of the glans sufficiently to facilitate manual reduction.
  — If tissue edema can be successfully compressed, the foreskin may be able to be manually reduced. Manual reduction is accomplished by pushing with the thumbs on the glans (to push it back through the prepuce), while the index and middle fingers try to pull the prepuce back over the glans.
- **VERTICAL INCISION/DORSAL SLIT:** If arterial compromise is suspected or has occurred, local infiltration of the constricting foreskin band with 1% plain lidocaine followed by superficial vertical incision of the band will decompress the glans and allow foreskin reduction.
  — Make a 1-2cm longitudinal incision at the 12-o'clock position on the foreskin (between two straight hemostats placed parallel near the 12-o'clock position for hemostasis)
  — Reduce the paraphimosis and repair the foreskin using 4-0 nylon sutures.
- Last resort is an emergent circumcision by a urologist.

DISPOSITION

- Admit any patient with phimosis and urinary obstruction.
- Most cases of paraphimosis are admitted to urology.
- Consider discharge if symptoms are relieved and there is no concern for urinary obstruction, recurrence, or skin infection.
- RETURN IF: Your symptoms return, you are unable to urinate, you are unable to reduce the foreskin, you have severe pain, fevers, or any other new or concerning symptoms.

Source
Ma OJ, Cline D, Tintinalli J et al. Emergency Medicine Manual. McGraw-Hill; 2003.

Notes

4 ▶ Scrotal Emergencies

- Acute scrotum: Inflamed and tender scrotum and its contents. Act quickly! You cannot miss or delay a diagnosis of torsion or a necrotizing infection.

EVALUATION

Ddx
Torsion (testicular or appendage)
Epididymitis
Epididymo-orchitis
Orchitis
Inguinal hernia
Abscess
Cellulitis
Necrotizing infection (Fournier's)
Testicular cancer
Hydrocele
Varicocele
Trauma

- A useful approach to the history is to inquire about the pain as you would normally (cardinal features, etc.) then add a directed review of symptoms to make more or less likely the "can't-miss" diagnoses.
- **High Yield History:** Time of onset (torsion does not go on steadily for days or weeks), past medical history(diabetes or immunocompromised puts pt at risk for Fournier's), sexual activity (STIs), trauma, duration, and associated systemic symptoms (nausea/ vomiting, abdominal pain, or fevers/chills).
- **Exam** (both when standing and supine): High riding testicle or transverse lie (torsion), edema, erythema, tenderness of the epididymis (epididymitis), isolated nodularity of the superior pole of the testicle, "blue dot sign" which is an isolated tender blue nodule on the upper pole of the testis or epididymis (appendage torsion), positive transillumination of scrotal fluid (hydrocele).
- **Special tests** (Note: Both poorly sensitive and **cannot** rule out torsion.)
    — **Cremasteric Reflex:** Using the handle end of a swab stick or a gloved finger, trace a line on the medial aspect of the thigh very close to the testicles – this should elicit ipsilateral contraction of the testes. Do this before touching the scrotum to get the best response. Note: This is non-specific, as not all healthy pts have a cremasteric reflex.
    — **Prehn's Sign**: Relief of pain with scrotal elevation
- **Diagnostics**
    — Imaging: Testicular US! This will rule out torsion. If deeper infection is considered you may order CT or MRI; do not delay surgery or urology consultation for this imaging, however. Note: If you are seriously considering torsion, you should call urology while getting the US, as this is a time-sensitive urological emergency.
    — Labs: CBC to screen for systemic infection and UA to look for an associated UTI.

MANAGEMENT

- Pain control, anti-emetics, and IVF. Time is a factor.
- Urology consult – If high suspicion for torsion do not delay – surgical exploration provides definitive diagnosis and treatment and will decrease subsequent atrophy; time is testicle!
- **Torsion: Manual detorsion**
    — "Open the book": Medial to lateral (but note that 30% of torsions are lateral to medial) with endpoint of pain relief; this should still be followed by surgical exploration.

- **Epididymitis: Antibiotics**
  — STD suspected: Doxycycline 100mg PO BID x 10 - 14 days AND Ceftriaxone 250mg IM x1 (Azithromycin 2gm x 1 if PCN allergic)
  — STD not suspected: Ciprofloxacin 500mg BID or Levofloxacin 750mg PO QDx 10 - 14 days
- **Appendage Torsion: NSAIDs**, will self-resolve after 1-2 weeks
- **Necrotizing Infection or Fournier's Gangrene: Early surgical consult** and broad-spectrum antibiotics (Ciprofloxacin 400mg IV and Clindamycin 1.2gm IV +/- Vancomycin 1gm IV)
- **Inguinal Hernia: Gentle reduction** and consult surgery if concern for incarceration (painful, non reducible, symptoms of SBO) or strangulation (incarcerated and toxic)
- **Cellulitis**: Ensure that not a necrotizing infection. Then treat as you would cellulitis of other areas with scrotal support/elevation.

DISPOSITION

- Testicular torsion, Fournier's, an incarcerated hernia, and serious trauma will likely end in the OR with urology or surgery (both services will ALWAYS need to be consulted).
- Most patients with epididymitis, orchitis, or appendage torsion can be discharged home with appropriate antibiotics and pain control. Consider observation for pain control or first dose IV antibiotics.
- RETURN IF: You develop high fevers, severe pain, difficulty urinating, or any other new or concerning symptoms.

BEWARE...

(!) Get the ultrasound started early on these patients; you may have your answer before you do your full history and physical.

(!) Consider the very wide differential; ultimately your first thought should be to rule out an acute scrotum that could result in loss of testicle or life.

Notes

5 ▶ Urinary Tract Infection and Pyelonephritis

- **UTI:** Infection with any one or a combination of organisms anywhere along the urinary tract, from the kidneys to the urethra.

- Extremely common and can affect men and women of all ages, but most common in women, infants, and patients with indwelling catheters or recent urologic procedures.

- Pyelonephritis is a UTI that affects the kidney.

- Asymptomatic bacteriuria describes a situation where bacteria are discovered on laboratory testing in the absence of any clinical symptoms.

- Offending organisms typically ascend the urethra, but seeding can occur from a distant site of infection through hematogenous or lymphatic spread.

Ddx
Urethritis
Vaginitis
PID
Nephrolithiasis
Iterstitial cystitis
Prostatitis
Mechanical irritation of the urethra
Epididymitis
Diverticulitis can cause dysuria

CLASSIFICATION

- **Uncomplicated** UTIs occur in patients with normal urinary tract structure and function. Typically respond to standard treatment.

- **Complicated** UTIs occur in patients with abnormal urinary tract structure and function, including patients with indwelling catheters, obstructing stones, prostatic hypertrophy, pregnancy, neurologic diseases affecting the ability to void, or diabetes.

EVALUATION

- **High Yield History:** Hematuria (cystitis/stone), prior or recent UTIs, urologic procedures or instrumentation, urethral or vaginal discharge and constitutional symptoms such as rigors (pyelonephritis), altered mental status, fevers, anorexia, back pain (pyelonephritis)

- **Classic symptoms**
  - Urgency, frequency, dysuria, suprapubic pain, hematuria, nausea, emesis, fever. **Infants or elderly patients may present with altered mental status or irritability.**
  - Pyelonephritis often presents with any of the UTI symptoms as well as pain in the costo-vertebral angle (CVA tenderness).

- **Exam:** In men, consider a genital exam and prostate exam to evaluate for prostatitis (boggy, tender prostate), prostatic hypertrophy, sexually transmitted infection, epididymitis. In women, consider a pelvic exam to evaluate for PID/STI symptoms.

- **Labs**
  - Urine sample: In women, a clean-catch urine may be obtained, but often is contaminated, making results difficult to interpret. A specimen obtained by sterile catheterization is the most reliable (especially for elderly). In men, it is usually not necessary to perform catheterization.
  - Urine dip: Evaluate for leukocyte esterase, nitrites, and hematuria.
  - Urine microscopy: Evaluate for leukocytes, bacteria, red cells, casts.

- Urine C&S: Consider obtaining in patients with complicated UTIs, male patients, pregnant women, children, patients with systemic symptoms, and symptomatic patients with negative urinalysis. A positive culture is defined as 10^5 CFU/mL.
- Consider **imaging** of the urinary tract and/or abdomen with CT or ultrasound when concerned for structural abnormalities, abscess, possible obstruction, or to evaluate for other etiologies of symptoms. Note: This is not routinely needed.
- **Most common organisms:** Enterobacter enterococcus, Escherichia coli, Staphylococcus saprophyticus, Proteus, and Klebsiella

UA Results	
Nitrite	50% sensitive, 90% specific. + E.coli (- in enterococcus, pseudomonas, acinobacter)
Leuk Esterase	70% sensitive, 50% specific
WBC	>5/HPF highly sensitive
Bacteria	>1/HPF 95% sensitive, 60% specific
Epithelial cells	>2-3 confounds above results

MANAGEMENT

- **Asymptomatic Bacteriuria:** Unless pregnant, patients with asymptomatic bacteriuria do not require treatment.
- **Antibiotics:** Depends on complicated vs. uncomplicated infections, severity of infection, ability of patient to tolerate oral antibiotics, and local resistance patterns. For patients who cannot tolerate PO regimens or are extremely ill, start parenteral antibiotics and transition to enteral options as clinically able.
- **Supportive care:** Patients with severe infections or certain associated symptoms may require intravenous fluids, anti-emetics, and in cases of sepsis, respiratory and hemodynamic support.
- **Symptom relief:** Pyridium (phenazopyridine) may be used for symptomatic control. Patients must be warned that this medication may give their urine and tears an orange color.
- **Consults and follow-up:** Patients with a UTI in the setting of obstruction or abscess require a prompt urology consult. Men with UTIs, patients with recurrent or unresolved UTIs should follow up with an urologist as an outpatient.

Antibiotic Regimens	
Uncomplicated	**Complicated**
Nitrofurantoin 100mg twice daily for 5 days	Ciprofloxacin 500mg twice daily for 5-14 days
Ciprofloxacin 250mg-500mg, twice daily for 3 days. 500mg in men	Levofloxacin 750mg once daily for 5-14 days
Levofloxacin 250mg-750mg, once daily for 3 days. 750 mg in men	Ceftriaxone 1 gram daily
Bactrim 160/800, twice daily for 3 days. Do not use if Bactrim use in prior 3 months	
Fosfomycin 3grams, single dose	

DISPOSITION

- Determined based on their clinical status and cause of UTI.
- Patients with obstruction, severe infection, inability to tolerate PO, hemodynamic instability, or other systemic symptoms require admission.
- Most uncomplicated UTI and early pyelonephritis can be treated on an outpatient basis.
- RETURN IF: You develop high fevers, chills, back pain, persistent vomiting, stop urinating, have blood in your urine, or any other new or concerning symptoms.

BEWARE...

- (!) UTI should be at the top of your differential in a nursing home patient with altered mental status.
- (!) Evaluate men complaining of dysuria for STIs and prostatitis.
- (!) If patient has signs and symptoms of UTI or pyelonephritis and a normal urinalysis, consider obstruction.
- (!) A positive nitrite test suggests Gram negative bacteria. Leukocyte esterase can yield false positives if the patient has consumed beets or is using phenazopyridine.
- (!) Consider fungal infection in diabetic patients.
- (!) Failing to consider contributing factors such as stones/urinary retention.
- (!) Treating positive UAs in patients with a neobladder; they may be colonized, not infected.
- (!) If hypotensive or in shock with recurrent pyelonephritis and persistent symptoms, consider imaging to rule out stone or perinephric abscess.

Sources

Gupta, K et al. International Clinical Practice Guidelines for the Treatment of Acute Uncomplicated Cystitis and Pyelonephritis in Women: A 2010 Update by the Infectious Diseases Society of America and the European Society of Microbiology and Infectious Diseases. *Clinical Infectious Diseases* 2011; 52 (5): e103-120.

Hooton, T et al. Diagnosis, Prevention and Treatment of Catheter-Associated Urinary Tract Infections in Adults: 2009 International Clinical Practice Guidelines from the Infectious Diseases Society of America. *Clinical Infectious Diseases* 2010; 50: 625-663

Notes

6 ▶ Vaginal Bleed Quick Guide

- ALWAYS: IV, O2, monitor, COMPLETE VS (including temperature and pulse oximetry), EKG, pelvic exam, HCG .
- Can't-miss diagnoses in first 2 minutes: Ruptured ectopic, septic abortion, or any hemodynamically significant bleed.

EVALUATION

- **High Yield History:** Duration, quantity/number of pads/hour (helps risk stratification), lightheadedness/ shortness of breath/chest pain (anemia), clots/tissue (spontaneous abortion), last menstrual period (pregnancy), trauma (foreign body), hot flashes (perimenopausal), cramping (adenomyosis, fibroids), association with intercourse (cervical lesion), cocaine use, history of C-sections (uterine abruption if pregnant), vaginal discharge/ pelvic pain/fever (PID), abdominal pain (ectopic)

Ddx	
Pregnant	**Not Pregnant**
Spontaneos abortion	Dysfunctional uterine bleeding
Molar pregnancy	Polycystic ovarian syndrome
Ectopic pregnancy	Fibroids
Placenta previa	Physiologic
Vasa previa	Post-coital
Placental abruption	Anovulation
Uterine rupture	Uterine leiomyomas
Implantation bleed	Thyroid dysfunction
Cervical polyp	Cervicitis/STIs
Cervical cancer	Uterine/cervical polyps
Post-coital	Endometrial cancer
	Exogenous hormone use
	Coagulopathy

- **Past medical history:** Clotting/bleeding disorders, spontaneous abortions/miscarriages, STIs, liver disease
- **Meds:** Coumadin, beta blocker (can mask tachycardia, 1st sign of hemodynamic instability)
- **Exam:** FULL VITALS!
  — Speculum: Os open/closed, blood in vault, clots, products of conception, consider cervical swabs if concern for infection
  — Bimanual: Softness/patency of os, cervical motion tenderness (PID), adnexal tenderness (ectopic)
  — If >20wks GA need to US before speculum exam to ensure no placenta previa.
  — Full abdominal exam (including enlarged uterus/masses – fibroids)
- **Initial Workup:** Urine HCG, CBC, type+screen (Rh), type+crossmatch 2 units if unstable, serum HCG, coags, pelvic US

MANAGEMENT

- Hemodynamically unstable: 2 large bore IVs, STAT OB/GYN consult. If need to transfuse blood use O negative.
  — Non-pregnant women:
    ▪ Consider Premarin (25mg IV) in non-pregnant women without contraindication
    ▪ Pediatric foley inserted into Os, with balloon inflated to tamponade the bleeding
    ▪ Patient may require urgent dilation and curettage with GYN

- — Pregnant women:
  - Emergent delivery
  - Supportive care with IVF and O negative blood
  - RhoGam 300 mcg IM in Rh (-) women
- Hemodynamically stable:
  - — Non-pregnant women:
    - Short term hormones (allows endometrium to stabilize). Consider OCP with or without progesterone based on the patient's risk factors.
    - Outpatient pelvic ultrasound to assess endometrial stripe and for anatomic etiology for bleeding
    - Some patients may require endometrial biopsy prior to initiation of hormonal therapy.
  - — Pregnant women
    - Specific management based on where the patient is in her pregnancy.
    - If early in pregnancy determine presence of IUP, if not visualized must work up for ectopic pregnancy.
    - If after 1st trimester, perform bedside US to assess FHR. Do not perform cervical exam unless location of placenta is known.
    - All patients should have a UA obtained.
    - RhoGam for Rh negative patients
    - If abruption is considered the patient warrants urgent evaluation by OB/GYN.
    - If bleeding thought to be from placenta previa or vasa previa patients should be admitted to the labor and delivery floor.

Sources

Zane RD, Kosowsky JM, et al. Pocket Emergency Medicine. 2nd ed. Philadelphia, PA: Lippincott Williams & Wilkins; 2011.

Ma OJ, Cline D, Tintinalli J, et al. Emergency Medicine Manual. 6th ed. New York, NY: McGraw-Hill Professional; 2003.

Marx J, Hockberger R, Walls R. Rosen's Emergency Medicine: Concepts & Clinical Practice. 5th ed. Maryland Heights, MO: Mosby; 2002.

Hans L, Mawji Y. The ABCs of Emergency Medicine. 12th edition. Toronto, Canada: University of Toronto; 2012.

Medscape News & Perspective. New York, NY: http://emedicine.medscape.com.

7 ▶ Non-Pregnant Vaginal Bleeding

- ED management of non-pregnant vaginal bleeding: Assess whether patient is stable/unstable, exclude pregnancy, ensure appropriate follow-up for patients able to be discharged.

EVALUATION

- **High Yield History:**

  — Nature of bleeding: Frequency, duration, volume, relationship to menstrual cycle and coitus

  — Irregular, heavy periods (anovulation) and whether the patient is pre- or post-menopausal

  — Changes in bowel or bladder function (mass)

  — New headache, nipple discharge, hot flashes, changes in skin/hair (endocrine disorder)

  — Obesity and hirsutism (polycystic ovarian syndrome)

  — Personal or family history of excessive bleeding, coumadin use (coagulopathy)

  — Recent pregnancies or gynecologic procedures

  — Last pap smear by OB/GYN, history of HPV, smoking history

Ddx
Neoplasm
Trauma
Fibroids
Retained POCs
Polycystic ovarian syndrome
Anovulatory cycle (mid cycle, lasting 2 wks)
Coagulopathy
Polyps
Rectal/GI bleed
Endometritis
Foreign body
Vaginitis
Thyroid
Urinary tract bleeding
STIs

- **Exam:** Vitals (signs of clinically significant hemorrhage), fever, abdominal tenderness. On speculum exam assess for amount of bleeding and presence of clots tissue or any visible traumatic injury. Have suction nearby in case of significant bleeding.

- **Diagnostic tests:**

  — Pregnancy test (exclude pregnancy-related bleeding), CBC, coags +/- type and screen (or cross), consider LFTs

  — Consider US in patients with painful or hemodynamically significant bleeding to assess for etiologies such as fibroids, ruptured ovarian cyst, or retained products of conception (POCs).

  — GCC if suspect infection,

MANAGEMENT OF UNSTABLE PATIENT

- 2 large bore IVs, IV NS, transfusion PRN, and emergent OB/GYN consult.
- Consider hormonal management with OB/GYN input (high dose estrogen therapy).
- Consider Foley catheter with 30cc balloon inserted through cervical os and inflated to tamponade bleeding.

DISPOSITION

- Majority of patients can be discharged with outpatient OB/GYN follow up.
- If concerned for retained products of conception consult OB/GYN for possible admission as well as treatment (expectant management vs. medical management with misoprostol vs. dilation and evacuation).
- May prescribe combined OCP taper (with at least 35mcg estrogen) or medroxyprogesterone if suspect dysfunction uterine bleeding in reproductive age women who have no contraindication to hormonal therapy (history of breast, uterine cancer, acute liver disease, hypertriglyceridemia, DVTs, PEs, endometriosis, fibroids).
- Patients should follow up with OB/GYN to have a TVUS to assess for fibroids or thickened endometrial stripe. Postmenopausal should have outpatient biopsy due to higher risk of endometrial carcinoma.
- RETURN IF: You have increased bleeding, lightheadedness, shortness of breath, fevers, severe pain, or any other concerning symptoms.

BEWARE...

- ⚠ Always obtain an HCG on patients with vaginal bleeding.
- ⚠ HCG can remain positive for weeks after a miscarriage or termination. It can also be negative in patients with retained POCs.
- ⚠ Always assess patient for non-vaginal source of bleeding (can be urethral or rectal).
- ⚠ Always consider sexual abuse in prepubertal girls presenting with vaginal bleeding, especially if trauma is to posterior fourchette (straddle injuries are more common to the mons or labia).

Notes

8 ▶ First Trimester Vaginal Bleeding

Key Steps:

1) Confirm pregnancy with urine or serum HCG.

2) Confirm the presence of an intrauterine pregnancy.

Many patients can be discharged with only a thorough history and physical and a bedside ultrasound.

Ddx
Spontaneous abortion
Ectopic pregnancy
Implantation Bleeding
Subchorionic hemorrhage
Infection
Hemorrhagic cystitis
Cervica/vaginal lesions (polyps, neoplastic lesions)
Trauma
Maternal coagulopathy
Thrombocytopenia

EVALUATION

- **High Yield History**: Characterize bleeding (onset, # of pads, blood only vs. clots or tissue), abdominal pain/contractions, weakness, dizziness, or other symptoms of anemia or hypovolemia, trauma (includes intercourse, but only for small bleeds).

- **Exam**: Tachycardia, hypotension, pallor, orthostatic hypotension or other positional features, abdominal tenderness, other mucosal bleeding (mouth, rectum).

  — Speculum exam to evaluate source of bleeding (os vs other), presence of clots / tissue (remove with scopettes), friable cervix. If POCs visible in vault or os save in specimen jar and send to pathology.

  — Cervical exam to determine if os is open or closed.

- If unstable, consider OR to locate source of bleeding.

- If stable:

  — Bedside US: Assess for IUP and fetal heart rate.

  — Formal US if unable to visualize IUP or obtain fetal heart rate.

- Ultrasound **findings associated with increased risk of failed pregnancy:**

  — Abnormally sized yolk or gestational sac

  — Slow fetal HR (<100bpm)

  — Subchorionic hematoma

- **Labs:** Based on presentation and stability. Consider CBC, type and screen, coags. If patient stable, minimal bleeding, and is known to be Rh + generally no need for labs other than UA or HCG.

Abortion Classifications	
Threatened	Patients present with vaginal bleeding but os is closed on exam and there is appropriate FHR on ultrasound.
Inevitable	Vaginal bleeding with an open os but have not passed any POCs and gestational sac can sometimes be seen on US.
Incomplete	Similar to inevitable but some tissue has passed.
Complete	The entire uterine contents have been expelled. US with empty uterus. Os may be open or closed,
Missed	Intrauterine fetal demise. May or may not have bleeding. Os generally closed. US with absent fetal heart rate.

MANAGEMENT

- Resuscitation and emergent OB/GYN consultation if unstable.
- RhoGAM in pts who are Rh negative.
- If ectopic pregnancy suspected → see ectopic chapter
- Incomplete, inevitable, or missed abortions can be managed expectantly, medically (generally misoprostol), or surgically (dilation and curettage /evacuation).

DISPOSITION

- Unstable patients are admitted.
- Patients with inevitable, incomplete, or missed abortions can generally be discharged home with close OB/GYN followup.
- Patients who are Rh+ and have threatened miscarriage can safely be discharged home without further intervention.
- Patients with subchorionic hematoma should be discharged with counseling and expectant management. No clear evidence to recommend bed rest. In one meta-analysis this finding on ultrasound was associated with an 18% risk of spontaneous abortion vs. 9% in those without this finding.
- RETURN IF: You have severe pain, heavy bleeding, lightheadedness, shortness of breath, high fever, or any other concerning symptoms.

BEWARE...

(!) Do not confuse empty uterus with completed abortion, if patient did not have a previously documented IUP this may still be an ectopic.

(!) Remember to treat asymptomatic bacteriuria in pregnant women.

Sources

Tannirandorm Y, Sangsawang S, Montoya S, Uerpairojkit B, Samritpradit P, Charoenvidhya D. Fetal loss in threatened abortion after embyryonic/fetal heart activity. *Int J Gynaecol Obstet.* 2003; 81 (3);263

Tuuli MG, Norman SM, Odibo AO, Macones GA, Cahill AG Perinatal outcomes in women with subchorionic hematoma: a systematic review and meta-analysis. *Obstet Gynecol.* 2011;117(5):1205.

Notes

9 ▶ Ectopic Pregnancy

- Occurs in up to 2% of all pregnancies, most common 6-10 wks after LMP.
- Symptoms variable based on location of pregnancy (majority in fallopian tube) and whether it is ruptured.
- A ruptured ectopic pregnancy can lead to a life-threatening hemorrhage.

Ddx
Spontaneous abortion
Threatened abortion
Ovarian torsion
Ruptured / hemorrhagic ovarian cyst
Appendicitis
Salpingitis
UTI
Nephrolithiasis
PID
Implantation bleed
Molar pregnancy

EVALUATION

- **High Yield History:**
  - Assess for risk factors: IUD, previous ectopic, fertility treatment, PID, tubal ligation, DES exposure.
  - Majority of patients present with abdominal pain (most common), vaginal bleeding, and positive HCG.
  - There is no bleeding pattern or description of the pain that is pathognomonic for an ectopic. Some patients may be asymptomatic.
- Exam: Vitals (tachycardia, hypotension). Lower abdominal tenderness. Speculum exam to quantify amount and source of bleeding. Bimanual exam: Assess if os is open/closed. Assess for unilateral adnexal tenderness.
- Labs: Quantitative and urine HCG (should double every 48hrs), CBC, ABO and Rh, coags.
  - Ultrasound: Start with bedside ultrasound to assess for IUP and FAST if concerned for ruptured ectopic. If bedside is FAST negative, no IUP is seen, and patient is hemodynamically stable, obtain TVUS.
  - To confirm an IUP, must visualize both a gestational sac and a yolk sac (generally present around 5 weeks).
  - A gestational sac alone does not rule in an IUP. Some ectopics can have a pseudogestational sac in the uterus.
    - Discriminatory zone: The HCG level above which an IUP, if present, should be seen:
    - Transvaginal US: roughly 1500-2000 IU/ml
    - Transabdominal US: 4,000-6,500 IU/ ml
    - Yolk sac generally seen at 5 weeks; fetal cardiac activity at 5.5 - 6 weeks after LMP.

Initial Management of Unstable Patient

- 2 large bore IVs, IVF, type and cross match 2 units of O negative blood, monitor, STAT OB consult for surgical management.

Initial Management of Stable Patient

- All patients who are pregnant, bleeding, and are Rh negative should receive Rhogam 300mcg.
- If below the discriminatory zone, consult OB/GYN to arrange follow up and have repeat HCG in 48-72hrs. Inappropriate rise in HCG and failure to visualize presence of yolk sac once above the discriminatory zone is considered an abnormal pregnancy.

- If above the discriminatory zone and no IUP seen and no clear ectopic visualized on TVUS, the patient has a pregnancy of unknown location vs. a failed early pregnancy. These patients also require OB/GYN consult for further management but generally are discharged home.
  - If visualized ectopic pregnancy, obtain OB/GYN consult for decision around treatment (surgical vs. medical therapy) and admission decision. All treatment decisions, especially methotrexate, should be made in conjunction with an OB/GYN. However, you should note the indications and contraindications in order to advocate for your patient.
    - **Methotrexate (MTX)**: A folate antagonist that interferes with DNA synthesis
    - Must check BUN/creatinine, LFTs, CBC before administering.
    - Contraindications: Unstable patients or ruptured ectopic pregnancies, quant HCG >15,000 IU/L, fetal cardiac activity, or free fluid on US, gestational sac > 3.5cm, liver or renal disease, patient is breastfeeding or is unable to comply with follow up monitoring.
  - Need follow-up serum HCG days 4 and 7.
  - Surgical Management: Often the treatment of last resort. Indicated in ruptured ectopic, hemodynamic instability, contraindications to methotrexate, or failed medical therapy.

DISPOSITION

- If unstable or plan for surgical admit to OB/GYN or to OR.
- Many patients can be discharged home but must ensure they have close OB/GYN follow up and ability to return.
- Patients receiving MTX need to be counseled regarding risk of rupture, not to consume alcohol, use NSAIDs, and avoid folate-containing vitamins.
- RETURN IF: You have abdominal pain, high fever, fainting, shortness of breath, increased vaginal bleeding, or other concerning symptoms.

BEWARE...

(!) Do not be reassured by stable vital signs. These patients are generally younger and have good physiologic reserve.

(!) Ectopic can present with ANY HCG level. Do not be fooled by a very low quantitative HCG level.

(!) Heterotopic pregnancies are exceedingly rare, but also keep it on the differential in in-vitro fertilization patients.

Notes

10 ▶ Preeclampsia/Eclampsia

Thought to be spectrum of similar disease process; generally happens after 20wks, and can occur up to 6wks in the postpartum setting.

- **Preeclampsia**: BP>140/90 with edema, proteinuria (1+ on dipstick is suggestive and 300mg in 24hrs diagnostic).

- **Eclampsia**: Preeclampsia with seizure (generally generalized tonic-conic) or coma.

- **HELLP Syndrome**: Hemolysis (microangiopathic), Elevated liver enzymes (LDH >600IU/L, AST >70, Tbili>1.2mg/dL) and Low Platelets (<100K). Controversy whether this is a severe form of preeclampsia or a separate entity.

Ddx
Hypertension – Chronic vs. Gestational
CVA
Seizure disorder
Meningitis
Drug use
Hypoglycemia
TTP
Reversible posterior leukoencphalopathy syndrome
Space occupying lesion

EVALUATION

- **High Yield History:** Assess for risk factors including parity, previous preecplampsia.
  - Common symptoms include headache, visual changes (scotoma or blurred vision), AMS, abdominal pain, nausea, vomiting, shortness of breath, and focal neurologic complaints.

- **Exam:** Hypertension, hyperreflexia, RUQ tenderness, and lower extremity edema

- **Labs:**
  - Fingerstick glucose
  - CBC
  - Thrombocytopenia or elevations in ALT/AST, BUN, creatinine, uric acid, +/- coags are concerning.
  - Consider urine protein or protein/Cr ratio (>0.18 is positive) in any pregnant pt with HTN.

  Eclampsia is seizure in these patients. Look for a gravid uterus in any seizing female.

- **Imaging:** Consider head CT to evaluate for alternative etiology or MRI to evaluate for PRES or CVA.

- **Transfusion:** Patients with HELLP should receive platelet transfusion if they are bleeding.

MANAGEMENT

- **ABCs:** If seizing, must protect airway (place oral airway or intubate as needed) and provide supplemental O_2.
  - Seizure management:
  - Prevention (Mg 2-4g IV load over 30 minutes then 1g/hr)
- Treatment (Mg 2-4g IV q5-10min; Diazepam 5mg IV q 5 min or phenytoin 15-20mg/kg IV x1)
  - Control BP: To prevent cerebral hemorrhage. Don't drop BP more than 25% in first 30min. Goal BP 140-155/90-105 within the first several hours.
  - Labetalol 10-20mg IV x1 and then double dose Q10min up 80mg to max 200mg.

- Hydralazine 5-10mg IV q20min as needed.
- Call OB immediately. Delivery and removal of the placenta is the only definitive treatment.
- If patient is post-partum, goal is aggressive seizure and blood pressure management.
- Complications of eclampsia include DIC, acute renal failure, acute pulmonary edema, intracranial hemorrhage, and ultimately cardiac arrest. Must be aware of these potential complications and treat as you would any other patient as you move toward emergent c-section.

DISPOSITION

- OR for STAT cesarean section if eclampsia.
- If preeclampsia, can admit to OB/GYN for further management.
- ICU for BP control and airway monitoring if postpartum.

BEWARE...

(!) Monitor for magnesium toxicity: diminished deep tendon reflexes, somnolence, dilated pupils, decreased respiratory drive, hypotension, and bradycardia.

(!) Remember, fetal well-being depends on maternal well-being. Do not be distracted by a fetal ultrasound and forget maternal ABCs.

Source

Steegers EA, Von dadelszen P, Duvekot JJ, Pijnenborg R. Pre-eclampsia. *Lancet*. 2010;376(9741):631-44.

Notes

11 ▶ Nausea and Vomiting in Pregnancy

- Common complaint in the first trimester and occurs in up to 70% of patients. New onset of nausea or vomiting after the first trimester is suspicious for other etiologies and should prompt further workup.

- **Hyperemesis Gravidarum** is a severe form of nausea and vomiting that causes starvation and metabolic derangements.

- Goal is to treat dehydration, electrolyte imbalances, and maternal malnutrition.

Ddx
Normal pregnancy
Hyperemesis Gravidarum
Gastroenteritis
DKA
Appendicitis
Cholecystis
Ovarian torsion
Nephrolithiasis
Intracranial process

EVALUATION

- **High Yield History:** Broad multi-system history is warranted (GI, urinary, neurologic).
  — Ask about pre-pregnancy weight, quantity and frequency of vomiting, inciting events (food, change in position, sick contacts, nausea earlier in pregnancy or in previous pregnancies).
  — Association with abdominal pain is suspicious for intra-abdominal process (appendicitis, cholecystitis, pancreatitis, SBO, gastroenteritis, food-borne illness).
  — Association with headache is common, but should raise suspicion of intracranial process.
  — Inquire about PO history and urine output.

- **Exam:** Tachycardia and hypotension can occur if very dehydrated. Assess mucus membranes, skin turgor, flow murmurs, thorough abdominal exam (localization and characterization of abdominal tenderness), neurologic exam if headache present.

- **Labs:**
  — BMP for assessment of electrolyte status and glucose if truly vomiting (comprehensive panel including LFTs if abdominal pain present)
  — CBC if systemic infection suspected. Also provides info on dehydration status/volume contraction.
  — UA for specific gravity and ketones.
  — TSH if hyperemesis gravidarum (HG) suspected.

MANAGEMENT

- Fluid resuscitation. Consider dextrose source if ketonuria is present.

- Antiemetic: Consider ondansetron or metoclopramide—both category B. Prochlorperazine is sometimes used but not first line agent. Recent literature has linked ondansetron to a possible increase in fetal cardiac malformations, so caution is advised. Vitamin B6 25-50mg.

- Correct metabolic derangements: Replete potassium.

- If non-pregnancy related etiology identified, treat as indicated with attention to radiation and medication teratogen concerns.

DISPOSITION

- Refractory nausea and inability to tolerate POs is criteria for admission.

- Patients who have relief of nausea and corrected electrolyte imbalances may discharge home following PO challenge.

- For suspected hyperemesis gravidarum, 25mg B-6 and 12.5mg doxylamine TID is effective prophylaxis in most cases and is now considered first line treatment for outpatients, according to ACOG.

- For non-hyperemesis cases, dietary modifications, famotidine PO, and follow up w/ OB/GYN. PO ondansetron (8mg Q8hrs PRN nausea) is effective but again, caution is advised as previously mentioned. Metoclopramide 5-10mg PO Q8 PRN nausea or promethazine 12.5mg PO Q4 PRN nausea are also effective.

- Patients should be counseled to see primary OB within 2-3 days.

- RETURN IF: Your vomiting persists and are unable tolerate and food or liquids, any severe abdominal pain, high fevers, vaginal bleeding, lightheadedness, palpitations, or any other new or concerning symptoms.

BEWARE...

⚠ Perform a careful abdominal exam in these patients; they are at higher risk for biliary disease, and the normal anatomic location of the intrabdominal organs will change with the growing uterus. The appendix could be anywhere!

⚠ Ensure a careful neurologic exam and carefully think through intracranial etiologies of symptoms, especially if headache also present.

Sources

McCarthy FP, Lutomski JE, Greene RA Hyperemesis gravidarum: current perspectives. *Int J Womens Health.* 2014 Aug 5; 6:719-25

Matthews A, Haas DM, O"Mathuna, Dowswell T, Doyle M Interventions for nausea and vomiting in early pregnancy. Cochran Database Syst Rev 2014 Mar 21;3.

Notes

12 ▶ Vaginitis

- Vaginitis is a term used to describe disorders of the vagina resulting in discomfort, increased discharge, odor, or pruritus.
- The most common causes are bacterial vaginosis, candida, and trichomoniasis.

Ddx	
Infectious	**Non Infectious**
Vaginal source	Physiological
Candida	Puberty
Trichomoniasis	Pregnancy
Bacterial vaginosis	Neoplasm
Cervical Source	Post-menopausal
Gonorrhea	Non-physiological
Chlamydia	Foreign body
Herpes simplex	Chemical irritant
	Med side effect

EVALUATION

- **High Yield History:** Nature of discharge (see table), abdominal pain, dyspareunia, vulvar pain, blisters, lesions, urinary symptoms, medications already tried. Pelvic pain and fever are atypical and suggest other etiology.
  - History of STIs, sexual history (number of partners, new partners, partner with symptoms) point toward infectious etiology.
  - Foreign bodies (such as tampons), personal hygiene practices (eg, douching), new soaps, lotions, or condoms make chemical irritation more likely.
  - Last menstrual period and if menopausal → decreased estrogen leads to atrophic changes.
  - Timing (duration, association with menstrual cycle) → physiologic discharge heaviest mid-cycle.
- **Exam:** Fever, abdominal or pelvic tenderness, vaginal exam including speculum and bimanual, looking for discharge, lesions, CMT (PID) , atrophic changes (thin, loss of elasticity, friable)
- **Diagnostics:** Urine HCG, urine/cervical GCC. If recurrent candida, consider FSGS to rule out DM.

MANAGEMENT

- Management based on etiology: Patients with unclear diagnosis or non-infectious etiology can generally follow up with OB/GYN for further diagnostics and treatment.
- Atrophic vaginitis: Follow up with OB/GYN to discuss topical estrogens.
- Chemical irritation: Stop the offending agent. If unclear irritant, advise symptom journal.
- If herpetic lesion seen on exam → Acyclovir 400mg TID
- If concern for GCC or PID → Ceftriaxone 250mg IM x1 AND Doxycycline 100mg BID x14 days; may add Metronidazole

Signs and Symptoms of Infective Causes of Vaginal Discharge			
Signs/Symptoms	Bacterial Vaginosis	Candida	Trichomoniasis
Discharge	Thin	Thick-white	Scanty to profuse
Odor	Offensive/fish	Non-offensive	Offensive
Itch	None	Vulvar	Vulvar
Other	Usually asymptomatic	Soreness, superficial dyspareunia, dysuria	Dysuria, lower abdominal pain
Signs	Discharge coating the vagina and vestibule, no vulvar inflammation	Normal OR vulvar erythema, fissuring with satellite lesions	Frothy discharge, vulvitis, vaginitis, cervicitis, strawberry cervix
Vaginal pH	> 4.5	<4.5	>4.5

- Trichomoniasis: Metronidazole 500mg BID x7 days OR Metronidazole 0.75% gel 5gm daily x 5 days. Gel is best for pregnant pt.

- Bacterial vaginosis: Metronidazole 500mg BID x 7-14 days, and partner should seek treatment.

- Candidiasis: Treat only if symptomatic. Uncomplicated: Fluconazole 150mg PO x1. Complicated: If poorly controlled DM or recurrent infections → Fluconazole 150mg PO x2 (day 0 and day 3). If pregnant use topical cream i.e. miconazole x 7 days

Dispostion

- Home with Abx as described, with close GYN follow up.

- If treating for GCC or PID, patient should follow up outpatient to have HIV testing and should inform their partners to be treated.

- RETURN IF: You develop fevers, pelvic pain, or symptoms get worse despite treatment.

BEWARE...

(!) If discharge is serosanguinous and patient has pelvic pain, have high suspicion for malignancy.

(!) If prescribing metronidazole, ensure you counsel patient regarding potential disulfiram-like reaction.

Sources

Zane RD, Kosowsky JM, et al. Pocket Emergency Medicine. 2nd ed. Philadelphia, PA: Lippincott Williams & Wilkins; 2011.

Ma OJ, Cline D, Tintinalli J, et al. Emergency Medicine Manual. 6th ed. New York, NY: McGraw-Hill Professional; 2003.

Marx J, Hockberger R, Walls R. Rosen's Emergency Medicine: Concepts & Clinical Practice. 5th ed. Maryland Heights, MO: Mosby; 2002.

Hans L, Mawji Y. The ABCs of Emergency Medicine. 12th edition. Toronto, Canada: University of Toronto; 2012.

Medscape News & Perspective. New York, NY: http://emedicine.medscape.com.

13 ▶ Pelvic Inflammatory Disease

- Pelvic inflammatory disease (PID) is an infection of upper female genital tract (uterus, fallopian tubes, and pelvic structures).

- If untreated, it can lead to tubo-ovarian abscess, peritonitis, or Fitz-Hugh-Curtis syndrome (infection of periphepatic structures).

- Most often caused by chlamydia; however, can also be caused by *Neisseria gonorrhoeae*, *Gardnerella vaginalis*, *Haemophilus influenzae*, and anaerobes such as *Peptococcus* and *Bacteroides* species.

- **Diagnostic criteria**: Women with uterine or adnexal tenderness AND cervical motion tenderness.

Ddx
Appendicitis
Cervicitis
UTI
Endometriosis
Adnexal tumors
Ectopic
Ovarian cysts

EVALUATION

- **High Yield History:** Symptoms are generally dull, achy, crampy bilateral lower abdominal pain, nausea, vomiting, post coital bleeding, and low grade fever.
  - Risk factors: Multiple sexual partners, menstruating, does not use contraception, lives in an area with high STI prevalence.

- **Exam:** Patients can have cervical motion tenderness (CMT), adnexal or uterine tenderness and mucopurulent cervicitis.
  - Systemic symptoms such as fever may be present
  - Adnexal fullness or disproportionate unilateral adnexal tenderness is suggestive of tubo-ovarian abscess (TOA).
  - RUQ tenderness, especially if associated with jaundice, may indicate Fitz-Hugh-Curtis.

- **Diagnostics**
  - Labs: Urine/cervical GCC, HCG, and UA. Others are most often not necessary. Can consider CBC and BMP systemically ill or help exclude alternate diagnoses.
  - TVUS: The absence of findings does not exclude PID, therefore should not delay treatment. Always treat, even with small suspicion. Can help evaluate for TOA, especially in patients who are febrile or systemically ill.

MANAGEMENT

- If systemically ill, resituate with IVF.

- If patient has an intrauterine device (IUD), the evidence is not clear regarding need for removal, but this patient needs close follow up.

- CDC guidelines for antibiotic choice:
  - Outpatient regimens
    - Ceftriaxone 250mg IM x 1 *PLUS* doxycycline 100mg PO BID x 14 days
      - Add metronidazole 500mg BID x 14 days if pt recently had GYN instrumentation or concern for vaginitis

      OR

- Cefoxitin 2gm IM x 1 with probenicid 1gm PO x 1 (administered at same time) *PLUS* doxycycline 100mg PO x 14 days
  - Add metronidazole 500mg BID x 14 days if pt recently had GYN instrumentation or concern for vaginitis
— Inpatient regimens (see criteria for admission)
  - Cefoxitin 2 gm IV every 6 hrs or cefotetan 2 gm IV every 12 hrs *PLUS* doxycycline 100 mg orally or IV every 12 hrs

DISPOSITION

- Discharge home with close PCP or GYN follow up (48 hrs) and recommend assessment of sexual partners.
- Admit if patient is pregnant (high maternal morbidity and preterm delivery), immunodeficiency, has failed oral antibiotics, inability to tolerate PO, severe illness, or has a tubo-ovarian abscess.
- RETURN IF: Your pain increases, you have persistent vomiting, fevers, you pass out, have heavy vaginal bleeding, or any other new or concerning symptoms.

BEWARE...

- ⚠ Do not assume all CMT is PID, and do not fail to appreciate lateralizing tenderness, which could suggest appendicitis or ectopic pregnancy.
- ⚠ Get a pregnancy test, as this WILL change your management.
- ⚠ Have a low index of suspicion for treatment. PID will affect future fertility, and there are variable clinical presentations.

Sources

Zane RD, Kosowsky JM, et al. Pocket Emergency Medicine. 2nd ed. Philadelphia, PA: Lippincott Williams & Wilkins; 2011.

Ma OJ, Cline D, Tintinalli J, et al. Emergency Medicine Manual. 6th ed. New York, NY: McGraw-Hill Professional; 2003.

Marx J, Hockberger R, Walls R. Rosen's Emergency Medicine: Concepts & Clinical Practice. 5th ed. Maryland Heights, MO: Mosby; 2002.

Hans L, Mawji Y. The ABCs of Emergency Medicine. 12th edition. Toronto, Canada: University of Toronto; 2012.

Medscape News & Perspective. New York, NY: http://emedicine.medscape.com.

Notes

Section XVII.
Weak and Dizzy

1 ▶ Weak and Dizzy Quick Guide

- **Syncope:** The sudden, transient loss of postural tone and consciousness generally due to cerebral hypoperfusion. Events are generally of short duration and have a spontaneous recovery. **Near syncope** is similar process but without the loss of consciousness.

- **Vertigo:** The inappropriate experience of motion (meaning the patient is still) due to vestibular dysfunction. Can be peripheral in origin, affecting the semicircular canals, vestibule, or the vestibular nerve. Or it can be central in origin, affecting the CNS - specifically the cerebellum or brainstem.

- **Dizziness:** This is an extremely vague term many patients will use to describe a variety of symptoms from fatigue, weakness, disequilibrium, near syncope to vertigo.

Near syncope, vertigo, and dizziness have significant overlap. It can be difficult for your patients to find the words to describe their symptoms. Concentrate on the patient's risk factors as well as the timing, onset, and precipitants of symptoms rather than just the patient's characterization of symptoms. These presentations mandate a careful and thorough history and physical to evaluate for potentially life-threatening conditions. (See vertigo and wyncope chapters for more detail.)

- ALWAYS: IV, monitor, COMPLETE vital signs, **fingerstick glucose**.

- Can't-miss diagnosis in first 2 minutes: Hypoglycemia, hypoxemia, dissection (aortic and carotid/vertebral), CVA, massive PE, arrhythmia, SAH, ACS, or ruptured ectopic. Don't forget about head/C-spine trauma or other injuries after fall.

- Stratify by: Focal weakness vs. syncope vs. pre-syncope vs. vertigo, VS (HR, hypotension), mental status, EKG. This takes precedence over moving onto anything else!!

EVALUATION

- **High Yield History:** History of arrhythmia, CHF, GI bleed, anemia, age >45yrs old. Meds and any recent changes, QT prolonging meds, family history of sudden cardiac death, first episode, any prodrome (more likely neuro than cardiac)? **Exertional** or while seated (think cardiac), within 2min of standing? (orthostatic), tonic-clonic activity (non-specific, not always a seizure!)/post-ictal period? (more specific for seizure) What did bystanders see?

- **Exam:** VS! Orthostatics, full neuro and cardiovascular exam (keys: aortic stenosis murmur, equal pulses, signs of heart failure), signs of trauma, bitten tongue, incontinence, guaiac, FAST. No patient should be discharged without evaluating their gait.

- **Initial workup:** CBC, BMP, CXR, UA/HCG (all generally low yield). Consider troponin if suspected cardiac etiology. Consider head CT/CTA if suspect stroke/dissection and echo if indicated by murmur, history of cardiac disease, or new EKG changes.

DISPOSITION

- Big Picture: Pts with obvious etiology also tend to have an obvious management and disposition (eg, arrhythmias are admitted to cardiology). For everyone else, we don't have good tools to know who to send home and who to admit. Use observation if available.

- Low-risk causes of syncope: Post-tussive, post-micturition, vasovagal, anxiety/panic d/o, breath-holding, pain-associated.

- In the absence of clear diagnosis, risk stratification guides dispo. Generally, young otherwise healthy patients without CHF, VS abnormalities, EKG changes, concerning family history, or neuro findings can discharge home with follow up.

Ddx (*note, large amount of overlap)		
Syncope	Vertigo	Dizziness
Cardiac Arrhythima Valvuar disease (specifically AS) Heart failure Tamponade **Neurologic** Seizure TIA SAH ICU Vertebrobasilar insufficiency **Other** Pulmonary embolism Aortic dissection Hypoglycemia **Neurocardiogenic (Vasovagal)**	**Central** Posterior circulation CVA TIA Vertebrobasilar insufficiency Migraine Neoplasm Multiple Sclerosis Parkinson's C-spine pathology **Peripheral** Benign positional vertigo Labrinthitis Meiniere's disease Infection (Otitis Media) Medication effect (aminoglycosides)	Non-specific term and encompasses near-syncope and vertigo Includes any of the etiologies in the first 2 columns, plus: Infection Hypoglycemia Hypthothyroid Anxiety or depression Hyperventilation Fatigue ACS Anemia Hypotension

2 ▶ Vertigo

- Disruption of the vestibular, visual or proprioceptive system leading to the perception of spinning even while at rest.
- Affects approximately 20-30% of the general population; becomes more prevalent with increasing age, rarely seen in children.

EVALUATION

- Goal is to determine if this is central or peripheral vertigo.
- **High Yield History:** Define symptoms in own words (environment is moving vs. lightheadedness or about to pass out). Onset, provoked or constant, worse with certain positioning.
  - Any associated symptoms such as hearing loss (Meniere's disease), weakness (TIA), visual changes, headache, or vomiting
  - Medication history and any significant past medical history, including recently viral illnesses or previous vertigo
  - Any head trauma or prodromal symptoms
- **Exam:** Complete vital signs and full physical and neurologic exam (including visual acuity)
  - Assess for any cardiac murmurs or arrhythmias
  - Any nystagmus, dysmetria, ataxia, diplopia, or focal weakness
- If peripheral vertigo is suspected (see differential):
  - Lab tests or imaging are not typically necessary
  - Perform the Dix-Hallpike maneuver to assess for BPPV. This test does not need to be performed rapidly to be effective.
- If central vertigo is suspected (see differential):
  - CBC, BMP, and coags may be beneficial
  - Expeditious CT/CTA or MRI/MRA of head and neck
  - Neurology consult
  - Neurosurgical consult for all patients with suspected hemorrhage, space-occupying lesion, brainstem compression, or edema

Common Presentations of Peripheral vs. Central Vertigo		
	Peripheral	**Central**
Onset	Sudden (sec to min)	Gradual
Severity	Intense	Less intense
Pattern	Paroxysmal	Constant
Nausea/Vomiting	Frequent	Variable
Diaphoresis	Frequent	Variable
Aggravated by position/movement	Yes	Variable
Fatigue of signs and symptoms over course of day	Yes	No
Hearing loss tinnitus/fullness	May occur	Does not occur
Nystagmus	Usually rotary or horizontal	Usually vertical
Disequilibrium	Frequent	Variable
CNS symptoms/signs	Absent	Usually present
Life-threatening	Not typically	Possibly

- Other causes of vertigo should be individually assessed based on history and physical exam.
- Most patients should at least have an EKG and a fingerstick glucose.

MANAGEMENT

- If suspected central vertigo, see relevant chapter. Can consider migraine treatments but continue investigation for other etiology.
- If suspect peripheral vertigo:
  — Symptomatic relief: Meclizine 25mg PO vs. Benadryl 25mg PO or IV, Valium 5mg IV, Ondansetron 4mg IV, and IVF as needed
- If suspect BPPV:
  — Canalith repositioning (Epley maneuver) can be performed at the bedside. Goal: Move the otoliths out of the posterior semicircular canal and back into the utricle, where they belong and provide curative relief (note: keep patient in each position for 30 seconds)
    - Determine affected side based on results of the Dix-Hallpike maneuver.
    - Seat patient and turn head 45 degrees toward affected ear.
    - Pt is gently brought to the recumbent position with the head hanging 30-45 degrees below the examining table.
    - Head is gently rotated 45 degrees to the midline.
    - The head is then rotated another 45 degrees to the unaffected side.
    - Pt rolls onto the shoulder of the unaffected side while rotating the head another 45 degrees.
    - Pt is returned to the seated position and head returned to midline.
  — Refer for vestibular rehabilitation.
  — BPPV is often self-limiting and can be managed by a PCP with watchful waiting.
- If suspect Meniere's disease:
  — A short course of prednisone can help reverse tinnitus and hearing loss.
  — Diuretics and diuretic-like medications (Acetazolamide and hydrochlorothiazide) may help prevent future attacks but do not help treat active disease.

> ### Dix Hallpike Maneuver
>
> 1. Begin with the patient seated and head turned 45 degrees to one side.
> 2. Gently lower patient to a supine position with head hanging over the edge of the bed while you assess for nystagmus.
> 3. Return patient to seated position and repeat on the patient's other side.
> 4. Rotary nystagmus is a positive test for BPPV. The ear toward which the fast phase of the rotary nystagmus is beating is the affected ear.

Ddx		
	Disease	**Characteristics**
Peripheral Vertigo	Benign Paroxysmal Positional Vertigo (BPPV)	Likely caused by otoconial particles, fatigues over the course of the day. Frequent distinct attacks throughout day may make pt think vertigo is constant Very sensitive to head movement
	Ménière's disease	Lasts for hours, roaring tinnitus, sense of aural fullness, and decreased hearing; diagnosis requires multiple attacks
	Vestibular Neuritis	Sudden and severe, lasting days to weeks, no associated hearing loss; may have concurrent URI
	Labyrinthitis	Viral or bacterial infection from otitis media, meningitis, and mastoiditis; +Hearing loss
	Acoustic Neuroma	Peripheral cause that can become central. An CN VIII schwannoma that typically presents with vertigo, sudden deafness, and tinnitus
Central Vertigo	Brainstem/Cerebral Infarction or Hemorrhage	Abnormal neurologic exam
	Cerebellar Hemorrhage	Often associated with truncal ataxia, abnormal Romberg, abnormal gait testing, headache, and vomiting
	Vertibrobasilar Insufficiency	Due to TIAs in patients with typical risk factors for CVD. May be sudden and does not last more than 24h. Rarely dependent on head movement
	Vertebrobasilar Migraine	Headache often associated with ataxia, tinnitus, decreased hearing, nausea and vomiting, diplopia, ataxia, bilateral paresthesias and AMS
Trauma	Post-concussive Syndrome	Symptoms may occur immediately or weeks to months after injury. Often associated with headache, hearing loss, blurred vision, sleep abnormalities, emotional liability, and impaired cognition.
Toxic/ Metabolic	Ototoxic Medications	Most often due to salicylates, aminoglycosides, quinidine, furosemide, antimalarial agents, and cytotoxic agents.
	Alcohol	Typically lasts minutes to hours and improves decreasing EtOH level
	Hyper/Hypoglycemia	Typically resolves with corrected blood sugar

— A low-sodium diet may also help prevent future attacks.
- If suspect vestibular neuritis:
  — Consider a 3-week course of methylprednisolone taper (starting dose of 100mg daily).
  — Watchful waiting.
- If suspect labyrinthitis:
  — Bed rest and hydration
  — Antibiotics should be reserved for cases with a positive culture result.

DISPOSITION

- Most patients with peripheral vertigo may be discharged home with PCP, ENT, or neurology clinic follow-up.

- Patients with intractable symptoms or inability to walk, irrespective of the cause of their vertigo, may require admission for IV anti-emetics, hydration, or PT.

- Patients with central vertigo should be admitted for emergent treatment and consultations.

- Posterior fossa hemorrhage is a true emergency and requires immediate neurology consultation in the ED.

- CVAs should be admitted under the care of a neurologist or neurosurgeon.

- TIAs may be placed in observation status dependent on the patient's presentation, ability to obtain follow-up, and neurology consultation.

- Suspected space-occupying lesions necessitate an urgent neurosurgical consultation.

- RETURN IF: Your symptoms return, you have a severe headache, persistent vomiting, changes in vision, focal weakness, difficulty walking, or any other new or concerning symptoms.

BEWARE...

(!) Focal neurologic deficits or decreased level of consciousness

(!) Patients with central vertigo, particularly those at high risk for CVA

(!) Intractable symptoms despite appropriate use of medications, hydration, and maneuvers for relief

Sources

Samy HM. Dizziness, Vertigo, and Imbalance. emedicine.com. July 28, 2014.

Epley JM. The canalith repositioning procedure: for treatment of benign paroxysmal positional vertigo. *Otolaryngol Head Neck Surg.* 1992;107(3):399-404.

Notes

3 ▶ Syncope and Near-Syncope

- Syncope is the sudden loss of postural tone and consciousness from cerebral hypoperfusion followed by a spontaneous recovery.
- Near syncope is similar but without the loss of consciousness.
- The etiologies of syncope range from the benign to the immediately life-threatening. Diagnostic and disposition decisions are generally straightforward for patients of the ends of the spectrum. Careful thought must be paid to those in the middle.

EVALUATION

- **High Yield History:**
  - Any triggers? What was the patient doing when event happened?
    - Patients with vasovagal syncope tend to have a trigger (the sight of blood, prolonged standing in a warm environment, etc.)
    - **Unheralded syncope** is highly concerning and suggests arrhythmia as etiology.
    - **Exertional syncope** is also concerning for structural heart disease (AS, HOCM) or ischemia induced arrhythmia (VF).
  - Any prodromal symptoms that guide you to a diagnosis?
    - Any associated chest pain, shortness of breath, palpitation, headache, abdominal, or back pain?
    - Patients with vasovagal syncope may describe a prodrome of tunnel vision, nausea, diaphoresis, and pallor.
  - How quickly did the patient return to baseline? Are they still symptomatic?
  - Past medical history: Any history of CHF, CAD, valvular heart disease, TIAs, risk factors for stroke or MI, any trauma, GI bleeds (ETOH use, hx of melena), any seizure disorders? Any PE risk factors? Infectious symptoms?
  - Family history of sudden death is a key question in younger patients.

Differential for Syncope/Near Syncope by Category				
Cardiovascular	**Neurologic**	**Neurocardiogenic (vasovagal)**	**Orthostatic Hypotension**	**Other**
Arrhythmias: AV blocks, SSS, VT. Brugada, WPW, long QT, pacemaker malfunction, pacemaker meditated tachycardia **Mechanical**: Aortic stenosis, HOCM, PE, tamponade, heart failure, MI, subclavian steal, aortic pathology	Ischemic stroke Hemorrhagic stroke Transient ischemic attack Subarachnoid hemorrhage Vertebrobasilar Insufficiency Vertebral dissection Migraine Seizure	**Associated with**: Cause Micturition (urination) Defecation Vomiting Carotid sinus sensitivity **Note that straining with defecation can also cause syncope from structural heart disease.	Hypovolemia Sepsis GI bleed Ruptured ectopic POTS Autonomic neuropathy Deconditioning Medications (diuretics and vasodilators)	Hypoglycemia Anemia Hypoxemia Narcolepsy Drug use Psychogenic Metabolic derangements (can also lead to arrhythmia)

- **Exam:** Full set of vitals. These patients should remain on telemetry.
  - —Cardiovascular exam for murmurs, volume status, signs of DVT, pulse exam (to check if each heartbeat is perfusing and if equal pulses)
  - — Neurologic exam: Full exam, but focus on any cerebellar signs (dysarthria, ataxia, dysmetria)
- **Labs:** In young, healthy patients with a clear neurocardiogenic story, reassuring exam and normal EKG, labs are generally not indicated. Otherwise, consider CBC (anemia, infection) BMP (derangements that can predispose to arrhythmia, dehydration), D-dimer (if concerned for dissection or PE) coags (if on anticoagulation and bleeding), UA, BNP, and trop. Note that acute primary plaque rupture rarely causes isolated syncope. An elevated troponin is more likely indicative of demand ischemia. Obtain an HCG in all women of childbearing age.
- **EKG:** Obtain ASAP! (looking for tachy/brady, long QT, short P-R +/- delta wave, Brugada, blocks, right heart strain for PE)
  - — All young patients with syncope should have EKG documented even if you think it is vasovagal. Look for:
    - Delta wave → WPW
    - LV hypertrophy → Hypertrophic obstructive cardiomyopathy
    - Prolonged QT
    - Brugada Syndrome (abnormal ST segment elevations in V1-V3)
    - Arrythmogenic right ventricular dysplasia (RBBB, epsilon wave- a terminal notch in the QRS)
- **Imaging:** Based on suspect etiology.
  - — Bedside US can help evaluate for RV strain (PE), positive FAST (in ectopic), tamponade, pulmonary edema, etc.
  - — CXR (pulmonary edema, widened mediastinum or PNA), CT head if concerned for ICH, MRI/MRA to evaluate posterior circulation
  - — Don't forget that syncope patients can sustain trauma with fall; image as indicated for traumatic injuries.

MANAGEMENT

- ABCs: Patients who are hypovolemic get IVF resuscitation and stabilization.
- All syncope patients should be monitored on telemetry while in the ED.
- For PE, ectopic, CVA, GI bleed, hypoglycemia, electrolyte derangement, or tamponade, see appropriate chapter.
- For arrhythmias, replete potassium and magnesium, stop any contributory medications (QT prolonging medications or nodal blockers). Keep pads nearby for pacing or cardioversion/defibrillation. Consider cardiology consult.
- For suspected neurologic etiology, consider head imaging and consult neurology.
- Patients with a murmur on exam should have an echo.

DISPOSITION

- Admit any patient with a history of cardiac disease, abnormal vitals, labs, or exam, or if concerning history - namely exertional or unheralded syncope.

- Consider ED observation (if available) in patient who may not be completely low risk (>45yo, mild hypovolemia) but still feel their presentation is low risk for life-threatening etiology.

- Discharge home low risk patients, meaning they are young, no concerning past medical history or family history, have a reassuring exam, and no EKG abnormalities.

- RETURN IF: You pass out again, have any chest pain, palpitations, chest pain, shortness of breath, severe headaches, changes in vision, focal numbness or weakness, any severe abdominal pain, any black, tarry stool, or any other new or concerning symptoms.

BEWARE...

⚠ Syncope with straining can be vasovagal but should raise suspicion for cardiac etiology in higher risk patients

⚠ Do not be falsely reassured by a younger patient. Obtain thorough family history, drug history, and screen for eating disorders

Sources

Huff JS, Decker WW, Quinn JV, et al. Clinical policy: critical issues in the evaluation and management of adult patients presenting to the emergency department with syncope. *Ann Emerg Med* 2007; 49: 431–44.

Hatoum T, Sheldon R. A Practical Approach to Investigation of Syncope. *Can J Cardiol.* 2014 Jun;30(6):671-4.

Notes

4 ▶ Posterior Circulation Stroke

Background

- Strokes involving the vertebral arteries, basilar artery, posterior cerebral arteries or their branches. Structures involved are the brainstem, cerebellum, midbrain, thalamus, and areas of the temporal and occipital cortex.

- **Vessels:** Subclavian → vertebral arteries → C6-C2 vertebral foramina →foramen magnum > basilar artery → post cerebral arteries

- **Etiology:** Embolic 40% (cardioembolic > artery-artery emboli > mixed emboli), large artery stenosis (32%), other causes: dissection, migraine, fibromuscluar dysplasia, coagulopathy, drug abuse, subclavian steal

- **Location:** Vertebrobasilar 48% (pons > medulla > midbrain), cerebellum 7%, PICA territory 36%, multiple locations 9%

- **Risk factors:** Older age, male, HTN, DM, Afib, smoking, dyslipidemia, CAD, peripheral vascular disease, EtOH abuse, obesity, or OCPs. Others: Marfan syndrome, Fabry disease can cause dissections.

- Accounts for 20-30% of all strokes.

Ddx
BPPV
Peripheral vertigo
Acute intracranial hemorrhage
SAH
Tumor
Migraine
Hypoglycemia
Central pontine myelinolysis
PRES

EVALUATION

- **High Yield History:** Most commonly: dizziness (vertigo, less severe than BPPV), unilateral limb weakness (weakness, clumsiness, paralysis), dysarthria, gait ataxia, unilateral limb ataxia, headache, nausea and vomiting ("the gastroenteritis that kills"), nystagmus, blurred vision, facial palsy, altered level of consciousness (lethargy to coma).

- **Exam:** Classically will have:
  — Cranial nerve deficits,
  — Cross deficits (CN deficits on one side of the face, with sensory/motor tract deficits on the opposite side)
  — Cerebellar deficits (dizziness, ataxia)
  — Multiple findings (rarely, presents with just vertigo)

- **Labs:** CBC, BMP, FSBS, coags, EKG (evaluate for Afib)

- **Imaging:**
  — CT (non-con, initially), will evaluate for ICH and can detect CVA 6-12 hrs old (16% sensitivity)
  — MRI (with diffusion weighted and perfusion weighted images, up to 80-95% sensitive)
  — Vessel imaging: CTA (100% sensitive, caution use in renal failure) vs MRA (87% sensitivity)

- STAT neurology consult

SYNDROMES

Vessel	Location	Symptoms
Posterior cerebral artery	Occipital lobe	Contralateral homonymous hemianopia (from occipital infarct), Hemisensory loss (all modalities from thalamic infarction)
		Anton's syndrome: (bilateral pca) cortical blindness with denial of blindness/confabulation, visual hallucinations
Posterior cerebral artery	Lateral midbrain	Weber syndrome: Ipsilateral oculomotor palsy with contralateral hemiplegia
Proximal basilar	Pons	Locked in syndrome – quadriparesis, loss of speech, preserved awareness/cognition, sometimes preserved eye movements
Mid basilar	Lateral pons	Ipsilateral loss of facial sensation/motor, ipsilateral dysmetria
	Medial pons	Ipsilateral dysmetria, contralateral arm/leg weakness, gaze deviation
Top of the basilar	Midbrain, thalamus, temporal/occipital lobes	Somnolent, confusion, bilateral vision loss
Posterior inferior cerebellar artery	Lateral medulla	Wallenberg syndrome, nystagmus, vertigo, ipsilateral Horner's syndrome, ipsilateral facial sensory loss, dysarthria, hoarseness, dysphagia, contralateral hemisensory loss in the trunk/limb (pain/temperature)
Vertebral artery	Medial medulla	Ipsilateral tongue weakness and later hemiatrophy of the tongue, contralateral hemiparesis of the arm/leg. Hemisensory loss (touch, proprioception)

MANAGEMENT

- BP control (only if SBP >220, DBP >120, MAP >130 or BP >185/110 and plan to undergo thrombolysis)
- IV TPA (if within 4.5 hrs of onset of symptoms, contraindicated in uncontrolled htn, history of intracranial hemorrhage, active internal bleeding, acute trauma, serious head trauma, intracranial or intraspinal surgery in past 3 months, bleeding disorder)
- Endovascular TPA (no better than IV TPA; however, can be considered up to 24 hrs from onset)
- IV heparin (if dissection does not extend intracranially)
- Neurosurgery consult, if large infarction of the cerebellum may cause delayed swelling, and need emergent posterior fossa decompression

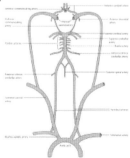

DISPOSITION

- Admit to neurology or the neuro ICU.

BEWARE...

(!) Be careful not to miss posterior circulation strokes in patients who are only lightheaded – sudden onset of lightheadedness, dizziness, or ataxia in the elderly is posterior circulation stroke until proven otherwise!

Sources

Markus HS, Van der worp HB, Rothwell PM. Posterior circulation ischaemic stroke and transient ischaemic attack: diagnosis, investigation, and secondary prevention. *Lancet Neurol.* 2013;12(10):989-98.

Merwick Á, Werring D. Posterior circulation ischaemic stroke. *BMJ.* 2014;348:g3175.

Nouh A, Remke J, Ruland S. Ischemic posterior circulation stroke: a review of anatomy, clinical presentations, diagnosis, and current management. *Front Neurol.* 2014;5:30.]

Notes

5 ▶ Stroke/Transient Ischemic Attack

- Ischemia to the brain from thrombosis (atherosclerosis), embolus (cardioembolic, embolism through a PFO, from carotid plaques, etc.), global hypoperfusion and injury to watershed areas. Ischemia can also occur due to hemorrhage or venous thrombosis (see relevant chapters).

- **Transient Ischemic Attacks** (TIA) are signs or symptoms of ischemia that completely resolve within 24hrs.

- **Large vessel**: Mixed sensory and motor symptoms. Usually with pathognomonic symptoms based on artery occluded.

- **Small vessel**: Also known as a lacunar infarct. Small and isolated motor or sensory symptoms.

Ddx
TIA (same presentation as stroke symptoms < 1hr), Hypoglycemia
Electrolyte derangement
Intracranial mass (tumor, abscess, hematoma)
Head bleed
Recrudescence
Complicated migraine
Infection
Seizure disorder
Bell's palsy
Benign positional vertigo
Labyrinthitis
Syncope (multiple etiologies)
Conversion disorder

EVALUATION

Evaluation

- **High Yield History:** Time last seen normal is KEY for tPA inclusion criteria (see figure). If symptom onset was noticed upon waking, time is when they went to bed, not when they woke up.

  — Amarosis fugax: Transient monocular vision loss due to occlusion of ophthalmic branch of the internal carotid artery

  — Risk factors include DM, HTN, HL, and atrial fibrillation

- **Exam:** Will often see elevated BP (must be < 185/110 for tPA). Neuro exam with attention to LOC, ataxia, aphasia, weakness, visual changes/deficits, hemi-neglect. Obtain a baseline NIH Stroke Scale.

- **Labs:** CBC, BMP, coags, fingerstick (>50 and <200 for tPA), urine HCG (tPA is pregnancy category C)

- EKG can evaluate for ACS masquerading as stroke (consider trop) as well as for stroke causes (Afib).

- **Imaging:**

  — Non-contrast head CT looking for bleed (blood = no tPA). Other explanation for symptoms may be seen (eg, mass effect or midline shift) but can't completely characterize ischemic stroke.

    ▪ Hyperdense artery sign can be an early finding of ischemia stroke on CT.

    ▪ Can also see loss of gray/white differentiation in first hours to days.

  — If high suspicion, go to MRI/MRA.

  — Echo or carotid duplex US can be done as inpatient to evaluate for embolic source.

Vascular Territory	Area of Brain Affected	Signs and Symptoms
Middle Cerebral Artery (MCA)	Posterior frontal, temporal, parietal	Contralateral hemiplegia (face and arms>leg), hemisensory loss, visual field cuts. If dominant hemisphere: Broca's, Wernicke's, or global aphasia Non-dominant: Spatial neglect, apraxia
Anterior Cerebral Artery (ACA)	Frontal	Contralateral hemiplegia(leg>face and arm weakness), hemisensory loss, confusion, apraxia, and frontal signs (eg, personality changes or disinhibition)
Posterior Cerebral Artery (PCA)	Occipital	Contralateral: homonymous hemianopia, +/- sensory loss (Wallenberg syndrome)

(For posterior stroke syndromes see posterior stroke chapter)

MANAGEMENT

- ABCs. Intubate for airway protection if needed. FSBS early because hypoglycemia can mimic a stroke.
- The approach to workup and treatment is to quickly determine likelihood of ischemic stroke and tPA eligibility while preventing complications (AIRWAY!). The ddx is very long and leads to a potentially time-consuming workup that could delay tPA if initiated while stroke is still a possibility. First rule out stroke (or at least tPA eligibility). Then work up alternate diagnoses.
- **Blood Pressure control:**
  - tPA candidates need BP < 185/110 (can give Labetalol 10-20mg IV Q10min or Nicardipine 5mg/hr infusion with titration)
  - Patients who are not a candidate for tPA, consider treating if sustained >220/120 or concerning comorbidities such as heart disease.
- **TPA** Is this patient eligible for tPA? Not generally recommended for minor/improving strokes or major strokes (large MCA stroke seen on head CT or NIHSS >22). Door to needle goal is <60min.
  - Time frame: <3hrs from symptom onset or last seen normal is encouraged.
    - 3-4.5hrs is acceptable, but with additional exclusion criteria (NIHSS > 25, age >80, combination of history of previous stroke and DM, or PO anticoagulants).
    - >4.5hrs is not widely practiced due to risk of bleeding tPA confers in the setting of hemorrhagic conversion of an ischemic stroke. No heparin or aspirin AFTER they get tPA.
    - Outside of 4.5hr window, pts may be candidates for intra-arterial tPA or mechanical clot retrieval. Time frame varies in reports. Discuss with local specialist.
  - Medications: Alteplase (tPA) 0.9mg/kg, max 90mg. 10% of dose given as bolus and remainder infused over 1hr.
- For TIA or minor strokes give aspirin 325mg PO.

- Very large stroke patients or patients presenting out of tPA window may be candidates for hemicraniectomy by neurosurgery to provide room for swelling brain tissue, thus reducing shift/compression.
- **TIA:** Goal of treatment in TIA is stroke prevention.
  — Antiplatelet therapy: daily aspirin or clopidogrel if aspirin allergy
  — Statin therapy for all patients
  — Consider anticoagulation if new onset Afib
  — Echocardiogram to evaluate for PFO or vegetations
  — Carotid duplex and ultimately carotid endarterectomy if >70% carotid stenosis

DISPOSITION

Contraindications to tPA
Any history of ICH
Seizure at stroke onset
Intracranial neoplasm
CVA or head trauma in prior 3months
MI within 3months
Major surgeries within 14days
Internal bleed within 3wks
Persistent BP>185/110 mmHg
Bleeding diathesis
Platelets <100,000
Anticoagulation
Non-compressible arterial puncture within 7days
Rapidly improving symptoms or low NIH stroke scale
FSBS <50
Age <18yo

- All patients who receive TPA are admitted to the ICU due to bleeding risk.
- Stroke pts who do not receive TPA are admitted to neuro ICU vs. floor depending on size of stroke, complications, and comorbidities.
- New onset TIA patients have significant short-term risk of stroke and should be admitted for workup unless the patient only has very minor symptoms; then work-up can be completed with close neuro follow up. Observation unit workup may also be possible, if available. The ABCD2 score was proposed to aid in identifying low risk patients, but numerous efforts have failed to validate it.

BEWARE...

- ⓘ Not quickly recognizing stroke and facilitating thrombolysis/neurosurgical intervention, particularly in altered patients.
- ⓘ Age is a risk factor for stroke, but don't forget pregnant and OCP related thrombosis and traumatic carotid and vertebral dissections in younger pts.
- ⓘ Do not forget other acute causes of neuro symptoms (eg, MI or hypoglycemia).
- ⓘ Have a low threshold to evaluate for a stroke. Over-calling is MUCH better than under-calling. A good starting point would be to consider ANY focal neuro complaint or acute change in mental status (without alternate explanation) a stroke until proven otherwise.
- ⓘ There is significant debate within the EM community regarding the safety and efficacy of tPA. Take the time to familiarize yourself with this topic.

Notes

6 ▶ Bradycardia

- Bradycardia HR <50bpm or inappropriate slow HR for clinical situation (eg, HR 60bpm in septic shock)
- First decision point: **Stable or unstable**? Check pulse. **ABCs if symptomatic, hypotensive or pulseless→ ACLS!!!** Frequently reassess.
- If stable, goal to determine etiology based on history, physical, and EKG in order to identify dangerous rhythms and reversible causes.

EVALUATION

Etiologies of Bradycardia
Hyperkalemia
Beta-blockers
Calcium channel blocker
Amiodarone
Digoxin
Vagal tone
Increased ICP
Infiltrative disease
Lyme disease
Chagas
Viral etiologies
Sick sinus syndrome
Ischemia (MI)
Hypothyroid

- **High Yield History:** Complete past medical history including thorough med review, history of CAD or CKD, last dialysis, infectious history, exercise history (marathon runner?), chart review for baseline HR, any signs or symptoms of any common etiologies. If patient has permanent pacemaker (PPM), why was it placed? Type of PPM, last battery check?

  — Assess for signs/symptoms of hypoperfusion, syncope, chest pain, shortness of breath

- **Exam:** Obtain complete set of vital signs; may be hypotensive or hypothermic.

  — Signs of volume overload, murmurs, goiter, abdominal tenderness, peripheral perfusion

- **Diagnostics:**

  — EKG to assess for specific rhythms and/or ischemia, pacer spikes.

  — Labs: BMP including K, Mg and glucose +/- TSH to assess for etiology. Consider trop, BNP, digoxin level

  — CXR: If concerned about CHF or if has a PPM to check for lead positioning or fractures.

  — Other: Based on findings on history or physical if concerned for increased ICP→head CT

MANAGEMENT

- Initial steps: Check pulse, ABCs, IV access, place on monitor, and defibrillator pads (pacing) ideally placed anterior-posterior. Obtain early EKG and rhythm strip.
- If becomes unstable, ACLS, treat as below. Treat the patient, not the rhythm.
- When stabilized, analyze EKG for specific rhythms.

  — Sinus Dysfunction (Sick Sinus Syndrome)

    ▪ Sinus bradycardia: HR <60 Every P followed by QRS, every QRS preceded by P wave. Upright P wave in lead II, inverted in lead AvR.

    ▪ Sinus arrest: Sinus rhythm with the intermittent absence of atrial depolarization for a period of time, associated with older age.

  — AV Blocks

- 1st degree AV block: PR >200
- 2ND degree AV block: **Mobitz I**: Progressively prolonged PR until a blocked sinus impulse. Looked for grouped beating; PR prolongation can be subtle; PR interval following the dropped QRS should be the shortest; QRS usually narrow. **Mobitz II**: Consistent PR interval with intermittent blocked sinus p wave. Unable to differentiate between Mobitz I and II if patient is in 2:1 block.

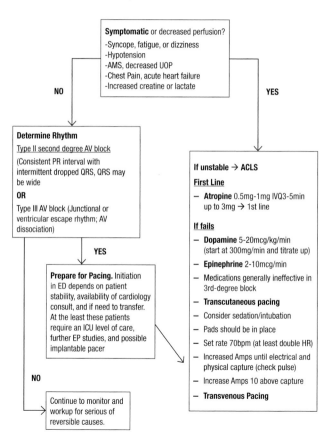

Symptomatic or decreased perfusion?
-Syncope, fatigue, or dizziness
-Hypotension
-AMS, decreased UOP
-Chest Pain, acute heart failure
-Increased creatine or lactate

NO

YES

Determine Rhythm

<u>Type II second degree AV block</u>

(Consistent PR interval with intermittent dropped QRS, QRS may be wide

OR

Type III AV block (Junctional or ventricular escape rhythm; AV dissociation)

YES

If unstable → ACLS

<u>First Line</u>

— **Atropine** 0.5mg-1mg IVQ3-5min up to 3mg → 1st line

<u>If fails</u>

— **Dopamine** 5-20mcg/kg/min (start at 300mg/min and titrate up)

— **Epinephrine** 2-10mcg/min

— Medications generally ineffective in 3rd-degree block

— **Transcutaneous pacing**

— Consider sedation/intubation

— Pads should be in place

— Set rate 70bpm (at least double HR)

— Increased Amps until electrical and physical capture (check pulse)

— Increase Amps 10 above capture

— **Transvenous Pacing**

Prepare for Pacing. Initiation in ED depends on patient stability, availability of cardiology consult, and if need to transfer. At the least these patients require an ICU level of care, further EP studies, and possible implantable pacer

NO

Continue to monitor and workup for serious of reversible causes.

- 3rd degree AV block: Failure of the SA node impulse to propagate to the ventricles. On EKG p-wave with consistent P-R interval. Also have ventricular escape rhythm; consistent R-R interval. No association between the two and thus variable PR interval.
  - Junctional rhythm: Loss of atrial conduction and the AV pacemaker takes over at 40-60bpm.
  - Idioventricular rhythm: Loss of both sinus and AV node activity. Impulses arise from bundle of His or Purkinje fibers resulting in a pseudo-bundle branck block with QRS >120.
- Assess EKG for signs of ischemia or other indications of etiology (eg, peaked T waves in hyperkalemia or scooped ST segments with digoxin)
- Treat based on perceived etiology:
  - Ischemia → cath lab (many of these are transient bradycardia)
  - Hyperkalemia → hyperkalemia treatment and emergent hemodialysis
  - Toxicological causes → specific antidote and consultation with toxicology
    - Digoxin → Digoxin Immune FAB
    - Calcium channel blockers→ Calcium, glucagon
    - Beta blocker → Hyperinsulinemic euglycemia
  - Hypothermia → warm patient, do not pace, and caution not to jostle patient and induce VF (see hypothermia)

DISPOSITION

- If paced or unstable rhythm, admit to ICU.
- Hemodynamically stable but symptomatic pts with new bradycardia should be admitted to telemetry floor.
- If stable, nothing concerning on exam or labs, and this is patient's baseline HR can be discharged home.
- RETURN IF: Any chest pain, dizziness, shortness of breath, you pass out, or have any other concerning symptoms.

BEWARE...

(!) Being distracted by bradycardia and missing ST changes in ischemia-induced bradycardia.

(!) Note that atropine will not have an effect on a transplanted heart.

(!) In unstable patient, if preparing to give atropine, should simultaneously be setting up to pace in case there is no effect from medications.

(!) In trauma patients, do not be reassured by lower HRs; may be inappropriate bradycardia from pain-induced vagal stimulation or med effect.

Sources
Deal N. Evaluation and Management of Bradydysrrythmias in the Emergency Department. *Emergency Medicine Practice*. March 2013;15(9).

7 ▶ Hypoglycemia

- Symptomatic glucose <55-70 relieved by administration of a glucose source
- **Hypoglycemic agents**: Sulfonylureas (chlorpropamide, glipizide, glyburide) increase insulin secretion, augment insulin activity, and stimulate insulin release, causing prolonged duration of action (12-24 hrs). There is hepatic metabolism and renal excretion of an ACTIVE metabolite and are the agents most likely to cause PROLONGED hypoglycemia.

Ddx
CVA
Intoxication
Sepsis
Metabolic disarray
Toxic ingestion
Seizure
Endocrine disorders
Depression

- **Antihyperglycemic agents:** Biguanides (metformin/glucophage) decrease hepatic production and intestinal absorption of glucose, increase insulin sensitivity, and decrease the glucose level of diabetic patients. Does not affect glucose level of non-diabetic patients. Treatment of metformin overdose is supportive, with possible hemodialysis for massive ingestion.

EVALUATION

- **High Yield History:** Obtain accurate medication history, including diabetic medication and if on any long-acting medications. Assess for possible ingestions or intentional overdose that could precipitate hypoglycemia. Changes in diet? Any infectious symptoms?
  — Adrenergic symptoms (glucose <70): Tremor, diaphoresis, weakness, tachycardia, anxiety, parasthesias, nausea
  — Neuroglycopenic symptoms (glucose <55): Headache, mental slowing, confusion, gait instability, visual changes, seizures
- **Etiologies:** Diabetes medications, beta blocker or calcium channel blocker overdose, EtOH, sepsis, malnutrition, renal failure, thyroid dysfunction
- **Exam:** Vital signs, helpful in determining etiology
  — Assess for adrenergic or neuroglycopenic signs
  — Search for signs or infection, and perform full neurologic exam
- **Diagnostics:** Based on suspected etiology, at minimum fingerstick glucose. Consider infections and ischemia workup.
  — Obtain C-peptide if concerned about factitious hypoglycemia (elevated in endogenous hyperinsulinemia).

MANAGEMENT

- 1 amp of $D_{50}W$, followed by D_5W infusion to keep glucose >100 until pt. can eat. If alert enough, can give oral glucose tablets or food.
- If altered and unable to obtain IV access can give glucagon 1mg IM.
- When treated, obtain a more complete history.
  — Overdose:
  — Sulfonylureas: 24hr admission, treat with octreotide and obtain Q1H fingerstick

- Asymptomatic pediatric ingestion of sulfonylureas →8hr observation; most sulfonylureas reach their peak effect in <8hrs.
  - Special agents:
  - **Octreotide:** Somatostatin analog that suppresses the secretion of insulin and helps counter the hyperinsulinism resulting from both the sulfonylurea and the paradoxical release of insulin created by treatment of hypoglycemia with dextrose.
  - **Diazoxide:** Nondiuretic vasodilator that is most commonly used for treatment of hypertensive emergency but also has been efficacious in the treatment of hypoglycemia.
  - **Glucagon:** A hormone that elevates serum glucose by recruiting hepatic glycogen stores and inducing gluconeogenesis. Glucagon should be used as a temporizing measure for those in whom intravenous access cannot be established expediently for the administration of dextrose.
- Treat underlying etiology such as infection, ischemia, or medication overdose. If due to poor PO intake may need decreased insulin dose.

DISPOSITION

- Admit if overdose on sulfonylurea or long-acting insulin, significant medical comorbidities, if cause unknown, recurrent hypoglycemia in ED, unable to tolerated PO, or if concerned for intentional overdose.
- If concern that patient is unable to administer their own hypoglycemic, consider case management involvement.
- Discharge if full recovery and able to eat, with identified cause and plan to prevent, and can monitor at home in a reliable patient.

RETURN IF: You are unable to tolerate food, recurrent low blood sugars, lightheadedness, tremors, palpitations, you have a seizure, or have any other new or concerning symptoms.

BEWARE...

(!) Patients with long-standing DM and previous hypoglycemic events may develop hypoglycemia unawareness. These patients may not manifest symptoms until even lower glucose levels (may lose their glucagon response) and their presenting symptoms may be seizure or altered mental status.

Sources

Zane RD, Kosowsky JM, et al. Pocket Emergency Medicine. 2nd ed. Philadelphia, PA: Lippincott Williams & Wilkins; 2011.

Ma OJ, Cline D, Tintinalli J, et al. Emergency Medicine Manual. 6th ed. New York, NY: McGraw-Hill Professional; 2003.

Marx J, Hockberger R, Walls R. Rosen's Emergency Medicine: Concepts & Clinical Practice. 5th ed. Maryland Heights, MO: Mosby; 2002.

Hans L, Mawji Y. The ABCs of Emergency Medicine. 12th edition. Toronto, Canada: University of Toronto; 2012.

Medscape News & Perspective. New York, NY: http://emedicine.medscape.com.

8 ▶ Electrolyte Abnormalities: Sodium

Hypernatremia *Mild: Na$^+$ > 146 mEq/L; Severe: Na$^+$ > 155 mEq/L*

EVALUATION

- **High Yield History:** Symptoms are variable based on rate of rise In Na and the serum osmolarity. They include irritability, headache, tremors, ataxia, lethargy, coma, and ultimately seizures. With rapid rise in serum Na may develop severe headache. Many symptoms are related to the underlying etiology of hyponatremia.

- **Exam:** Assess volume status. Exam can correlate with underlying etiology. Hypotension and tachycardia (if hypovolemia), pulmonary or LE edema (if hypervolemic) and AMS, hyperreflexia, or generalized weakness.

- Free water deficit = 0.6 x wt(kg) x (([Na+]/140) − 1); urine Osm >700 (likely non-renal: GI loss, insensible loss, hypodipsia) if <700 (renal: diabetes insipidus)

- Estimate deficit: (Serum Na-140)/3 = free water deficit in liters

- Consider head CT if concerned for complications such as SAH, SDH, or ICH.

- PO free water, IV D$_5$W. Consider NGT free water boluses if altered or unable to meet PO needs.

Etiologies of HyperNa
Hypovolemic: Decreased water intake (unconscious, AMS, sedation, lack of access, impaired thirst),
Euvolemic: Excessive free water loss (diarrhea, vomiting, hyperpyrexia, excessive sweating, diabetes insipidus),
Hypervolemic: Excessive Na intake (supplements, salt pills, hypertonic saline, Cushing syndrome, Aldosteronism)

Etiologies of HypoNa
Hypovolemic (common): poor PO intake, GI losses, pancreatitis, thiazides, adrenal insufficiency
Euvolemic: Hypothyroid, adrenal insufficiency, primary polydipsia, decreased intake (tea/toast diet), SIADH (diagnosis of exclusion once rule out abnormal thyroid and adrenal function in setting of CNS, lung, or carcinoma disease
Hypervolemic: CHF, cirrhosis, nephrotic syndrome, renal failure

- Don't lower Na more than 10 mEq/L per day (~0.5 mEq/L/hr to prevent cerebral edema).

- NS for perfusion deficits, monitor UOP, and switch to ½ NS after UOP is 0.5cc/kg/h; can try furosemide 20-40mg IV to lose excess sodium.

- If concerned for central diabetes insipidus, use desmopressin 0.05mg PO Q12hrs.

HYPONATREMIA: *Na+ < 135 mEq/L*

EVALUATION

- **High Yield History:** Symptoms correlate with rate of decrease and absolute Na level. They include headache, abdominal pain, muscle cramps, agitation, AMS, hallucinations, lethargy, coma, and seizures.

- **Exam:** Determine volume status. Perform full neuro exam, looking for global weakness, ataxia, mydriasis, and in severe cases, signs of herniation.

- Calculate Na+ deficit: weight(kg) x 0.6 x (140-measured [Na+]) = sodium deficit (mEq)
- **Urine Na**: <10-20 suggests intravascular volume depletion (hypovolemia, CHF, cirrhosis); urine Na>20 suggests hypothyroidism, adrenal insufficiency
- **Urine osm**:<100-200: decreased ADH (polydipsia, poor PO intake); >300: high antidiuretic hormone (hypothyroid, adrenal insufficiency - not necessarily SIADH!)

MANAGEMENT

- If hypovolemic, give just NS to restore adequate perfusion.
- If euvolemic, fluid restrict and admit.
- If severe hyponatremia (Na<120) that developed rapidly with CNS changes (seizures/coma), give hypertonic saline 3% NS at 25-100 mL/hr.

DISPOSITION

- Admit all patients with severe derangements, are symptomatic, and those with concerning etiologies or etiologies that are likely to persist after discharge.
- Consider discharge in patients with mild lab derangements (or are at their baseline hypo or hypernatremia), are asymptomatic, corrected in the ED, and have good follow up for lab checks and determination of underlying etiology.
- RETURN IF: You experience any return of your symptoms, are unable to follow up with your doctor, or have any other concerning symptoms.

BEWARE...

(!) Rapid correction can cause CHF or central pontine myelinolysis →AMS, dysphagia, dysarthria, paresis. Max correction: 12 mEq/L/day (0.5 mEq/hr).

(!) Acuity or chronicity impacts rate of correction; If acute (<48hrs) can correct quicker.

(!) Consider pseudohyponatremia in hyperglycemia (correct Na=2.4 mEq/L ↓ per 100 ↑ in glucose over 100), hyperlipidemia, hyperproteinemia.

(!) Treat the symptoms, not the lab value.

(!) Morbidity and mortality for hypernatremia are highest in infants and elderly who may be unable to respond to increased thirst.

Sources

Adrogué HJ, Madias NE. Hypernatremia. *N Engl J Med.* 2000;342(20):1493-9.

Adrogué HJ, Madias NE. Hyponatremia. *N Engl J Med.* 2000;342(21):1581-9.

Yeates KE, Singer M, Morton AR. Salt and water: a simple approach to hyponatremia. *CMAJ.* 004;170(3):365-9.

9 ▶ Electrolyte Abnormalities: Potassium

HYPERKALEMIA: K$^+$ > 5.5 mEq/L

EVALUATION

- **High Yield History:** Usually asymptomatic and noted only on labs or EKG changes. When diagnosed, assess for etiology.

- **Exam:** May have vague complaints of weakness, paralysis, GI upset. Look for signs that point to etiology, such as a fistula to suggest renal failure.

- **ECG:** Peaked T waves, prolonged PR/short QT, QRS widened and flattened P waves. Eventually a sine-wave pattern develops → PEA arrest, asystole, VF, or heart block. However, ECG doesn't always correlate with K$^+$ level.

Etiologies of hyperkalemia
Renal failure (most common)
Acidosis
Increased intake
Addison's disease
Hypoaldosteronism
Spironolactone
Hyperglycemia
Succinylcholine
Renal tubular acidosis type 4

Etiologies of hypokalemia
Loop diuretics (most common)
GI loses (vomiting, diarrhea, laxatives)
Medication effect
Alkalosis
Insulin
Renal tubular acidosis (RTA)
Hyperaldosteronism

MANAGEMENT

- All patients should be on cardiac monitor due to risk of arrhythmia.

- Next, provide cardiac membrane stabilization if EKG changes, specifically QRS widening, are noted: Give calcium chloride (5mL 10% solution) or calcium gluconate (1-2g IV) (caution if patient is on digoxin).

- Shift K$^+$ intracellular

  — Glucose and insulin (1-2 amps D$_{50}$W + 10-20 units regular insulin **use less insulin in CKD)

  — Bicarbonate (1-2 amps sodium bicarb); highest utility is if patient is acidotic.

  — Can also use albuterol nebs to lower K$^+$ but effect is transient.

- Promote K+ excretion using diuretics (furosemide 40mg IV) and dialysis in severe cases (if from renal failure, consult renal for dialysis). Poor data to support sodium polystyrene sulfonate (2% risk of bowel necrosis with 50% case-fatality rate!), but still sometimes used (1gm binds 1mEq K$^+$ over 10 min). Give 30-90gm PO with 50 mL 20% sorbitol (sodium polystyrene sulfonate alone is constipating). Avoid in post-op pts who are at highest risk for bowel necrosis.

- If not contraindicated, give IVF to promote dilution and excretion.

- Recheck electrolytes Q2-4 hrs.

HYPOKALEMIA: K^+ < 3.5 MEQ/L

EVALUATION

- **High Yield History:** Symptoms include weakness, fatigue, cramps, hyporeflexia, constipation, and parasthesias. Assess for etiology.
- **Exam:** May be hypertensive (if due to hyperaldosteronism, etc.) or hypotensive (dehydration). Neuro exam with generalized weakness and hyporeflexia. Assess for signs of etiology (eg, dental enamel erosion in bulimia or ileostomy with high output).
- **EKG:** Dysrhythmias, sinus bradycardia, premature atrial contractions (PACs)/premature ventricular contractions (PVCs), U waves, ST-segment depression, prolonged QT interval, ventricular ectopy, VT/VF
- Always check serum Mg.

MANAGEMENT

- Oral KCl 40 mEq/L or KCl IV Q4H: can give 10mEq/h peripherally or 20mEq/hr centrally. Expected increase: 0.1mEq/L per 10mEq given
- Recheck K Q4H and always replete magnesium, otherwise K repletion is ineffective.

DISPOSITION

- Always admit patients with EKG changes, persistent symptoms, failure to respond to treatment, or any concerning etiology.
- Discharge patients with mild hyper or hypokalemia, who respond to treatment, are without EKG changes, and without a concerning etiology. Patients should have close follow up for repeat labs in 2-3 days.
- RETURN IF: You have any chest pain or palpitations, you pass out, are unable to have your labs rechecked, or have any other new or concerning symptoms.

BEWARE...

- ! For hypokalemia, oral replacement rapid and safer than IV and avoid glucose containing IVF, which can promote intracellular shift of K^+.
- ! Be aware of total body potassium levels and physiology that can cause falsely low values (eg, hyperventilation in anxiety attack).
- ! If patient is in the ED for a prolonged period of time, may require re-dosing of medications as K^+ moves back into the extracellular space.
- ! If the potassium level does not fit the clinical picture, repeat the blood work. K^+ will be falsely elevated with hemolysis.

Sources

Nyirenda MJ, Tang JI, Padfield PL, Seckl JR. Hyperkalaemia. *BMJ*. 2009;339:b4114.

Groeneveld JH, Sijpkens YW, Lin SH, Davids MR, Halperin ML. An approach to the patient with severe hypokalaemia: the potassium quiz. *QJM*. 2005;98(4):305-16.

10 ▶ Electrolyte Abnormalities: Calcium

Hypercalcemia *Ca >10.5 mEq/L or ionized >2.7 mEq/L*

EVALUATION

- **High Yield History:** Symptoms include stones (renal calculi), bones (bone destruction), groans (abd pain, N/V, constipation, polyuria, polydipsia, pancreatitis), and psychic overtones (lethargy, weakness, fatigue, confusion). Assess for etiology (eg, any bony tenderness, medication history, or family history).

- **Exam:** Vital signs may demonstrate bradycardia, hypo or hypertension, and may have hyporeflexia on exam.

- **EKG** (depressed ST segments, wide T waves, short QT, heart block)

- Measure total serum calcium, ionized calcium, albumin, phosphate, renal function, and PTH.

  — Check PTH: if inappropriately normal or high, send 24hr urine Ca → likely parathyroid problem.

  — If PTH low (appropriate), continue with malignancy workup.

Etiologies of HyperCa
Malignancy most common
Small cell carcinoma
Multiple myeloma
Bony metastases
Alkalosis
Low albumin
Addison's disease
Paget's disease
Sarcoidosis
Excess Vit D
Milk-alkali syndrome
Lithium
Thiazide diuretics
Hyperthyroidism

MANAGEMENT

- Treat patients who are symptomatic, have a Ca>12, and/or have abnormal renal function.

- IVF for hydration – may need up to 5-10L (goal to increase urinary Ca+ excretion) +/- furosemide 20-60mg IV

- Bisphosphonates inhibit osteoclastic bone resorption: 4mg zoledronic acid (or pamidronate); ensure patient has replete 25D stores.

- If not effective, add calcitonin 0.5-4units/kg IV over 24hrs or IM divided Q6h with hydrocortisone 25-100mg IV Q6hr – can use with bisphosphonates.

- Hemodialysis for refractory cases (consult renal).

Etiologies of HypoCa
Hypoparathyroidism
Vitamin D deficiency
Hypomagnesemia
Sepsis
Severe burn
Pancreatitis
Hungry bone syndrome
Certain malignancies
Medications including bisphosphonates, cisplatin, colchicine, phenytoin and phenobarbital, and PPIs

HYPOCALCEMIA: *CA <10.5 MEQ/L OR IONIZED >2.7 MEQ/L*

EVALUATION

- **High Yield History:** Signs and symptoms include perioral paresthesias, increased DTRs, cramps, weakness, confusion, seizures.

- **Exam:** On vital signs can see hypotension or bradycardia. On neuro exam may see hyperreflexia, muscle spasms, and tetany. Patients may also have chorea or Parkinson's symptoms.
  - Chvostek's sign: Twitch of corner of mouth with tapping of finger on CN VII at zygoma
  - Trousseau's sign: Carpopedal spasm when BP cuff inflated at pressure above the SBP longer than 3min.
- **EKG:** Bradycardia, prolonged QT (can lead to Torsades!), T wave changes, and heart block.
- Corrected Ca = [(4.0 - albumin) x 0.8] + measured calcium

MANAGEMENT

- If asymptomatic, give calcium gluconate 1-4 gm/day PO divided Q6h with vitamin D OR calcium carbonate or calcium citrate (1-3gm/day in divided doses).
- If symptomatic, treat as a medical emergency. Give IV Ca gluconate (1-2g) or IV CaCl 10 mL 10% solution IV slowly and check Ca levels Q1-2hrs. Consider continuous infusion and titrate to EKG or symptom improvement.
- Treat concurrent hypomagnesemia.

DISPOSITION

- Admit all patients with severe derangements, EKG changes, and those with concerning etiologies or those that are likely to persist after discharge and result in return of symptoms.
- Consider discharge in patients with mild lab derangements, are asymptomatic, corrected in the ED, and have good follow up for lab checks and determination of underlying etiology.
- RETURN IF: You experience any return of your symptoms, are unable to follow up with your doctor, or have any other concerning symptoms.

BEWARE...

- (!) If alkalotic, ionized calcium may be very low even with normal total calcium. Also, always correct Ca for albumin level.
- (!) Caution with Ca supplementation in hyperphosphatemia, rhabdomyolysis, or tumor lysis syndrome because it can precipitate Ca-Phos crystals.
- (!) In hypocalcemia, make sure to correct concurrent hypokalemia or hypomagnesemia.
- (!) **DO NOT** use thiazide diuretics, as they can worsen hypercalcemia.

Notes

11 ▶ Electrolyte Abnormalities: Magnesium

HYPERMAGNESEMIA *MG > 2.1 MEQ/L (> 1.05 MMOL/L)*

EVALUATION

- **High Yield History:** Symptoms include weakness, dizziness, nausea, vomiting, and somnolence. Also ask about ingestions, particularly laxative and antacids, which can contain large amount of magnesium.

- **Exam:** Can see decreased respiratory rate, hypotension, bradycardia, weakness, decreased deep tendon reflexes.

  — Exam findings roughly correlate with Mg level: DTRs disappear at approximately >3.5 mEq/L, muscle weakness at approximately >4 mEq/L, hypotension at approximately >5mEq/L, and respiratory paralysis occurs at > 8 mEq/L.

- **EKG:** Bradycardia, wide QRS, long QT, and heart block

Etiologies of Hypermagnesemia
Renal failure
Hyperparathyroidism
Iatrogenic (i.e. Mg infusion in preeclampsia)
Excess laxative
Excess antacids

Etiologies of HypoMag
EtOH
Total parenteral nutrition
Acute pancreatitis
GI losses
Diuretics
Antimicrobials (aminoglycosides, amphotericin)
Tacrolimus
PPIs
Inherited renal tubular defects
Hyperaldosteronism
Hypercalcemia

MANAGEMENT

- Rehydrate with NS and give furosemide 20-40 mg IV to promote excretion.

- Correct acidosis with ventilation and sodium bicarb 50-100 mEq, if needed.

- If symptomatic, give calcium (CaCl 10% solution IV or 1 amp Ca gluconate) to antagonize Mg's effects (Mg can act as a physiologic calcium channel blocker).

HYPOMAGNESEMIA *MG < 1.4 MEQ/L (< 0.70 MMOL/L)*

EVALUATION

- **High Yield History:** Primarily a lab diagnosis. Symptoms are generally neurologic and include depression, vertigo, ataxia, and seizures. Assess for etiologies.

- **Exam:** Full neuro to evaluate for ataxia, increased DTRs, nystagmus, or carpopedal spasms.

- **EKG:** Prolonged QT and PR, peaked or inverted T waves. May have a variety of arrhythmias.

MANAGEMENT

- Correct potassium, calcium, and phosphate levels first.

- Oral repletion: 1-3 tabs magnesium oxide per day of 240mg / 400mg tablet (can cause diarrhea).

- IV repletion: If Mg slightly low, give 2-4gms MgSO4.
- Check DTRs Q15min; stop infusion when hyperreflexia disappears.

DISPOSITION

- Admit in cases of severe dysrhythmias, significant symptoms, or concerning etiology.
- Patients with mild derangements that are asymptomatic and easily corrected may be discharged home.
- RETURN IF: You have any palpitations, lightheadedness, unexplained sleepiness, tremor, seizures, or any other new or concerning symptoms.

BEWARE...

- ⚠ In hypermagnesemia, suspect coexisting hyperkalemia and phosphate or calcium abnormalities.
- ⚠ The diagnosis should not be based on Mag levels because total depletion can occur before any significant lab changes, so must be suspected clinically.
- ⚠ As with many electrolyte abnormalities, the rate of change is often more concerning than the absolute lab value.

Source
Iannello S, Belfiore F. Hypomagnesemia. A review of pathophysiological, clinical and therapeutical aspects. *Panminerva Med.* 2001;43(3):177-209.

Notes

Section XVIII.
Procedure Guide

1 ▶ Procedure Quick Guide

This chapter covers some of the most common EM procedures.

The table lists the procedures required by the ACGME. This can be used to track your procedures and serve as a reminder of which procedures you should be logging.

Procedure Requirements		Number Performed
Adult Medical Resuscitation	45	
Adult Trauma Resuscitation	35	
Cardiac Pacing	6	
Central Venous Access	20	
Chest Tube	10	
Cricothyrotomy	3	
Dislocation Reduction	10	
ED Bedside Ultrasound	150	
Intubations	35	
Lumbar Puncture	15	
Pediatric Medical Resuscitation	15	
Pediatric Trauma Resuscitation	10	
Pericardiocentesis	3	
Procedural Sedation	15	
Vaginal Delivery	10	

The following chapters are not a complete list of procedures or the definitive approach to any single procedure. This guide should serve as a reference. If you are new to or uncomfortable with a procedure, we recommend that you familiarize yourself with either of the following two resources and always have a senior resident or attending involved.

1) Roberts, J. *Roberts & Hedges' Clinical Procedures in Emergency Medicine*. 6th. Philadelphia: Elsevier, 2014.

2) **NEJM Procedural Videos** are a great resource for viewing step-by-step instructions prior to performing a procedure. Search "NEJM" and whatever procedure you are attempting (eg, arterial line, paracentesis)

FOR ALL PROCEDURES, YOU SHOULD ENSURE:

1) Right patient, right procedure, correct side

2) Consent signed and in chart if not emergent

3) Appropriate labs and imaging have been reviewed

4) Answered patient's questions

5) Comfortable positioning for both you and the patient, as well as adequate lighting

6) All supplies in room or immediately available

7) Time out is performed

8) Follow universal precautions

9) You have adequate supervision and the ability to get help if needed

10) Anticipated possible complications and have contingency plans

Sources

Roberts J. Roberts & Hedges' Clinical Procedures in Emergency Medicine, 6th ed. Philadelphia:Elsevier, 2014.

Videos in Clinical Medicine, keyword search to specific procedure. *N Engl J Med.*

Notes

2 ▶ Arterial Line

INDICATIONS

Blood gas sampling or continuous blood pressure monitoring

CONTRAINDICATIONS

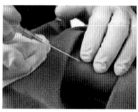

Inadequate circulation, Raynaud's, Buerger's disease, full thickness burns, coagulopathy, skin infection at the site, inadequate collateral flow (positive Allen's test)

SUPPLIES

Antiseptic, local anesthetic, needles, syringe, IV catheter, guide wire, transducer cable and tubing, arm board, tape, suture material or other method to secure to arm, gloves, and sterile drape

PROCEDURE

- There are several approaches to a radial A-line placement. Your hospital may have different supplies, necessitating an alternative approach.
    — Position the wrist in extension and supinated, prep skin, drape, and palpate radial pulse.
    — Use lidocaine to place a wheal over entry site.
    — Holding the syringe at 45° with bevel up, palpate the artery with the index and middle finger of your non-dominant hand. Puncture the skin distal to your fingers, and slowly advance toward pulsating vessel.
    — When you achieve pulsatile blood flow, insert needle slightly farther, to go through the back wall of the artery.
    — Holding the catheter with your non-dominant hand, remove the needle and grab the guidewire with your dominant hand.
    — Lower the catheter so it's parallel to skin and slowly pull the catheter back, until pulsatile flow starts again, and then advance the guidewire. The guidewire should advance freely and easily. DO NOT FORCE.
    — After the guidewire has easily advanced, advance the catheter over the wire and into the artery.
    — Remove the wire and attach the catheter hub to the transducer, and secure to skin.

TIPS

- The radial artery is more superficial distally. Start distally; if you miss and there is resultant vasospasm, you can try again more proximally.
- Ensure that you palpate the pulse across the wrist to clearly delineate the artery's position.
- If unable to accurately palpate pulse, you can use ultrasound.
- Check to make sure you are not using a filtered angiocatheter, which will not allow passage of the guidewire.

COMPLICATIONS

Hematoma formation, infection, bleeding, ischemia, thrombosis/embolism, AV fistula formation, pseudoaneurysm formation

Source

Tegtmeyer K, Brady G, Lai S, Hodo R, Braner D. Videos in Clinical Medicine. Placement of an arterial line. *N Engl J Med.* 2006;354(15):e13.

Notes

3 ▶ Arthrocentesis

INDICATIONS

To obtain synovial fluid for analysis

CONTRAINDICATIONS

Overlying cellulitis, bleeding diathesis

SUPPLIES

Antiseptic, sterile gauze, sterile gloves and
drape, lidocaine 1%, 25g needle, 18g needle,
5cc syringe, 30-60cc syringe, appropriate
test tubes

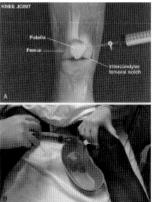

PROCEDURE

- Position the patient, either extended fully
  or flexed at 15-20 degrees, with a towel
  under the knee.

- Can use the medial or lateral approach.
  Identify the middle or superior portion of the patella.

- Don sterile gloves, clean and drape patient.

- Anesthetize the skin and down to the area of the joint capsule with local anesthetic.

- Using 18-20g needle attached to large syringe (30-60cc), enter at 45°, aiming under the patella,
  and aspirate while advancing until fluid is obtained.

- Remove as much fluid as possible.

FLUID ANALYSIS

Cell count with differential, protein, glucose, crystals, gram stain, and culture

	WBC/µL	PMNs	Glucose
Normal	<200	<25%	serum glucose
Non-Inflammatory (OA, trauma, etc.)	<2,000	<25%	serum glucose
Inflammatory (RA, crystals)	>2,000	>50%	<25
Septic	Generally >50,000	>95%	<25

CRYSTALS

- Gout – monosodium urate crystals, negative birefringent, needle shaped
- Pseudogout – calcium pyrophosphate crystals, positive birefringent, rhomboid

COMPLICATIONS

Infection, bleeding, pain

Source

Thomsen TW, Shen S, Shaffer RW, Setnik GS. Videos in clinical medicine. Arthrocentesis of the knee. *N Engl J Med*. 2006;354(19):e19.

Notes

4 ▶ Central Venous Line

INDICATIONS

Central venous pressure monitoring, resuscitation, emergency access, repetitive blood sampling, insertion of PA catheters (a cordis is also used for PA catheter placement).

Remember, 2 large bore IVs (18G) are better for rapid infusion of IVF or blood. Also, during a code it is generally better to start with an intraosseous line rather than interrupt chest compressions to place a central line.

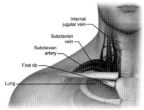

CONTRAINDICATIONS

Infection over site, distortion of landmarks by trauma, coagulopathy, venous thrombosis in target vessel, prior vessel injury

SUPPLIES

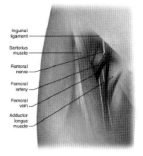

- Central line kit (sterile drape, antiseptic, lidocaine, syringes, 22g and 25g needle, scalpel with No. 11 blade, venipuncture syringe, 18g needle, dilator, triple lumen catheter, guidewire, suture)
- Cordis if using for volume replacement
- Sterile gloves, mask, hat, eye protection, gown
- US machine, probe cover, sterile lubricant

PROCEDURE

- Gown and glove, prep the area, apply full body drape.
- Patient should be on telemetry due to possibility of arrhythmia.
- Flush triple lumen catheter and make sure only the brown port is open.
- Cover ultrasound probe with sterile sheath, identify anatomic structures on ultrasound.
- Anesthetize tissues overlying vein with local anesthetic.
- Insert needle and syringe while slowly advancing and applying negative pressure, following needle tip along on ultrasound, until vein is entered and blood enters the syringe.
- Remove the syringe and advance the guidewire.
- Remove the needle over the guidewire *(DON'T LET GO)*. Confirm you are in vein with US prior to dilating. Can also use manometry prior to guidewire placement to confirm position.
- Make an incision at the site of the wire to facilitate dilator and catheter passage.

- Thread the dilator over the guidewire into the skin and subcutaneous tissue (⅓ of length), and then remove.
- Advance the catheter over the wire and into the vessel; the guidewire will emerge from your open brown port. Remove the wire, cap the open port.
- Confirm that all ports draw back, and then flush all ports with saline.
- Suture the catheter in place, clean the area around the site, and place a simple dressing.
- CXR to confirm placement and assess for pneumothorax in IJ/subclavian lines.

COMPLICATIONS

Arterial puncture (call vascular surgery if you dilate artery), pneumothorax, hemothorax, vessel injury, air embolism, cardiac dysrhythmia, nerve injury, infection, thrombosis

Source

Graham AS, Ozment C, Tegtmeyer K, Lai S, Braner DA. Videos in clinical medicine. Central venous catheterization. *N Engl J Med.* 2007;356(21):e21.

Notes

5 ▶ Intubation

For more detailed information, please see airway management chapter.

INDICATIONS

Failure to oxygenate, failure to ventilate, inability to protect airway, or expected clinical course

CONTRAINDICATIONS

Most are relative, as this is an emergent procedure. Anticipate a difficult airway (infection, oral or facial trauma, tumor, or airway edema). Keep inline stabilization if concern for c-spine trauma.

SUPPLIES

- Medications
    - Pretreatment option: Lidocaine 1.5mg/kg IV, fentanyl 3μg/kg IV, atropine 0.02mg/kg IV
    - Induction agents: Etomidate 0.3mg/kg IV, propofol 0.5-1.5mg/kg IV, ketamine 1-2mg/kg IV
    - Paralyzing agents: Succinylcholine 1.5mg/kg IV, rocuronium 1mg/kg IV
- Bag-valve-mask attached to oxygen source (15L/min)
- Tracheal tube (7.0 – 9.0) with stylet in place, syringe to check/inflate balloon
    - Pediatric: Uncuffed tube size = (age in years/4) + 4
    - Always have a second tube ready for back up
- Tape or tube stabilizer
- Laryngoscope with working light source
    - Mac (3,4), Miller
    - Videoscope such as C-mac or Glidescope is preferred if available
- Oral suction device (Yankauer)
- Capnography
- Respiratory therapist with ventilator
- **Backup plan** and adjuncts (eg, bougie, LMA, etc.)

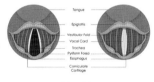

VOCAL CORD

PROCEDURE

- Preoxygenate – provide maximal FiO2 with non-rebreather for 3-5min, plus a nasal cannula under the NRB mask to decrease risk of desaturation during the procedure.
- Assess airway (see airway chapter)
- Elevate patient's head, aligning ear with sternal notch, or tilt foot of the bed down in patient who requires cervical spine immobilization. Scissor open mouth with right hand (thumb pushing lower jaw down, index finger pushing upper jaw up).
- Taking the laryngoscope in left hand, insert into right side of patient's mouth, sliding along to displace tongue to the left.

- Move the tip of the blade toward the base of the tongue, pulling the laryngoscope up and forward until you see the epiglottis. The vector of force should err toward the ceiling corner in front of you.
    — If using a MAC blade, insert into the tip into the vallecula and continue to elevate, exposing the vocal cords.
    — If using a MILLER blade, insert tip slightly beyond the epiglottis and directly lift it up.
    — If using a videoscope, placement of the blade is based on the model. Center the cords in the middle of the screen.
- With your right hand, insert the tube through the vocal cords.
- Remove the blade, and while holding the tube in place, inflate balloon and verify placement:
    — Bilateral breath sounds, chest rise, and end-tidal CO2.
    — CXR to assess placement.
- Place OGT.

COMPLICATIONS

Esophageal intubation, right mainstem intubation, laryngospasm, bradycardia, and oral trauma

Source
Kabrhel C, Thomsen TW, Setnik GS, Walls RM. Videos in clinical medicine. Orotracheal intubation. *N Engl J Med.* 2007;356(17):e15.

Notes

6 ▶ Tube Thoracostomy

INDICATIONS

Pneumothorax, hemothorax, empyema, traumatic arrest

For an unstable patient with tension pneumothorax, can quickly needle decompress with 14-16g needle in anterior second intercostal space in the midclavicular line, or the anterior axillary line in the fourth or fifth interspace.

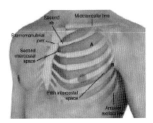

CONTRAINDICATIONS

Significant coagulopathies, concern for pleural adhesions, prior thoracic surgeries on that side, or the presence of a large diaphragmatic hernia

SUPPLIES

- Chest tube kit: sterile drapes, syringe and needles, 1% lidocaine, antiseptic, scalpel, large clamps (Kelly), needle holder, suture, forceps, scissors
- Chest tubes (28F or larger, based on indication; minimum of 36F for hemothorax)
- Chest tube drain with sterile water for water seal and sterile tubing
- Occlusive dressing

PROCEDURE

- Identify your site; most common is midaxillary to anterior axillary line in the fourth or fifth intercostal space (nipple level). Position the patient on the unaffected side, and abduct the arm of the affected side over the patient's head.

- Wearing gown, gloves, mask, and eye protection, clean and drape the patient.

- Clamp the distal end of the tube so drainage from the chest cavity does not get out.

- Use generous local anesthesia (up to 5mg/kg 1% lidocaine), injecting over the superior aspect of the rib, and down to the pleura (the most painful part).

- Cut a transverse incision 3-5cm through the skin and subcutaneous tissue with a No. 10 blade.

- Insert a large Kelly clamp to push and spread the deeper tissues. Bluntly dissect a tract over the rib (vessels and nerves run on inferior margin of each rib).

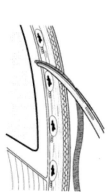

- Firm resistance will be felt when the parietal pleura is met. Close the clamp and push it forward to penetrate the pleura ("pop"), and then spread the clamp to make an adequate hole.

- Slide a finger into the pleura and withdraw the clamp, then pass the tube into the pleural space, passing the tube posteriorly, medially, and superiorly until the last hole of the tube is in the thorax.

- Secure the tube to the chest with sutures, and place an occlusive dressing.

COMPLICATIONS

Infection, laceration of intercostal vessel, laceration of lung, intraabdominal or solid organ placement of chest tube, subcutaneous air

Source

Dev SP, Nascimiento B, Simone C, Chien V. Videos in clinical medicine. Chest-tube insertion. *N Engl J Med.* 2007;357(15):e15.

Notes

7 ▶ Lumbar Puncture

INDICATIONS

Diagnosis of meningitis, SAH, or detect opening pressure to assess for idiopathic intracranial hypertension

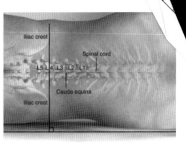

CONTRAINDICATIONS

Skin infection over puncture site, elevated ICP, hydrocephalus, mass, severe bleeding diathesis, platelets <50. Consider head CT prior to LP in patients who are elderly, immunocompromised, have a history of CNS pathology (CVA or tumor), or have focal findings on neurologic exam.

SUPPLIES

- LP kit
- Extra LP needles (3.5 inch 20g for adults, 2.5 inch 22g for children)
- Sterile gloves, hat, mask, eye protection

PROCEDURE

- Position patient:
  - Use L4/L5 (level of iliac crests), or one level above/below (spinal cord ends at L1/L2).
  - Lateral position (to obtain opening pressure): Patient is in fetal position, spine is parallel to bed and curls, pushing low back toward provider.
  - Upright position: Patient sits on bed, leans over side table with low back arched, perpendicular to bed.
- Open kit. Put on sterile gloves. Organize kit, and make sure tubes are in order and open.
- Sterilize area and drape.
- Anesthetize with 1% lidocaine, first with superficial wheal, then deeper with large bore needle.
- Orient bevel 90° from patient's head. (To ceiling in lateral position, to side in upright.)
- Insert needle, and then advance slowly toward umbilicus with needle parallel to ground. Remove stylet frequently to check for CSF flow.
- Once flow is established, manometer can be used to check opening pressure.
- Collect tubes 1-4, 1-2cc per tube.

Tube	Lab	Tests
1 (1 mL)	Heme	CSF cell count
2 (1 mL)	Chem	Total protein, glucose
3 (3-5 mL)	Micro	Gram stain and culture. +/- HSV PCR, cryptococcal antigen, viral culture, AFB stain, VDRL.
4 (1 mL)	Heme	CSF cell count, hold for further testing

- Replace stylet and withdraw needle after tubes collected. Place bandage.

COMPLICATIONS

- Tonsillar herniation: Immediately replace stylet into needle and **call neurosurgery.** Protect airway, and hyperventilate if needed.

- Spinal epidural hemorrhage: Serious bleeding leading to significant complications like cauda equina. More frequent in coagulopathic patients.

- Nerve root injury: Shooting pains down legs, usually transient. Stop advancing. If pain continues, withdraw needle/stylet.

- Post-LP headache: Reported incidence between to 1-70%. Typical onset within 28hrs, lasting 1-2 days (rarely up to 2 weeks). To minimize risk, use smaller gauge needle. IV caffeine is the drug of choice. If persistent, call anesthesia/pain service for epidural blood patch. No data to support hydration or lying recumbent after lumbar puncture for reducing post-LP headache.

CSF INTERPRETATION

	Pressure	WBC per µL	Predominant Cell Type	Glucose (mg/dL)	Protein (mg/dL)
Normal	9-18	0-5	Lymph	50-75 (0.6:1, CSF:serum)	15-40
Bacterial Meningitis	20-30	100-10,000+	>80% PMNs	<40	>50
Viral Meningitis	9-20	6-1000	Lymph or PMNs	Normal or low	Normal or slightly elevated

Source

Ellenby MS, Tegtmeyer K, Lai S, Braner DA. Videos in clinical medicine. Lumbar puncture. *N Engl J Med.* 2006;355(13):e12.

8 ▶ Paracentesis

INDICATIONS

New onset ascites, to assess for SBP, to relieve tense ascites (up to 5-6L in chronic ascites), emergently in patient who is experiencing dyspnea/hypoxia secondary to ascites.

CONTRAINDICATIONS

Coagulopathy with fibrinolysis and/or DIC (no official INR or platelet cutoff), bowel dilation or obstruction, pregnancy, superficial infection at puncture site, abdominal hematoma

**US can detect as little as 100-250cc of fluid.

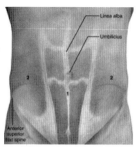

SUPPLIES

- Paracentesis kit: sterile drape, lidocaine, 18-22g needle, 60cc syringe, sterile vacuum bottles for large volume paracentesis
- Sterile gloves, eye protection
- Ultrasound

PROCEDURE

- Place the patient in the supine position; some clinicians prefer the lateral decubitus position. Wear sterile gloves and clean and drape the patient.
- Preferred sites are 2cm below the umbilicus in the midline, and in the right or left lower quadrant, approximately 4-5cm cephalad and medial to the anterior superior iliac spine. US guidance is recommended to find the largest volume of fluid.
- Anesthetize the skin and subcutaneous tissue with 1% lidocaine.
- Pull the skin approximately 2cm caudad to the deep abdominal wall while slowly inserting the paracentesis needle, then release the skin when the needle has penetrated the peritoneum (z-tract). Insert in 5mm increments to avoid puncturing the bowel.
- Once fluid is flowing, stabilize the needle; take fluid sample (diagnostic vs. large volume). Can use an angiocatheter and leave catheter in while you remove fluid. If performing a large volume paracentesis (LVP), use the needle and catheter as directed on the kit.
- After fluid removal is complete, remove needle/catheter and place adhesive bandage over site.

Fluid analysis: Cell count and differential, albumin, LDH, protein, glucose, gram stain & culture

** Spontaneous bacterial peritonitis is diagnosed if neutrophils >250mm^3.

SERUM-ASCITES ALBUMIN GRADIENT

High ≥ 1.1 Secondary to Portal Hypertension	Cirrhosis, CHF, acute hepatitis, liver metastases, HCC, Budd-Chiari syndrome, portal vein thrombosis, myxedema
Low < 1.1	Spontaneous or secondary bacterial peritonitis, TB peritonitis, peritoneal carcinomatosis, malnutrition, biliary, pancreatitis, nephrotic syndrome

COMPLICATIONS

Ascitic fluid leak, abdominal wall hematoma, local infection, hyponatremia, renal dysfunction, hepatic encephalopathy, hemodynamic compromise, bleeding, perforation of vessels, generalized peritonitis, abdominal wall abscess

** For large volume paracentesis (>4-5L), 6-8g of albumin per liter of fluid removed (up to 50g) can be given for colloid replacement via 25% or 5% albumin as appropriate.

Source

Thomsen TW, Shaffer RW, White B, Setnik GS. Videos in clinical medicine. Paracentesis. *N Engl J Med.* 2006;355(19):e21.

Notes

9 ▶ Procedural Sedation

PREPARATION

- Safety/risk assessment: History and exam, including airway evaluation (see airway section), ASA class (may not be safe if 3+), time patient has been NPO (*Note: ACEP guidelines say NPO not needed, but hospital policies differ*). Perform airway assessment.
- Get consent, do paperwork, arrange personnel (minimum: EM attending, RN, MD doing procedure). The person running the sedation should not be the same person performing the indicated procedure.
- Decide on level of sedation and meds/doses. In general, you want analgesia AND sedation, though you can do sedation only for short procedures with adequate pre-procedure analgesia.
- Place patient on monitor, pulse ox, ETCO2. Pre-oxygenate. Place in position that allows for easy intubation and access to the head of the bed.
- Ensure reversal meds and airway meds/equipment are in the room and working (eg, BVM, nasal/oral airway, suction, LMA, ETT).

LEVEL OF SEDATION

- Moderate: Patient is awake and responds to verbal commands. Use for some reductions, LP/I&D in certain patients.
- Deep: Patient reacts purposefully to repeated painful stimuli. Use for most reductions or elective cardioversion.

Med	Dose IV (typical)*	Kinetics IV	Side effects	Best for	Not for	Comments
			Sedation			
Midazolam (Versed)	0.02-0.05 mg/kg (1-2 mg) q3-5min [Nasal: 0.2-0.5 mg/kg]	Onset 1-3m Peak 5-7m Duration 20-30m	Respiratory and Cardiovascular depression	Peds, Short procedures		Do not redose too quickly
Propofol	0.5-1 mg/kg (20-40 mg), then 0.5 mg/kg (20 mg) q1-2min	Onset 30s Duration 10-15m	Hypotension, bradycardia	Short procedures	Soy/milk/egg allergy, hypotensive	More if thin, less if obese
Etomidate	0.1-0.15 mg/kg (5-10 mg), then 0.05 mg/kg q2-3min	Peak 1m Duration 5-15m	Myoclonus, emesis	Hypotensive		

Med	Dose IV (typical)*	Kinetics IV	Side effects	Best for	Not for	Comments
Analgesia						
Fentanyl	1-2 mcg/kg, then 1 mcg/kg (25-50 mcg) q3-5min	Onset 1-2m Peak 10-15m Duration 30-60m	Hypotension, respiratory depression			Do not redose too quickly
Dissociation						
Ketamine	1 mg/kg, then 0.5 mg q2-5m (peds 1.5-2 mg/kg) [IM: 4-5 mg/kg]	Onset 1-2m Duration 15-30m	Emergence reaction, increased HR +BP, emesis, hypersalivation, laryngospasm	Peds, longer procedures, difficult airway, hypotensive	<3 month age, Severe HTN, psychiatric history,	Analgesia and sedation

*Use lower doses in elderly

EXAMPLES

- Fentanyl/Versed: Usually for moderate sedation
- Fentanyl/propofol or fentanyl/etomidate: Deep
- Ketofol: Deep, mix 1:1 in same syringe or give ketamine 1st, 0.5 mg/kg of each to start, then more propofol prn. i.e.
  — Ketamine 50 mg/mL, empty 2cc from a 10cc flush, draw up 2cc drug → 10mL of 10mg/mL = 100mg total
  — Propofol 10 mg/mL, draw up 10mL → 10mL of 10mg/mL = 100 mg total

Troubleshooting: ETCO2 beeping, desaturations or oversedation

Try (roughly in this order): stimulation (sternal rub), head tilt/jaw thrust, suction, laryngospasm notch pressure (bilateral firm pressure behind earlobe b/w mastoid process and condyle of mandible), nasal airway, BVM at 1 breath every 5-6 seconds, consider naloxone (start 0.4mg) for opioid reversal, consider flumazenil for benzo reversal (start with 0.2mg, max 1mg), LMA, and ultimately intubation if needed.

DISPOSITION

- Patients can be discharged after they are cleared from their other medical issues and are awake and able to ambulate independently.
- Patient will need a ride home or to wait approximately 6hrs for medications to wear off before it is safe for them to operate a car.

10 ▶ Intraosseus Access

INDICATIONS

Limited or no vascular access and/or the
need for rapid access for the administration
of drugs or fluids (as may be the case in
quickly decompensating patients, cardiac or
respiratory arrest, or those requiring urgent
intubation or sedation).

CONTRAINDICATIONS

Fracture in the targeted bone; previous
orthopedic procedures near the insertion
site, such as joint or limb prosthetics; I/O
attempt or insertion in that targeted bone
within the past 24 hrs; infection at the
insertion site; vascular injury; iatrogenic fracture risk: osteoporosis or osteogenesis imperfecta;
inability to locate the landmarks or excessive soft tissue.

*Acutely burned skin is **not** a contraindication.

SUPPLIES

- Antiseptic or alternate sterilizing supplies and gloves
- Lidocaine (for conscious patients; 1% or 2% lidocaine without preservatives or
  epinephrine is recommended) and a saline flush
- Intraosseous needle set-up:
  — Manual: needle with the central trochar
  — Impact driven: FAST1 (sternal only); Bone Injection Gun (humerus, tibia)
  — Power driven (EZ-IO): comes in 15mm/15g, 25mm/15g, 45mm/15g with internal trochar
- Needle driver (if using EZ-IO)
- Connecting tubing, securing device

PROCEDURE

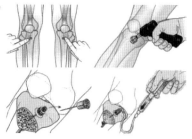

- Determine your IO site and
  identify landmarks.
  — **Preferred:** Proximal tibia,
    distal tibia and proximal
    humerus
  — **Alternate:** Sternal, distal
    radius, distal ulnar and iliac
    crest intraosseous sites are

used in some circumstances with either the manual IO or FAST1, but these sites should be avoided with the driver-assisted EZ-IO.

- Needle size selection: You need 5mm (or one black line) of needle to enter the bone.
  — Estimate soft tissue depth with your finger and visualize where the black line will be after penetration of the skin.
  — Take into consideration excessive adipose or muscle tissue or edema.
- Prime the connective tubing with either lidocaine or saline.
- Clean site with antiseptic.
- Stabilize the extremity with your non-dominant hand.
- Insert needle at a 90 degree angle to the bone, then push steadily downward until the needle touches bone.
- When your needle hits the cortex, start drilling gently with no more than 5 to 8 lbs of pressure (for adults).
- Stop drilling when you feel a "pop" or "give."
- Remove any trochar and stabilize the needle.
- Attach the already primed tubing and a saline-filled syringe.
- Aspirate marrow to confirm placement, and flush with saline and/or lidocaine.
- Discard the trochar in the sharps container.

COMPLICATIONS

Osteomyelitis (0.6%; associated with prolonged use), abscess (0.1%); extravasation (0.8% leading to compartment syndrome) and/or leakage around the insertion site; failed placement, dislodgement, or difficulty removing the device

LENGTH OF USE

In austere environments, IO access have been used for up to 96hrs, but to minimize the risk of infection, the recommended time is no longer than 24hrs.

Sources

Day MW. Intraosseous devices for intravascular access in adult trauma patients. *Crit Care Nurse*. 2011 Apr;31(2):76-89.

Luck RP, Haines C, Mull CC. Intraosseous access. *J Emerg Med*. 2010 Oct;39(4):468-75.

Weiser G, Hoffmann Y, Galbraith R, Shavit I. Current advances in intraosseous infusion – a systematic review. *Resuscitation*. 2012 Jan;83(1):20-6.